Handbook of
Veterinary Anesthesia

Handbook of
Veterinary Anesthesia

Third Edition

William W. Muir III
DVM, PhD, Dipl ACVA, ACVECC
Professor

John A. E. Hubbell
DVM, MS, Dipl, ACVA
Professor

Roman T. Skarda
Dr. Med Vet, PhD, Dipl ACVA
Associate Professor

Richard M. Bednarski
DVM, MS, Dipl ACVA
Associate Professor

All of the Department of Veterinary Clinical Sciences
The Ohio State University College of Veterinary Medicine
Columbus, Ohio

Illustrations by Tim Vojt

with 141 illustrations

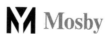 Mosby

St. Louis Baltimore Boston Carlsbad Chicago Naples New York
Philadelphia Portland London Madrid Mexico City Singapore
Sydney Tokyo Toronto Wiesbaden

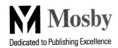

Mosby

Dedicated to Publishing Excellence

Editor: John A. Schrefer
Executive Editor: Linda L. Duncan
Senior Developmental Editor: Teri Merchant
Project Manager: Linda McKinley
Project Specialist: Rich Barber
Designer: Judi Lang

THIRD EDITION

Printed in the United States of America
Composition by Clarinda
Lithography/color Film by Clarinda Company
Printing/binding by Fairfield

Mosby, Inc.
A Harcourt Health Sciences Company
11830 Westline Industrial Drive
St. Louis, Missouri 64146

Library of Congress Cataloging in Publication Data

International Standard Book Number 0-323-00801-1

00   01   02   03   04   /   9 8 7 6 5 4 3 2 1

Contributors

Nancy Anderson, DVM
Department of Veterinary Clinical Sciences
The Ohio State University
Columbus, Ohio

Raymond Wack, DVM, MS
Department of Veterinary Clinical Sciences
The Ohio State University
Columbus, Ohio
Director of Veterinary Services
Columbus Zoo
Columbus, Ohio

Preface to the First Edition

The purpose of this preface is to serve as a dedication, prologue, and means of expressing gratitude. Briefly, this handbook of veterinary anesthesiology is dedicated to the veterinary student and practicing veterinarian. It was designed to be used by veterinary students, residents, and veterinary practitioners requiring an immediate source of information relating to the practice of veterinary anesthesia, cardiopulmonary emergencies, and euthanasia. Recent versions have been completely rethought, rewritten, and expanded.

The present edition is the result of the labors of the Section of Anesthesiology of the Department of Veterinary Clinical Sciences at The Ohio State University.

The material contained within this handbook is based upon the collective clinical experiences, research, and teaching activities of each of the contributors. Technical advice and suggestions were offered by Mary Ferguson, Sarah Flaherty, Earl Harrison, William Sheehan, Tom Sherman, Peter Hellyer, and Mark Leonard. Ideas and contributions to earlier versions of this final document were provided by Elaine Robinson, Cheryl Buchanan, and Karen Rosenberry Spenser. The final version is principally due to the concentrated and combined efforts of myself, Richard Bednarski, John Hubbell, Roman Skarda, Clifford Swanson, and Diane Mason. Our individual interests and dedication to teaching have made this work enjoyable. We have attempted to summarize and simplify what has become a very large and oftentimes confusing topic. It is not our intent to have this handbook replace more comprehensive textbooks of veterinary anesthesia, but to supplement them.

William W. Muir, III
John A.E. Hubbell

Preface to the Second Edition

The first edition of this handbook was designed to provide a ready reference on clinical veterinary anesthesia for students, practicing veterinarians, animal health technicians, and researchers who use animals in their experiments. Since its publication 5 years ago, new anesthetic drugs, equipment, and monitoring devices have appeared. This edition incorporates information on these advances and provides an update on the drugs and techniques previously described.

In addition to adding new information, we have attempted to increase the readability and utility of the text. Our goals were to clarify, but not oversimplify and to provide interested students and others with an information base on which to build a more complete and comprehensive understanding of the practice of clinical veterinary anesthesia. As Thomas Mann said, "Order and simplification are the first steps toward mastery of a subject—the actual enemy is the unknown."

Edition two is the result of the labors of the Section of Anesthesiology of the Department of Veterinary Clinical Sciences of The Ohio State University. Advice from Dr. Ann Wagner, Earl Harrison, Jennifer Ford, Diane Hurley, Stephen Drab, and Beverly Ventura is greatly appreciated. Significant contributors to this edition include Roman Skarda, Rich Bednarski, Diane Mason, Julie Smith, Nancy Anderson, and Ray Wack. Our thanks to Frances Crowell for typing the manuscript.

William W. Muir, III
John A.E. Hubbell

Preface to the Third Edition

Like previous editions of this handbook, we designed it to provide a readily available and clinically useful source of information for producing chemical restraint and anesthesia in animals. Emphasis has been placed on those animals that are commonly seen by veterinarians, although specific attention and chapters have been dedicated to anesthesia in exotic species and birds. We have retained and updated chapters that encompass the full spectrum of the anesthetic experience, including anesthetic equipment, ventilators and ventilation, acid-base and fluid therapy, cardiopulmonary resuscitation, shock therapy, and euthanasia. Special emphasis and an independent chapter have been added describing drugs and techniques, including acupuncture for the treatment of pain.

This third edition is the result of the advice and labors of the Section of Anesthesiology of the Department of Veterinary Clinical Sciences at The Ohio State University. Recent critiques were provided by Dr. Tamara Grubb, Dr. Phillip Lerche, Jennifer Gadawski, Jennifer Ford, Gladys Karpa, Earl Harrison, and Tirina Miller.

William W. Muir, III
John A.E. Hubbell

Preface to the Third Edition

Like previous editions of this handbook, we designed this edition to provide a readily available and clinically useful source of information for producing chemical restraint and anesthesia in animals. Emphasis has been placed on those animals that are commonly treated by veterinarians, although specific attention and chapters have been dedicated to anesthesia in exotic species and birds. We have retained and updated chapters that encompass the full spectrum of the anesthetic experience, including anesthetic equipment, ventilators and ventilation, acid-base and fluid therapy, cardiopulmonary resuscitation, shock therapy, and euthanasia. Special emphasis and an independent chapter have been added describing drugs and techniques, including acupuncture for the treatment of pain.

This third edition is the result of the advice and labors of the Section of Anesthesiology of the Department of Veterinary Clinical Sciences at The Ohio State University. Recent critiques were provided by Dr. Tamara Grubb, Dr. Phillip Lerche, Jennifer Gadawski, Jennifer Ford, Gladys Karpa, Earl Harrison, and Tirina Miller.

William W. Muir, III
John A.E. Hubbell

"To look back is to relax one's vigil."
BETTE DAVIS

*"It's what you learn after
you know it all that counts."*
JOHN WOODEN

*"Order and simplicity are the first steps
toward mastery of a subject."*
THOMAS MANN

Contents

CHAPTER ONE

Introduction to Anesthesia

"There are no safe anesthetic agents; there are no safe anesthetic procedures; there are only safe anesthetists."

ROBERT SMITH

OVERVIEW

The art and practice of anesthesia are based on a general understanding of (1) the terms that describe the effects of anesthetic drugs in animals, (2) the pharmacology of anesthetic drugs and their antagonists, (3) the correct methods of anesthetic drug administration, and (4) appropriate therapy for anesthetic-related complications or emergencies. This chapter outlines commonly used terms, the general uses for anesthetics, the routes of administration of anesthetic drugs, or drug combinations used to produce chemical restraint and anesthesia in animals.

GENERAL CONSIDERATIONS

   I. Anesthesia and/or chemical restraint is a reversible process; the purpose of anesthesia is to produce a convenient, safe, effective, yet inexpensive means of chemical restraint so that medical or surgical procedures may be expedited with minimal stress, pain, discomfort, and toxic side effects to the patient or to the anesthetist
   II. Criteria for selection of drugs and techniques
      A. Species, breed, age, and relative size of the patient
      B. Physical status and specific disease processes of the patient
      C. Concurrent medications
      D. Demeanor of the patient and the severity of pain
      E. Personal knowledge and experience
      F. Availability and training of assistants

G. Familiarity with available equipment

H. Length and type of operation or procedure to be performed

III. Patient responses can vary because dosages and techniques are for the "average, normal" healthy animal; thus it is essential that the practitioner know how to modify anesthetic techniques

IV. Definitions

A. Medical terms used in the practice of anesthesia:

Agonist: A drug that produces an effect by interacting with a specific receptor site (e.g., opioid agonist morphine)

Akinesia: Loss of motor response (movement) caused by paralysis of motor nerves

Analgesia: Loss of sensitivity to pain

Anesthesia: Total loss of sensation in a body part or in the whole body, generally induced by a drug that depresses the activity of nervous tissue either locally (peripherally) or generally (centrally)

Local anesthesia: Analgesia limited to a local area

Regional anesthesia: Analgesia limited to a local area produced by blocking sensory nerves

General anesthesia: Loss of consciousness in addition to loss of sensation; ideally includes hypnosis, hyporeflexia, analgesia, and muscle relaxation; can be produced with a single drug or by a combination of drugs

Surgical anesthesia: Loss of consciousness and sensation accompanied by sufficient muscle relaxation and analgesia to allow surgery to be performed without pain or movement by the patient

Balanced anesthesia: Surgical anesthesia produced by a combination of two or more drugs or anesthetic techniques, each contributing its own pharmacological effects; includes tranquilizers, opioids, nitrous oxide, muscle relaxants, and inhalants

Dissociative anesthesia: A central nervous system (CNS) state characterized by catalepsy, analgesia, and altered consciousness; produced by drugs like ketamine

Antagonist: A drug that occupies a receptor site but produces minimal or no effect (e.g., opioid antagonist Naloxone)

Catalepsy: State in which there is malleable rigidity of the limbs. The patient is generally unresponsive to aural, visual, or minor painful stimuli

Hypnosis: Artificially induced sleep or a trance resembling sleep from which the patient can be aroused by sufficient stimuli; patients cannot be aroused during general or surgical anesthesia

Narcosis: Drug-induced stupor or sedation in which the patient is oblivious to pain, with or without hypnosis

Neuroleptanalgesia: Hypnosis and analgesia produced by the combination of a neuroleptic drug and an analgesic drug

Sedation: Mild degree of CNS depression in which the patient is awake but calm; a term often used interchangeably with tranquilization; with sufficient stimuli the patient may be aroused; produces a dose-dependent depression of the cerebral cortex

Tranquilization, ataraxia, neurolepsis: State of tranquility and calmness in which the patient is relaxed, reluctant to move, awake, and unconcerned with its surroundings and potentially indifferent to minor pain; sufficient stimulation will arouse the patient

V. Clinical jargon

Bag: "The animal was bagged." The rebreathing bag on the anesthetic machine was squeezed to inflate the animal's lungs during anesthesia

Block: "The leg was blocked." Local anesthesia was produced at a specific site, locally or regionally

Bolus: "A bolus of thiobarbiturate was administered." A specified quantity of drug was rapidly administered intravenously

Breathed: "The animal was breathed six times a minute." The lungs were either manually or mechanically inflated

Crashed: "The animal crashed." The patient demonstrated marked CNS and cardiopulmonary depression following the administration of an anesthetic drug. "The animal was crash induced." Anesthesia was rapidly induced with an intravenous (IV) or inhalant anesthetic drug

Deep: "The animal is in a deep stage of anesthesia." The anesthetic drugs produced significant CNS depression. The greater the degree of CNS depression, the deeper the anesthesia. This term is used in direct contrast to the term *light,* which implies minimal CNS depression. Animals that are "light" demonstrate active corneal and palpebral reflexes, may develop nystagmus, and occasionally lift their heads or move a limb during surgery

Down: The animal was "knocked down" or "put down." The animal was given a drug or combination of drugs that produced recumbency. The term *put down* is also used to denote euthanasia

Dropped: "The animal was dropped." The animal received drugs that produce recumbency

Extubated: "The animal was extubated." The endotracheal tube was removed from the airway. The term is the opposite of "intubated"

Hit or stick a vein: "I hit the vein on the first attempt." A successful venipuncture was performed

Induced: "The animal was induced." The animal was given a drug or drugs that produced anesthesia

Intubated: "The animal was intubated." An endotracheal tube was placed through the nose or mouth into the trachea

IV drip: "The patient received an IV drip." A fluid with or without added drug(s) was administered intravenously

Mask induced: "The animal was mask induced." A face mask was used to facilitate delivery of anesthesia. Because face masks are used to supply gaseous or volatile anesthetics, the term also implies that an inhalation anesthetic was used

Pre or post: "A preanesthetic was administered." Anything administered or done before anesthesia is considered to be in the preanesthetic period. Occurrences following the discontinuation of anesthetic drugs are considered postanesthetic

Preemptive: "The patient received preemptive analgesia." The deliberate administration of therapy (in this case, analgesia) before the event requiring therapy. A form of prophylaxis

Pushed: "The thiobarbiturate was pushed." An IV drug or fluids were administered either rapidly or in amounts greater than usually given

Ran a strip: "I ran a strip on that animal." An electrocardiogram was obtained

Reversed: "The animal was reversed." A drug's effects were antagonized by administering a specific antagonist. For example, the opioid antagonist naloxone can be administered to reverse the effects of morphine

Spiked: "The animal spiked a fever," or "The fluids were spiked with potassium." Depending on the clinical situation, *spiked* may mean a sudden rapid increase or that some substance (K^+) or drug was added to a solution

Stabilized: "The animal is stable" or "The animal has been stabilized." Cardiopulmonary variables or the "depth" of anesthesia have been returned to or are within acceptable limits

Topped-off: "The animal was topped off with a thiobarbiturate." An additional drug was administered to produce the desired effect. The term implies that the original calculated dosage was insufficient to produce the desired effect

Tubed: "The animal was tubed." An endotracheal tube was placed in the trachea through either the mouth or nasal cavities (see also intubated)

USE OF ANESTHETICS

I. Restraint
  A. Radiography
  B. Cleaning, grooming, dental prophylaxis
  C. Biopsy, bandaging, splinting, cast application
  D. Capture of exotic and wild animals
  E. Transportation
  F. Manipulation
    1. Catheterization
    2. Wound care
    3. Obstetrics
  G. Assist or control breathing
II. Anesthesia (see Definitions: Anesthesia)
  A. To facilitate or permit medical and/or surgical procedures
III. Control of convulsions
IV. Euthanasia

TYPES OF ANESTHESIA (ACCORDING TO ROUTE OF ADMINISTRATION)

Acupuncture	Infiltration†	Intravenous†
Buccal	Inhalation†	Oral†
Controlled hypothermia	Intramuscular†	Rectal
Electroanesthesia	Intraosseous	Subcutaneous*
Epidural*	Intraperitoneal	Topical†
Spinal (subarachnoid)	Intratesticular	Transdermal*
Field block†	Intrathoracic	

*Epidural, subcutaneous, and transdermal
†Route commonly used in veterinary medicine

EFFECT OF ROUTE AND METHOD OF ADMINISTRATION OF ANESTHETIC DRUG

  I. Given intravenously (Figs. 1-1, 1-2): onset of action is immediate; peak effect is rapidly obtained; duration of action is short, and effects are generally more intense than with other routes
 II. Given intramuscularly or subcutaneously: onset of action may take 10 to 15 minutes; peak effect may not be obtained for many minutes to hours and depends on the blood supply to the tissues at the site of injection, drug absorption, and the rate of metabolism of the drug; duration of action is more prolonged than by the IV route
III. Given transdermally: peak system effects may not occur for many hours
 IV. Rapidity of injection: rapid injections generally cause more intense effects, especially true when cardiac output is low
  V. Concentrations of solutions
     A. Drugs should be administered on a unit/kg basis (e.g., mg/kg); most drugs list concentration as unit/ml (e.g., mg/ml) or percent (%); percent solutions can be converted

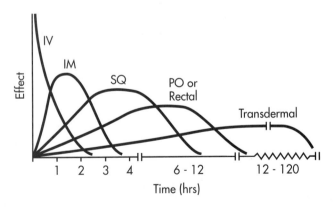

Fig. 1-1
Magnitude of effect and duration of action associated with various routes of administration.

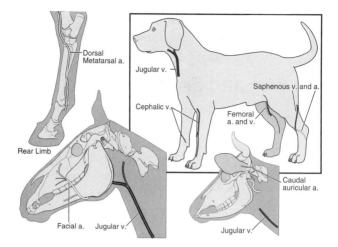

Fig. 1-2

The jugular, cephalic, femoral, and saphenous veins are used in dogs and cats for intravenous administration of fluids and drugs. The jugular vein is the most frequently used vein in horses, cattle, sheep, and goats. Various arteries are catheterized to directly monitor arterial blood pressure or anaerobically obtain blood samples for pH and blood gas analysis.

       to unit/ml (a 1% solution contains 10 mg/ml); therefore a 0.5% solution contains 5 mg/ml, and a 3% solution contains 30 mg/ml

  B. Increasing drug concentration increases the intensity and duration of the immediate drug effect

  C. Increasing concentrations may increase vascular irritation and cause pain on injection

  VI. Amount: the amount (dose) of drug administered should be reduced in sick or shocky patients

 VII. The onset of action of inhalation drugs requires absorption of gas from alveoli into the blood, then diffusion of anesthetic into the CNS

VIII. Duration of drug action is primarily determined by the pharmacokinetic characteristics of the drug (metabolism and elimination), but it is also influenced by the potency of the drug hemodynamics and the influence of drugs on cellular function

CHAPTER TWO

Patient Evaluation and Preparation

"For every mistake that is made for not knowing, a hundred are made for not looking."

ANONYMOUS

OVERVIEW

Anesthesia is more than just the delivery of anesthetic drugs to produce anesthesia. Safe anesthesia includes selecting the appropriate drugs for each procedure, assessing the physical status of the patient, noting the administration of concurrent medication, and a working familiarity with anesthetic drugs, their potential toxicities, and their treatment. This chapter outlines preoperative evaluation as it relates to subsequent anesthetic management.

GENERAL CONSIDERATIONS

I. The preanesthetic evaluation (history and physical examination) dictates the choice and dose of anesthetics to be used

II. The history and physical examination are the basis of patient evaluation; the need for further workup is indicated by abnormalities found during physical examination *or* historical information that suggests altered bodily functions

III. Laboratory tests are no substitute for a thorough physical examination

IV. A patent airway must be maintained in every patient

V. A patent intravenous route must be maintained for all high-risk patients

VI. Unexpected events must be anticipated
VII. An emergency cart with appropriate antidotes and antagonists should be maintained (see Chapter 28)

PATIENT EVALUATION

I. Patient identification
  A. Case number or identification
  B. Signalment
  1. Species
  2. Breed
  3. Age
  4. Sex
  C. Body weight
II. Client complaint and anamnesis (history)
  A. Duration and severity of illness
  B. Concurrent symptoms or disease
  1. Diarrhea
  2. Vomiting
  3. Hemorrhage
  4. Seizures
  5. Heart failure (cough, exercise intolerance)
  6. Renal failure
  C. Level of activity (exercise tolerance)
  D. Recent feeding
  E. Previous and current administration of drugs (see Chapter 13)
  1. Organophosphates
  2. Insecticides
  3. Antibiotics
    a. Sulfonamides
    b. Chloramphenicol
    c. Gentamicin, amikacin, polymyxin B
  4. Digitalis glycosides
  5. β-blockers
  6. Calcium channel blockers
  7. Diuretics
  8. Catecholamine-depleting drugs
  F. Previous anesthetic history and reactions

CURRENT PHYSICAL EXAMINATION

I. General body condition
   A. Obesity
   B. Cachexia
   C. Pregnancy
   D. Hydration
   E. Temperature
   F. Calm or excited
   G. Nervous or apprehensive (stress)
II. Cardiovascular
   A. Heart rate and rhythm (Table 2-1)
   B. Arterial blood pressure and pulse pressure quality and regularity
   C. Capillary refill time ($<$1.5 seconds)
   D. Auscultation (cardiac murmurs)
III. Pulmonary
   A. Respiratory rate, depth, and effort
      1. Usually 15 to 25 for small animals, 8 to 20 for large animals
      2. Tidal volume approximately 14 ml/kg
   B. Mucous membrane color
      1. Pallor (anemia or vasoconstriction)
      2. Cyanosis ($>$5 g/dl of unoxygenated hemoglobin)
   C. Auscultation (breath sounds)
   D. Upper airway obstruction
   E. Percussion

TABLE 2-1
NORMAL HEART RATE AND MEAN ARTERIAL BLOOD PRESSURE RANGES

ANIMAL	HEART RATE	ARTERIAL BLOOD PRESSURE
Dog	70-100	70-100
Cat	145-200	80-120
Cow	60-80	90-140
Horse	30-45	70-90
Colt	50-80	60-80
Sheep, goat	60-90	80-110
Pig	60-90	80-110

IV. Hepatic
    A. Jaundice
    B. Failure of blood to clot
    C. Coma, seizures

V. Renal
    A. Vomiting
    B. Oliguria/anuria
    C. Polyuria/polydipsia

VI. Gastrointestinal
    A. Diarrhea
    B. Vomiting
    C. Distention
    D. Auscultation of gut sounds
    E. Rectal palpation when appropriate

VII. Nervous system and special senses
    A. Aggression/depression
    B. Seizures
    C. Fainting
    D. Coma

VIII. Metabolic and endocrine
    A. Temperature (hypothermia, hyperthermia)
    B. Hair loss
    C. Hyperthyroidism/hypothyroidism
    D. Hyperadrenocorticism/hypoadrenocorticism
    E. Diabetes

IX. Integument
    A. Hydration
    B. Neoplasia (pulmonary metastasis)
    C. Subcutaneous emphysema (fractured ribs)
    D. Parasites (fleas, mites); anemia
    E. Hair loss
    F. Burns (fluid and electrolyte loss)
    G. Trauma

X. Musculoskeletal
    A. Muscle mass (% fat)
    B. Weakness
    C. Electrolyte imbalance (hypokalemia, hyperkalemia; hypocalcemia)
    D. Ambulatory or nonambulatory
    E. Fractures

PATIENT PHYSICAL STATUS

1. Class I: normal patient with no organic disease
2. Class II: patient with mild systemic disease
3. Class III: patient with severe systemic disease that limits activity but is not incapacitating
4. Class IV: patient with incapacitating systemic disease that is a constant threat to life
5. Class V: moribund patient not expected to live 24 hours with or without an operation. Designate emergency operation by an "E" after appropriate classification

---

PRESURGICAL LABORATORY WORKUP

I. Minimum laboratory evaluation (Table 2-2)
   A. Plasma protein (oncotic pressure)
   B. Packed cell volume
   C. Hemoglobin
II. Other laboratory tests (Tables 2-2 through 2-5)
   A. Complete blood count
   B. Blood gases and pH
   C. Hemostasis
   D. Albumin
III. Blood chemistry profile (Table 2-5)
   A. Electrolytes ($Na+$, $K+$, $Cl-$, Ca^{2+})
   B. Blood urea nitrogen
   C. Creatinine
   D. Aspartate aminotransferase (AST), alanine aminotransferase (ALT)
   E. Bile salts
IV. Urinalysis (normal findings given in parentheses)
   A. Specific gravity (1.01 to 1.03)
   B. Physiochemical evaluation
      1. pH (7.0 to 7.5, meat diet; 7.0 to 8.0, vegetable diet)
      2. Protein (negative)
      3. Acetone (negative)
      4. Bilirubin (negative)
      5. Blood (negative)

TABLE 2-2
NORMAL HEMATOLOGIC VALUES

	DOG	CAT	COW	HORSE	SHEEP	PIG
Plasma protein (g/dl)	6-7.5	6-7.5	6-7.5	6-7.5	6.3-7.1	6-7.5
PCV (%)	35-54	27-46	23-43	25-45	30-50	30-48
Hb (g/dl)	12.5-19	8.5-16	8-13	10-16	10-16	10-15
Total leukocytes ($\times 10^9$/L)	6.5-19	4.5-16.5	4-12	5-15	4-12	6.5-20
Neutrophil—segmented ($\times 10^9$/L)	3-11.5	3-13	1.4-6	2.3-8.5	1-6	3-15
Neutrophil—band ($\times 10^9$/L)	0-0.3	0-0.3	0-0.1	0-0.1	0-0.1	0-0.5
Lymphocytes ($\times 10^9$/L)	1.2-5.2	1.2-9	1.4-7	1-5	2-8	2-12
Monocytes ($\times 10^9$/L)	0.2-1.3	0-0.7	0-0.8	0-0.7	0-0.6	0-0.6
Eosinophil ($\times 10^9$/L)	0-1.2	0-1.2	0-2	0-0.8	0-1	0-0.6
Basophil ($\times 10^9$/L)	rare	rare	0-0.2	0-0.3	0-0.1	0-0.1

PCV, Packed cell volume, *Hb*, hemoglobin.

TABLE 2-3
SERUM CHEMISTRY

	UNITS	DOG	CAT	HORSE	COW	SHEEP	PIG
CO_2 combining	mEq/L	16-30	15-25	25-35	21-32	—	—
Calcium	mg/dl	9.8-12.8	9.1-12.3	11.6-13.4	8.9-11.6	8.1-9.5	—
Phosphorus	mg/dl	2.5-7.3	2.8-8.7	1.5-5.1	4.5-8.2	3.5-6.7	5.3-9.6
Glucose	mg/dl	66-120	70-175	78-140	45-90	50-80	60-100
Creatinine	mg/dl	0.7-1.3	0.7-1.8	0.9-1.4	0.8-1.5	—	1.0-2.7
Bilirubin (T)	mg/dl	0-0.2	0-0.2	0-1.1	0-0.3	—	—
Bilirubin (D)	mg/dl	0-0.2	0-0.1	0-0.8	0-0.2	—	—
Albumin	g/dl	2.6-3.6	2.5-3.9	2.2-3.4	2.8-4.1	2.4-3	—
Protein	g/dl	5.3-7.5	6.2-8.2	5.7-7.9	6.3-8.9	6.3-7.1	—
BSP		5% R	5% R	$2-3.7\ t_{1/2}$	$2.5-4\ t_{1/2}$	—	3% R
BUN	mg/dl	6-30	15-33	19-33	6-32	5-20	8-24
Cholesterol	mg/dl	106-330	50-275	50-105	60-240	—	—
ALP	IU/L	20-130	0-83	90-325	0-200	—	—
Amylase	IU/L	350-1950	700-1800	—	—	—	—
CK	IU/L	14-460	100-850	150-450	90-350	—	—
LDH	IU/L	?	?	?	?	—	—
SDH	IU/L	—	—	4-20	6-30	—	—
AST	IU/L	10-50	15-36	220-600	55-100	—	—

TABLE 2-3
SERUM CHEMISTRY—cont'd

	UNITS	DOG	CAT	HORSE	COW	SHEEP	PIG
ALT	IU/L	15-110	15-75	—	—	—	—
Na	mEq/L	145-155	150-170	137-143	137-148	140-145	139-152
K	mEq/L	4.0-5.4	3.7-6.0	3.2-4.5	3.5-5.1	4.9-5.7	4.4-6.7
Cl	mEq/L	104-117	111-128	98-105	84-102	—	100-105
Ca^{2+}	mg/dl	9.8-12.8	9.1-12.3	11.6-13.4	8.9-11.6	—	9.5-12.7
Mg	mg/dl	1.8-2.4	—	2.2-2.8	2.2-3.4	—	—
pH	Units	7.27-7.43	7.25-7.33	7.34-7.42	7.32-7.45	—	—
Po$_2$	mmHg	25-46	31-49	26-46	24-39	—	—
Pco$_2$	mmHg	28-49	35-49	39-53	34-53	—	—
HCO$_3$	mEq/L	18-25	18-22	23-31	23-31	—	—
Base excess	mEq/L	−6 to 0.5	−6 to −3	−1 to 5	−1 to 4.2	—	—
Cortisol 0 hr	μg/dl	1-4.8	—	1-4.4	1-2.7	—	—
Cortisol 2 hr	μg/dl	5-26	—	5.1-14.6 (8 hr)	2.7-6	—	—
IM ACTH							
T$_3$ (RIA)	ng/dl	50-200	60-200	—	—	—	—
T$_4$ (RIA)	μg/dl	1-4	1.5-5	—	—	—	—

ACTH, Adrenocorticotropic hormone; *ALP,* alkaline phosphatase; *ALT,* alanine aminotransferase; *AST,* aspartate aminotransferase; *BSP,* bromosulphalein; *BUN,* blood urea nitrogen; *CK,* creatine kinase; *LDH,* lactate dehydrogenase; *R,* retention; *SDH,* sorbitol dehydrogenase; *T$_{1/2}$,* half-life; *T$_3$,* triiodothyronine; *T$_4$,* thyroxine.

TABLE 2-4
ARTERIAL BLOOD GASES

	NORMAL VALUES (21% O_2)	VALUES ROUTINELY OBSERVED DURING ANESTHESIA
pH	7.4 ± 0.2	7.30-7.45
$PaCO_2$ mm Hg	40 ± 3	30-60*
PaO_2 mm Hg	94 ± 3	250 to 500 (100% O_2) up to 250 (50% O_2)
Base excess	0 ± 1	-4 to -10

*The development of respiratory acidosis during anesthesia is common; its degree of severity depends in part on the drugs used, the depth of anesthesia, the duration of anesthesia, and patient status.

    C. Microscopic evaluation of urine sediment
      1. Casts (negative or rare)
      2. Red blood cells (RBC) (negative)
      3. White blood cells (WBC) (negative); occasional red blood cells are seen depending on how sample is collected
      4. Epithelial cells (negative)
      5. Bacteria (negative)
      6. Crystals
        a. Oxalate (normal finding)
        b. Triple phosphates (normal finding)
        c. Urates (normal finding)
        d. Calcium carbonate (normally found in horses only)

FURTHER PRESURGICAL TESTS

  I. Electrocardiography
    A. Traumatized patients (myocardial trauma and arrhythmias)
    B. Irregular rhythm on physical exam
  II. Radiology
    A. Thorax
    B. Abdomen
  III. Ultrasonography

PATIENT PREPARATION

  I. Withhold food
    A. Withholding food is species dependent (see species-specific recommendations)

TABLE 2-5
HEMOSTASIS AND TEMPERATURE

	UNITS	DOG	CAT	HORSE	COW	SHEEP	PIG
Platelets	1000/μl	150-400	150-400	100-400	200-800	250-800	200-700
PT	seconds	10-12	6.5-9	15-19	23-28	13-17	—
APTT	seconds	18-24	14-20	55-110	55-80	35-50	—
Normal body temperature Fahrenheit		101.5-102.5 (small breed) 99.5-101.5 (large breed)	100-102.5	99.5-101.5 (foal) 99-100.5 (adult)	101.5-103.5 (calf up to 1 yr) 100-102.5 (ox)	102-104	102-104 (piglet) 100-102 (adult)
Centigrade		38.5-39.2 (small breed) 37.5-38.6 (large breed)	37.8-39.2	37.5-38.6 (foal) 37.2-38 (adult)	38.6-39.8 (calf up to 1 yr) 37.8-39.2 (ox over 1 yr)	38.9-4	38.9-40 (piglet) 37.8-38.9 (adult)

PT, Prothrombin time; *APTT,* activated partial thromboplastin time.

      B. Do not withhold food for excessive periods in neonates, toy breeds, animals weighing under 10 pounds, or birds

II. Correct or compensate for
    A. Dehydration (hypovolemia)
    B. Anemia, blood loss, or hypoproteinemia
    C. Acid-base and electrolyte abnormalities
    D. Cardiac dysfunction
    E. Respiratory distress
    F. Renal dysfunction
    G. Hemostatic defects
    H. Temperature

III. Specific preparation for intended procedure
    A. Thoracic
    B. Abdominal
    C. Orthopedic
    D. Ophthalmologic
    E. Neurologic

IV. Other considerations
    A. Fluid and caloric needs during and following anesthesia
    B. Special medications (inotropes, antiarrhythmics)
    C. Duration of surgery
    D. Needs of the surgeon

PLAN FOR ANESTHETIC MANAGEMENT

   I. Formulation of anesthetic care plan
      A. Surgical procedure (special requirements)
      B. Positioning
      C. Selection of drugs: emphasis on the control of pain during all phases of the preoperative, intraoperative, and postoperative periods
      D. Airway management
      E. Fluid management
      F. Body temperature management
      G. Monitoring
      H. Anticipation of possible untoward effects and response problems
  II. Assembling of emergency drugs and equipment (see Chapter 28)

CHAPTER THREE

Drugs Used for Preanesthetic Medication

"No patient should ever be anesthetized without the benefit of preanesthetic medications."

WILLIAM WALLACE MUIR, III, 1970

OVERVIEW

Preanesthetic medications are an essential part of safe anesthetic management. When used appropriately, they minimize stress, cardiopulmonary depression, and the deleterious effects associated with many intravenous and inhalation anesthetics.

Routine preanesthetic medications are classified into four categories. *Anticholinergics* limit excessive salivary secretions and prevent bradycardia. *Phenothiazine* and *butyrophenone tranquilizers* produce calming and decrease the amount of general anesthetic required to produce anesthesia. α_2-*Agonists* produce sedation, analgesia, and muscle relaxation without producing general anesthesia. *Opioids* produce analgesia and euphoria. The combination of an α_2-agonist or tranquilizer with an opioid, (neuroleptanalgesic), produces marked calming and analgesia and light stages of anesthesia in small animals.

GENERAL CONSIDERATIONS
Purposes of Preanesthetic Drugs

I. Aid in animal restraint by modifying behavior (produces a patient that is not interested in its surroundings and is reluctant to move)

II. Reduce stress

III. Prevent pain before, during, and after surgery

IV. Produce muscle relaxation

V. Decrease the amount of potentially more dangerous drugs used to produce sedation, muscle relaxation, analgesia, or general anesthesia

VI. Facilitate safe and uncomplicated induction, maintenance, and recovery from anesthesia

VII. Minimize the adverse and potentially toxic effects of concurrently administered drugs

VIII. Minimize autonomic reflex activity, whether of sympathetic or parasympathetic origin

DRUG CATEGORIES

I. Anticholinergics (e.g., atropine, glycopyrrolate, scopolamine)

   A. Competitively antagonize acetylcholine at sites innervated by postganglionic, parasympathetic (cholinergic) nerve fibers and on smooth muscles that are influenced by acetylcholine but lack innervation; referred to as parasympatholytics, anticholinergics, or antispasmodics

   B. Primarily used to limit salivary secretions and to prevent bradycardia or deliberately increase heart rate. Increases in heart rate generally increase arterial blood pressure and cardiac output (HR $\times$ SV = CO)

   C. Atropine and scopolamine may produce drowsiness and potentiate the effects of central nervous system (CNS) depressant drugs; large doses may stimulate cerebral areas, leading to restlessness, disorientation, and delirium, an effect more common in ruminants

   D. Glycopyrrolate, a quaternary ammonium drug, does not cross the blood-brain or placental barriers

   E. Reduce glandular secretions of the respiratory tract, gastrointestinal tract, oral and nasal cavities

      1. The accumulation of excessive secretions in the oral cavity of small animals (e.g., cats) may predispose to upper airway obstruction and laryngospasm

      2. Increased secretory activity may occur after parasympatholytic drug effects subside; this is known as a *post-parasympatholytic rebound phenomenon*

3. Gastric pH is increased (i.e., less acidic); gastrointestinal motility and contractions of the bladder and ureter are reduced; intestinal motility can be decreased for several hours in horses, an effect that could cause colic. Ruminal atony (bloat) can occur in ruminants

F. Produce bronchodilation (increased physiologic dead space) and mydriasis

G. Inhibit bradycardia caused by reflex increases in vagal tone (e.g., laryngeal or ocular stimulation and vagovagal reflexes)

   1. Increasing heart rate generally increases arterial blood pressure and cardiac output

   2. Parasympatholytics may induce a sinus tachycardia or occasionally precipitate ventricular arrhythmias. Anticholinergic drugs cause sinus bradycardia to progress through various stages of first- and second-degree atrioventricular block before the establishment of sinus rhythm (Fig. 3-1)

   3. Atropine sulfate may stimulate vagal nuclei in the medulla and thus induce an initial sinus bradycardia; glycopyrrolate does not cross the blood-brain or placental barrier and therefore is devoid of CNS or fetal effects

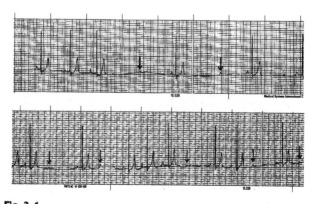

Fig. 3-1
ECG of sinus bradycardia with 2 atrioventricular block (P waves not followed by QRS complexes). Arrows indicate blocked P waves.

       4. Vagal reflexes produced by traction on visceral organs or during ocular surgery are not always successfully treated with parasympatholytic drugs

       5. General anesthetics, opioids, α2-agonists, digitalis glycosides, hyperkalemia, acidosis, and injection of calcium salts augment vagal effects and may precipitate bradycardia

          a. Halothane, methoxyflurane, sevoflurane, isoflurane, and barbiturates indirectly enhance parasympathetic effects by suppressing sympathetic tone

          b. Phenothiazine tranquilizers rarely produce a CNS-induced cholinergic effect and sinus bradycardia

H. Administer intramuscularly (IM) or subcutaneously (SQ) (intravenously [IV] for emergencies)

       1. Atropine sulfate (0.01 to 0.02 mg/lb) or glycopyrrolate (0.005 mg/lb) increases heart rate and dries secretions in small animals. The duration of action of atropine sulfate is 60 to 90 minutes; the duration of action of glycopyrrolate is 2 to 4 hours

       2. Parasympatholytics are of questionable value in horses and cattle because of side effects (colic) or lack of effect, respectively

          a. Horses: atropine, 0.02 to 0.04 mg/lb; glycopyrrolate, 0.0015 to 0.003 mg/lb

          b. Ruminants: not recommended for decreasing salivation; atropine temporarily decreases secretions, which can become more viscid; proper positioning of the head and neck is of the utmost importance to prevent pooling of saliva solution in the pharynx and subsequent aspiration

          c. Pigs: atropine (0.02 mg/lb); glycopyrrolate (0.0015 mg/lb)

I. Untoward reactions

       1. Atropine may cause an initial bradycardia after intravenous administration

       2. Cardiac arrhythmias, particularly sinus tachycardia and first- and second-degree atrioventricular block, are observed after intravenous administration of atropine or glycopyrrolate; ventricular arrhythmias may occur after intravenous atropine administration

    3. Sinus tachycardia increases myocardial oxygen consumption and can precipitate heart failure or pulmonary edema in patients with preexisting cardiovascular disease

    4. Atropine may cause depression in dogs and cats; it may cause restlessness, delirium, and disorientation in ruminants

    5. Colic in horses is due to ileus

II. Tranquilizers and sedatives (e.g., phenothiazines, butyrophenones, benzodiazepines, and α2-agonists) (Table 3-1)

  A. Phenothiazines (e.g., acepromazine, promazine), butyrophenones (e.g., droperidol)

    1. Mode of action

      a. Calming and neurologic effects appear to be mediated by depression of the reticular activating system and antidopaminergic actions in the CNS

      b. Suppression of the sympathetic nervous system (depresses mobilization of catecholamines centrally and peripherally)

      c. Phenothiazine tranquilizers may lower seizure threshold in animals with epilepsy; butyrophenones do not

      d. Phenothiazines and butyrophenones produce antiemetic effects by inhibiting dopamine interaction in the chemoreceptor trigger zone in the medulla

    2. Physical properties

      a. Water soluble

      b. Can be mixed with other water-soluble drugs

    3. Produce mental calming, decrease motor activity, and increase threshold for responding to external stimuli

      a. Not noted for analgesic activity, but improve the analgesic effects of drugs with analgesic activity

      b. Excessive doses of phenothiazines and butyrophenones can cause apparent involuntary (extrapyramidal) musculoskeletal effects and hallucinatory activity in some animals, particularly horses

      c. The calming effect can be temporarily reversed with an adequate stimulus; larger doses may be required in excitable or apprehensive animals

TABLE 3-1
INTRAVENOUS DOSAGES OF COMMONLY USED TRANQUILIZERS AND SEDATIVES (MG/LB)

AGENT	DOG	CAT	HORSE	COW	GOAT	PIG
Major tranquilizers						
Acepromazine*	0.05-0.2	0.05-0.3	0.01-0.04	0.02-0.04	0.02-0.04	0.1-0.3
Promazine	0.3-0.5	0.5-1.5	0.1-0.5	0.1-0.5	0.1-0.5	0.5-1.5
Minor tranquilizers						
Diazepam	0.1-0.2	0.1-0.2	0.01-0.004	0.01-0.04	0.01-0.04	0.1-0.2
Midazolam	0.1-0.2	0.1-0.2	0.01-0.02	—	—	—
Sedatives						
Xylazine	0.2-0.5	0.2-0.5	0.2-0.5	0.01-0.05	0.01-0.03	
Detomidine	—	—	5-10 μg/lb	1-5 μg/lb	—	—
Medetomidine	0.005-0.01	0.01-0.02	0.005-0.01	—	—	—
Romifidine	0.02-0.04	0.04-0.08	0.04-0.08	—	—	—
Chloral hydrate	—	—	10-15	20-30	15-25	20-30

*The maximum dose for acepromazine when used as a preanesthetic medication in dogs is 4 mg.

4. Cardiopulmonary effects
    a. α-Adrenergic blockade results in a decrease in arterial blood pressure (epinephrine administration may cause a paradoxic drop in blood pressure [BP] since alpha receptors are blocked)
        (1) Hypotension occurs more frequently in excited or apprehensive patients. Reflex tachycardia may occur in response to hypotension. Treated with IV fluids
        (2) Severe reactions include hypotensive crisis resulting in fainting and (rarely) bradycardia resulting in death
        (3) Phenylephrine (α-agonist) and fluids can be used to increase blood pressure if hypotension is severe
    b. Heart rate usually decreases as the patient becomes calm; however, reflex tachycardia may occur due to hypotension; centrally induced bradycardia (rare)
    c. Antiarrhythmic effects: phenothiazines produce quinidine-like effects; epinephrine-induced cardiac arrhythmias are prevented by quinidine-like effects and decreases in central sympathetic, ganglionic, and peripheral (adrenal) activity
    d. Dose-dependent depression of the myocardium and vascular smooth muscle
    e. Ganglionic blocking activity
    f. Reduces respiratory rate; may decrease tidal volume when administered in large doses; decreases respiratory center sensitivity to increases in CO_2
5. Potentiates the ventilatory and cardiovascular depressant effects of α_2-agonists, opioids, and drugs used to produce general anesthesia
6. Useful as antiemetics
7. Most have antihistaminic properties; phenothiazines and butyrophenones should be avoided when skin testing for allergies
8. Most phenothiazine tranquilizers cross the placental barrier relatively slowly
9. Many phenothiazine tranquilizers, including acepromazine and promazine, may cause erection (priapism)

in yearlings, and temporary or permanent prolapse of the penis in stallions. Potentially reversible by administering benztropine (0.01 mg/lb, IV)

10. Butyrophenone tranquilizers produce calming and prevent fighting and cannibalism in pigs
11. Primary organ of metabolism is the liver; should be avoided in patients with moderate to severe liver disease.
12. Clinical effects are present for 4 to 8 hours but may last up to 48 hours or longer in older animals or animals with liver disease (portal-caval shunts)
13. Commonly used phenothiazines include acepromazine and promazine; butyrophenone tranquilizers are rarely used in veterinary medicine, including droperidol (see Tables 3-1 and 3-2)
14. Dose (see Table 3-1)
15. Side effects
    a. Tachycardia or (rarely) bradycardia
    b. Hypotension
    c. Hypothermia
    d. Akathisia: restless condition in which the patient needs to be in constant motion
    e. Acute dystonic reactions: hysteria, seizures, ataxia
    f. Inhibits platelet aggregation
    g. Tranquilizers (e.g., droperidol) can cause excitement and extrapyramidal effects in old dogs and horses at relatively low doses

B. Benzodiazepines (e.g., diazepam, midazolam, zolazepam) are centrally acting muscle relaxants that are sometimes referred to as *minor tranquilizers* (Table 3-1)
    1. Mode of action
        a. Exert many of their pharmacologic effects by enhancing the activity of CNS inhibitory neurotransmitters (γ-aminobutyric acid, glycine) and opening chloride channels, thereby hyperpolarizing membranes; also produce their effects by combining with CNS benzodiazepine (BZ_1, BZ_2) receptors. Effects can be antagonized by the benzodiazepine antagonist, flumazenil

TABLE 3-2

INTRAVENOUS DOSAGES OF COMMONLY USED OPIOIDS AND NEUROLEPTANALGESICS (MG/LB)

AGENT	DOG	CAT	HORSE	COW	GOAT	PIG
Opioid agonists and partial agonists						
Morphine	0.2-0.5	0.05-0.1	0.02-0.05	—	—	0.2-0.4
Meperidine	0.2-0.5	0.1-0.2	0.2-0.5	—	—	0.2-0.5
Oxymorphone	0.05-0.1	0.05	0.01-0.05	—	—	—
Methadone	0.1-0.3	—	0.03-0.06	—	—	—
Fentanyl	0.001-0.003	—	0.03-0.06	—	—	—
Pentazocine	0.1-0.2	0.05-0.01	0.2-0.4	—	—	0.1-0.2
Butorphanol	0.1-0.2	0.1-0.2	0.005-0.1	—	—	0.1-0.2
Buprenorphine	0.01	0.01	0.005	—	—	—
Neuroleptanalgesics						
Acepromazine-oxymorphone	0.1-0.2 mg/lb (acepromazine)* 0.05 mg/lb (oxymorphone)*					
Xylazine-morphine	0.1-0.5 mg (xylazine) 0.1-0.3 mg (morphine)					

Intramuscular dose is two to three times the intravenous dose. Lower drug dosages should be used in sick patients.

*Dogs and cats only.

b. Depress the limbic system, thalamus, and hypothalamus (reducing sympathetic output), thereby inducing a mild calming effect

c. Reduce polysynaptic reflex activity, resulting in muscle relaxation

d. Cause minimal CNS depression and produce anticonvulsant effects in most animals; may cause disorientation and agitation after rapid intravenous administration, particularly in cats

e. Stimulate appetite and pica

2. Physical properties

a. Diazepam is solubilized by mixing with 40% propylene glycol, ethyl alcohol, sodium benzoate, or benzoic acid; in rare cases, produces hypotension, bradycardia, and apnea if administered too rapidly intravenously

b. Midazolam and zolazepam are water soluble

3. Recommended dosages produce minimal or no calming in normal animals; calming effects are observed in sick, depressed, or debilitated animals

a. Muscle relaxation

b. Anticonvulsant

c. Behavior modification

4. Cardiopulmonary effects

a. Minimal hypotensive effects are observed after intravenous administration

b. Bradycardia and hypotension have occurred after rapid intravenous administration

c. Respiratory rate and tidal volume are minimally affected

d. Some antiarrhythmic effects result from decreases in sympathetic nervous system activity

5. Produce excellent muscle relaxation in animals and reduce muscle spasms and spasticity; effects are additive or synergistic with other drugs used to produce general anesthesia (e.g., barbiturates, propofol)

6. Increase seizure threshold

7. Effects on gastrointestinal activity undetermined

8. Use in pregnancy not investigated

9. Diazepam is eliminated in the urine and feces after metabolism by the liver; duration of action is 1 to 4 hours

10. Diazepam increases appetite in domestic cats and ruminants (probably in all species)
11. Dose (see Table 3-1)
12. Side effects
    a. Ataxia, particularly evident in large animal species
    b. Paradoxical increase in anxiety leading to aggression in cats
    c. Possible CNS depression in neonates
    d. Diazepam painful if administered IM because of propylene glycol
    e. Bradycardia and hypotension if administered rapidly by IV
13. Antagonists: benzodiazepine effects can be antagonized by benzodiazepine antagonists (e.g., flumazenil: 0.005 to 0.01 mg/lb IV; Table 3-3)
C. Xylazine, detomidine, medetomidine, romifidine (see Table 3-1)
    1. Mode of action
        a. Produce CNS depression by stimulating presynaptic α_2-adrenoceptors in the CNS and peripherally; this decreases norepinephrine release centrally and peripherally; the net result is a decrease in CNS

TABLE 3-3
BENZODIAZEPINE, α_2-, AND OPIOID ANTAGONISTS*

AGENT	DOSE
Benzodiazepine antagonist	
Flumazenil	0.1 mg/lb
α_2- antagonist	
Yohimbine	1-2 mg/lb
Tolazoline	0.5-2 mg/lb
Atipamazole	0.05-0.2 mg/lb
Opioid antagonist	
Naloxone	15 μg/5 lb opioids

*Antagonists are used whenever drug reversal is desired. Analgesia may be reversed also.

sympathetic outflow and a decrease in circulating catecholamines and other stress-related substances; the CNS effects of α_2-agonists can be antagonized by α_2-receptor antagonists (e.g, yohimbine, tolazoline, atipamazole)

b. Comparative drug selectivity for α_2- vs. $\alpha 1$-receptors

DRUG	α2:α1-SELECTIVITY
Clonidine	220:1
Xylazine	160:1
Detomidine	260:1
Medetomidine	1620:1
Romifidine	200:1 ?

c. Polysynaptic reflexes are inhibited (centrally acting muscle relaxant), but the neuromuscular junction is not influenced; depress internuncial neuron transmission

d. Induce a sleeplike state comparable to phenothiazines, but it is more pronounced

e. Produce analgesia by stimulating CNS α_2-receptors

f. Effects are additive and may be synergistic when combined with other depressants and analgesic drugs used to produce chemical restraint or general anesthesia

2. General properties
   a. Produce calming effect/sedation, muscle relaxation, and analgesia
      (1) Xylazine: 20 to 40 minutes IV
      (2) Detomidine: 90 to 120 minutes IV
      (3) Medetomidine: 45 to 90 minutes IV
      (4) Romifidine: 45 to 90 minutes IV
   b. Can be administered epidurally or subarachnoidally to produce regional or segmental analgesia

3. Cardiopulmonary effects
   a. Decreased heart rate due to decreased CNS sympathetic outflow and increased parasympathetic activity; may initiate sinus bradycardia or first- or second-degree atrioventricular blockade; complete or third-degree atrioventricular block with escape beats occurs rarely

b. Increased cardiac sensitivity to catecholamine-induced arrhythmias during halothane anesthesia; this effect occurs early, is transient, and is caused by α_1- and possibly α_2-adrenoceptor stimulation; this effect coincides with the increase in arterial BP and is not observed after detomidine, medetomidine, or romifidine administration

c. Cardiac output may decrease by 30% to 50% and coincides with decreases in heart rate and increases in peripheral vascular resistance

d. Arterial blood pressure increases shortly after drug administration (α_1- and α_2-adrenoceptor stimulatory effect), then decreases to below control values because of decreases in CNS sympathetic outflow and a decrease in norepinephrine from sympathetic nerve terminals

e. Initially increase peripheral vascular resistance

f. Initial vasoconstriction may cause pale mucous membranes

g. Depress respiratory centers centrally

h. Decrease respiratory center sensitivity to increases in P_{CO_2}; decrease tidal volume and respiratory rate with an overall decrease in minute volume when administered in large dosages IV

i. Respiratory threshold to CO_2 increases when large dosages are administered, resulting in marked respiratory depression

j. May induce stridor and dyspnea in horses and brachycephalic dogs with upper airway obstruction

4. Other organ systems

a. Suppress salivation, gastric secretions, and gastrointestinal motility; may stimulate pica and appetite at low doses

b. Cause vomiting in dogs and cats and are suspected of predisposing to bloat in large-breed dogs

c. Depress swallowing reflex

d. Excellent for treating gastrointestinal pain (colic), although prolonged effects may delay surgery or mask the severity of disease

e. Suppress insulin release by stimulating presynaptic α_2-receptors in the pancreas, resulting in an increase in plasma glucose concentration and glucosuria

f. Promote diuresis with increases in water and sodium excretion

5. Absorption, fate, and excretion
   a. Rapidly absorbed after intramuscular, subcutaneous, or oral administration
   b. Relatively rapidly metabolized by the liver and excreted in the urine
   c. Active metabolites possible; more than 20 identified

6. Other
   a. Produce profound sleep in dogs, cats, foals, and small ruminants; this is partially reversible with doxapram hydrochloride (0.05 to 0.2 mg/lb IV)
   b. Crosses the placenta, but an abortifacient effect has not been noted in pregnant mares; neither were observable effects upon gestation or parturition; xylazine may induce premature delivery in cattle
   c. Effect is oxytocin-like in ruminants; this activity has not been reported in mares or small animals
   d. Highly excited or nervous animals may react adversely by becoming extremely ataxic, reacting violently or viciously when approached or touched, or showing inadequate response to the drug
   e. Clinical value in pigs is questionable because of their relatively rapid metabolism

7. Side effects
   a. Respiratory depression (respiratory acidosis)
   b. Bradyarrhythmias
   c. Hypotension
   d. Ataxia in large animals
   e. Sweating in horses
   f. Diuresis
   g. Occasional unpredictable effects
   h. Occasional severe inflammatory response if administered SQ in horses or cattle

8. α_2-Antagonists (Table 3-3)
   a. Yohimbine (0.25 mg/lb IV)
   b. Tolazoline (1 to 2 mg/lb IV)
   c. Atipamazole (0.05 to 0.2 mg/lb)

       d. Doxapram HCl, as noted above, although not a specific antagonist, is useful for reversing respiratory depression and mild sedation

III. Opioids (see Table 3-2)

  A. Mode of action

    1. Act by reversible combination with one or more specific receptors (opiate and nonopiate) in the brain and spinal cord to produce a variety of effects, including analgesia, sedation, euphoria, dysphoria, and excitement

    2. Referred to as opioid agonists, partial agonists, agonist-antagonists, and antagonists

      a. Represented by a variety of naturally occurring (opiate) derivatives and synthetically manufactured drugs

      b. Classified according to analgesic activity or addiction potential

      c. Commonly used opioids include morphine, meperidine, oxymorphone, and fentanyl; pentazocine, butorphanol, and buprenorphine are drugs with opioid agonist-antagonist (pentazocine, butorphanol) or partial agonist (buprenorphine) effects

      d. Analgesic potency

        (1) Morphine: 1

        (2) Meperidine: 0.5

        (3) Oxymorphone: 5 to 10

        (4) Fentanyl: 100^+

        (5) Pentazocine: 0.1

        (6) Butorphanol: 2 to 5

        (7) Buprenorphine: 3 to 5

    3. Senses are not significantly depressed by opioids

      a. Touch

      b. Vibration

      c. Vision

      d. Hearing

  B. Used before (preemptive), during, or after surgery for analgesia

Fentanyl, sufentanil, and oxymorphone are generally used during surgery as part of a balanced anesthetic technique

    1. Fentanyl patches can be used to provide analgesia. The fentanyl patch is a transdermal drug delivery system (see Table 3-2)

TABLE 3-4
COMMONLY USED ANALGESIC AND TRANQUILIZER COMBINATIONS FOR INTRAVENOUS USE*

ANIMAL	DRUGS	RECOMMENDED INTRAVENOUS DOSAGES	UNTOWARD EFFECTS
Dog	Acepromazine-meperidine	0.05-0.1 mg/lb 0.1-0.3 mg/lb	Hypotension
	Acepromazine-oxymorphone	0.05-0.1 mg/lb 0.05-0.1 mg/lb	Hypotension
	Acepromazine-butorphanol	0.05 mg/lb 0.1-0.2 mg/lb	Bradycardia Hypotension
	Diazepam-fentanyl	0.1-0.2 mg/lb 0.005 mg/lb	Bradycardia
Cat	Acepromazine-oxymorphone	0.1 mg/lb IM 0.04 mg/lb	Excitement
	Acepromazine-butorphanol	0.05 mg/lb 0.1-0.2 mg/lb	Bradycardia Hypotension

Horse	Xylazine-morphine†	0.3 mg/lb	Bradycardia
		0.1-0.3 mg/lb	Hypotension
	Xylazine-meperidine	0.3 mg/lb	Hypotension
		0.5 mg/lb	
	Xylazine-butorphanol	0.3 mg/lb	Ataxia
		0.01 mg/lb	
	Xylazine-acepromazine	0.3 mg/lb	Hypotension
		0.025 mg/lb	
	Meperidine-acepromazine	0.25 mg/lb	Hypotension
		0.025 mg/lb	
Ruminants			
Cow	Xylazine	0.02-0.05 mg/lb	Respiratory depression, bradycardia
Sheep	Xylazine	0.05-0.1 mg/lb	
Goat‡	Xylazine	0.005-0.05 mg/lb*	

*Lower doses should be used in sick patients
†Detomidine (1 to 5 µg/lb IV) can be substituted for xylazine in horses; medetomidine (0.003-0.01 mg/lb IV) or romifidine (0.01-0.04 mg/lb IV) can be substituted for xylazine in dogs and cats
‡Variable response

       2. Morphine is administered epidurally or subarachnoidally to produce regional or segmental analgesia

C. Produce analgesic action at doses lower than needed for sedation (dosage tailored to individual animal)

D. Effects in addition to analgesia
   1. Behavioral changes (e.g., sedation, euphoria, dysphoria, excitement)
   2. Change in response to external stimuli (animal may not recognize owner)
   3. Miosis in dogs and pigs; mydriasis in cats and horses
   4. Decreases in body temperature caused by panting; caused by resetting of the thermoregulatory center and panting in dogs
   5. Sweating, particularly in horses

E. Produce additive or synergistic effects when used with other depressants (e.g., tranquilizers, barbiturates, inhalation anesthesia)

F. May be used in combination with tranquilizers and sedatives to produce neuroleptanalgesia (see Tables 3-2 and 3-4)

G. Produce excellent sedation in dogs, but may cause excitement when given rapidly IV; cats and horses are particularly susceptible to the excitatory effect of opioids; this is typified by increased motor activity and pacing in horses

H. Use is strictly controlled; increased security and accurate record keeping are required

I. Cardiopulmonary effects
   1. Bradycardia caused by stimulation of medullary vagal nuclei
   2. Possible hypotension caused by release of histamine (morphine, meperidine)
   3. Positive inotropic action when used in low dosages (morphine only) caused by release of epinephrine and norepinephrine from the adrenal and sympathetic nerve terminals
   4. Respiratory depression is dose-dependent and rarely observed unless the patient is already depressed or unconscious (rate and tidal volume); raises the threshold of the respiratory center to increases in P_{CO_2}
   5. Reduced respiratory reserve capabilities

J. Gastrointestinal effects
   1. Salivation
   2. Nausea
   3. Vomiting in those species that can
   4. Nonpropulsive gastrointestinal hypermotility ("ropy guts"), increases in sphincter tone
   5. Defecation
K. Decrease in urine production as a result of increased ADH release
L. Cross the placental barrier relatively slowly; useful for cesarean section because depressant effects can be antagonized
M. Extensively metabolized by the liver, and metabolites are eliminated in the urine; the opioid agonists vary in biologic half-life, most with durations of action ranging from 30 minutes to 3 hours in most species; morphine may produce effects lasting 6 to 8 hours in horses
N. Tolerance develops with continued use
O. Opioid agonist-antagonists and partial agonists
   1. Pentazocine, butorphanol, and buprenorphine (partial agonist) antagonize some of the effects of other opioid agonists (e.g., morphine, meperidine, oxymorphone, fentanyl) but can produce mild CNS depression, euphoria, and analgesia when administered in therapeutic doses
   2. Butorphanol is an excellent cough suppressant
P. Opioid antagonists (see Table 3-3)
   1. Classification
      a. Pure antagonist (e.g., naloxone, nalmefene)
      b. Agonists-antagonists (e.g., pentazocine, butorphanol)
      c. Partial antagonists (e.g., buprenorphine)
      d. Opioid antagonists may possess many of the same properties as opioids; naloxone possesses the least narcotic agonist effects
   2. Mechanism of action
      a. Opioid antagonists compete with opioid drugs for specific receptor sites
      b. Partial antagonists act in a fashion similar to opioid antagonists

        (1) Can produce autonomic, endocrine, analgesic, and respiratory depressant effects

        (2) Are less potent than morphine as an analgesic

        (3) May add to existing respiratory depression

    3. Metabolized in the liver

    4. Dosage

      a. Naloxone: 1 to 15 μg/lb IV

      b. Nalorphine: 1 mg/5 lb IV

Q. Side effects

    1. Excitement, dysphoria

    2. Apnea

    3. Bradycardia

    4. Ataxia and incoordination

    5. Excessive vomiting

    6. Excessive sweating in horses

IV. Neuroleptanalgesia

A. A state of CNS depression and analgesia produced by the combination of a tranquilizer or sedative and analgesic drug; useful in dogs, cats, horses, and pigs (see Definitions, Chapter 1; Table 3-4)

B. The animal may or may not remain conscious and is responsive to auditory stimuli; many animals defecate, some vomit

C. Results of the drug combination

    1. Sedation-analgesia, ataxia, and/or recumbency

    2. Depression of ventilation (apnea may occur)

    3. Bradycardia

    4. Defecation and flatulence

    5. Analgesia for periods up to 40 minutes

D. Overdosages usually result in profound bradycardia and respiratory depression; respiratory depression can generally be reversed by an opioid antagonist (e.g., nalorphine, levallorphan, naloxone)

E. Most animals are premedicated with a parasympatholytic (e.g., atropine or glycopyrrolate) to prevent bradycardia and excessive salivation

F. Neuroleptanalgesics are used in combination with barbiturates in dogs to eliminate the stimulatory effect of loud noises and to produce better muscle relaxation

    1. Thiopental (1 mg/lb) after acepromazine-oxymorphone

G. Opioids and tranquilizers have been used to produce sedation and analgesia
1. Acepromazine (0.1 to 0.2 mg/lb) in combination with
morphine (0.2 to 0.4 mg/lb IV or SQ), meperidine (0.5
to 1 mg/lb IV), or oxymorphone (0.05 to 0.1 mg/lb IV)
is used to produce neuroleptanalgesia in dogs; diazepam
(0.1 mg/lb IV) and oxymorphone (0.04 mg/lb IV), or
acepromazine (0.1 mg/lb IM) and butorphanol (0.1 to
0.2 mg/lb IM) are used in dogs and cats
2. Alpha-2-agonists (xylazine, medetomidine) combined
with opioids (morphine, butorphanol) are also used to
produce neuroleptanalgesia in dogs and cats
   a. Medetomidine (1 to 5 μg/lb IM) combined with morphine (0.1 μg/lb IM)
3. The combination of xylazine (0.3 mg/lb IV) or detomidine (1 to 3 μg/lb IV) and morphine (0.1 to 0.3 mg/lb
IV), or butorphanol (0.01 to 0.02 mg/lb IV) are commonly used for horses
H. Useful for short operative procedures and for cesarean section in small animals
I. Side effects
1. Respiratory depression
2. Bradycardia
3. Ataxia
4. Excitement
5. CNS and behavioral abnormalities in some breeds of
dogs (e.g., Doberman Pinschers)
V. Nonsteroidal anti-inflammatory drugs (NSAIDs; see Chapter 18)
A. Reduce inflammation and produce analgesia primarily
through inhibition of prostaglandin synthesis
1. CNS actions not well characterized
2. Inhibit the activity of cyclooxygenase peripherally
B. Prostaglandins
1. During inflammation, prostaglandins:
   a. Cause vasodilation
   b. Increase vascular permeability
   c. Sensitize peripheral pain receptors
   d. Chronically new blood vessels and granulation tissue are produced

      2. Prostaglandins also help maintain tissues
        a. Protect gastric mucosa
        b. Facilitate platelet aggregation
        c. Regulate renal blood
      3. Currently available NSAIDs inhibit all prostaglandin formation

C. Minimal acute side effects

D. Toxicity associated with gastrointestinal ulceration and renal papillary necrosis

E. Currently used NSAIDs
      1. Phenylbutazone
        a. Widely used in horses (oral and IV)
        b. Used for a variety of musculoskeletal conditions
        c. Toxic in dogs, cats, and humans (gastric ulceration, renal necrosis, anemia)
      2. Flunixin meglumine
        a. Used in horses (oral, IV, IM)
        b. Used for musculoskeletal conditions and mild colic
        c. Counteracts the effects of absorbed endotoxins
        d. Toxic in dogs and cats (single dose occasionally used for ocular inflammation)
      3. Carprofen
        a. Used in dogs (oral)
        b. Indicated for chronic arthritis and mild perioperative pain
        c. Liver toxicity reported in Labrador Retrievers (resolves with drug withdrawal)
      4. Ketoprofen
        a. Approved for use in horses (IV)
        b. Used in dogs and cats for perioperative analgesic

CHAPTER FOUR

Local Anesthetic Drugs and Techniques

"And don't give me any of those local anesthetics. Get me the imported stuff."

FROM THE CARTOON "HERMAN" UNIVERSAL PRESS SYNDICATE

OVERVIEW

Local anesthetics produce desensitization and analgesia of skin surfaces (topical anesthesia), local tissues (infiltration and field blocks), and regional structures (conduction anesthesia, intravenous regional anesthesia). Local anesthetic techniques are an alternative or adjunct to intravenous and inhalation anesthesia in high-risk patients. A number of anesthetic drugs are available; they vary in potency, toxicity, and cost. The most commonly used local anesthetic drugs are lidocaine hydrochloride and mepivacaine hydrochloride; they have a rapid onset, produce an intermediate duration of action (90 to 120 minutes), and provide anesthesia over a wide field. Vasoconstrictors (epinephrine) are occasionally incorporated with or added to lidocaine to increase intensity and prolong anesthetic activity. Adding hyaluronidase increases tissue penetration in the region of infiltration and hastens the onset of anesthesia.

GENERAL CONSIDERATIONS

    I. Use sterile solutions and injection equipment
   II. Do not inject into inflamed areas
  III. Use undamaged needles

IV. Use as small a gauge of needle as practical
 V. Aspirate for blood before injecting
VI. Use lowest effective concentration of local anesthetic drug
VII. Use smallest possible amount of local anesthetic (consider the use of a vasoconstrictor)

LOCAL ANESTHETICS

I. Mechanism of membrane and impulse conduction
    A. Clinically used local anesthetics are membrane-stabilizing agents
    B. The drugs enter and occupy (by polar association) the membrane channels through which ions normally move
    C. The most immediate and apparent effect is the prevention of the inflow of Na^+ blocking subsequent ionic flow
    D. Nerve cell depolarization is prevented, thus retarding or stopping the conduction of nerve impulses
II. Uptake
    A. The salt of the anesthetic base is an ionizable quaternary amine with little or no anesthetic properties of its own
        1. Salts are not lipid soluble
        2. Salts are not absorbed into the nerve cell membrane
    B. Once the salt of the anesthetic base is deposited into tissues, it is buffered by the slightly alkaline tissue fluids, and the anesthetic base (RN) is liberated as follows:

$$RNH^+ \ Cl^- \Leftrightarrow Cl^- + RNH^+ \Leftrightarrow RN + H^+$$

    Salt   anion   cation   base

    C. The free anesthetic base is absorbed at the outer lipid nerve membrane, where the anesthetic action takes place
    D. Effect of tissue pH
        1. If sufficient local buffering capacity exists to remove the dissociated H^+, this reaction proceeds to the right to liberate a more active base and exert an anesthetic effect
        2. Infected or inflamed tissues are more acidic and lack buffering capacity; smaller amounts of the free base are produced, resulting in poor local anesthesia

III. Absorption
   A. Local anesthetics are poorly absorbed through intact skin
   B. Local anesthetics are variably absorbed from:
      1. Injured skin
      2. Mucous membranes
      3. Serosal surfaces
      4. Respiratory epithelium
      5. Intramuscular deposition
      6. Subcutaneous deposition
      7. Intravenous administration
IV. Classification and function of nerve fibers
   A. Myelinated A-fibers
      1. α (Alpha): motor, proprioception
      2. β (Beta): motor, touch
      3. γ (Gamma): muscle spindles
      4. δ (Delta): pain, temperature
   B. Myelinated B-fibers (preganglionic sympathetic)
   C. Nonmyelinated C-fibers transmit
      1. Pain
      2. Temperature
V. Priority of blockade (least resistant to most resistant)
   A. B-fibers, C-fibers, $>A_\delta$-fibers, $>A_\alpha$-fibers
   B. Sensation disappears in the following order: pain, cold, warmth, touch, joint, and deep pressure
VI. Blocking quality
   A. Potency: binding affinity to receptor protein (tetracaine $>$ lidocaine $>$ procaine)
   B. Latency is the time between injection and the peak effect
   C. Duration of action is related to the logarithm of the concentration (e.g., doubling the concentration increases the duration by only approximately 30%)
   D. Recovery time is the time it takes for normal sensation to return
      1. Dependent on outflow diffusion and gradual release of local anesthetic from the nerve membrane
      2. It may be 2 to 200 times longer than induction time
VII. Ampules of hydrochloride salts can be autoclaved at 120° C for 20 to 30 minutes without affecting potency

DRUGS USED FOR VASOCONSTRICTION

I. Epinephrine (adrenaline) or L-norepinephrine (Levarterenol)
    1:50,000 (1 mg/50 ml saline) or 1:200,000 (1 mg/200 ml saline)

II. Effects of vasoconstriction
    A. Maximal vasoconstriction is probably produced by the lower of these concentrations, but because of the instability of epinephrine, the higher concentration is used to increase shelf life
    B. Vasoconstrictors delay absorption, reducing toxicity and increasing the margin of safety
    C. Vasoconstrictors increase intensity and prolong anesthetic activity
    D. Vasoconstrictors can increase risk of cardiac arrhythmias and ventricular fibrillation

DRUGS USED TO HASTEN THE TIME OF ONSET OF ANESTHESIA

I. Hyaluronidase
    A. Increases the area of diffusion, resulting in a larger total area being desensitized
    B. Often produces rapid anesthesia
    C. Usually shortens anesthesia time because of increased absorption, unless a vasoconstrictor is also used
    D. Is not a substitute for precise, accurate technique; fascial planes are barriers to diffusion
    E. Use five turbidity-reducing units per milliliter of local anesthetic solution

II. Combinations

    Hyaluronidase + procaine → Doubles the area anesthetized

    Epinephrine + procaine → Increases duration of local anesthesia almost five times

SPECIFIC LOCAL ANESTHETIC DRUGS

I. Ester-linked drugs (Table 4-1)
    A. Cocaine (alkaloid of the leaf of *Erythroxylon coca*)

TABLE 4-1
LOCAL ANESTHETICS

AGENT (GENERIC NAME)	TRADE NAME (REGISTERED BY)	CHEMICAL NAME	POTENCY RATIO (PROCAINE = 1)
Procaine	Novocain (Winthrop Stearns)	Para-aminobenzoic acid ester of diethylaminoethanol	1:1
Chloroprocaine	Nesacaine (Wallace & Tiernan)	Para-amino-2 chlorobenzoic acid ester of B-diethylaminoethanol	2.4:1
Lidocaine	Xylocaine (Astra Pharmaceutical)	Diethylaminoacet-2,6 xylidide	2:1
Mepivacaine	Carbocaine (Winthrop Laboratories)	1-methyl-2',6'-pipecoloxylidide monohydrochloride	2.5:1
Tetracaine	Pontocaine (Winthrop Laboratories)	Parabutylamino benzoyl-dimethylaminoethanol-HCl	12:1
Hexylcaine	Cyclaine (Merck, Sharpe, and Dohme)	1-cyclo-hexamino 2-propylbenzoate	1-2:1
Dibucaine	Nupercaine (CIBA Pharmaceutical Products)	a-butyl-oxycin-choninic acid of diethylethylene-diamide	20:1
Bupivacaine	Marcaine (Breon Laboratories)	1-butyl-2',6' pipecoloxylidide-HCl	8:1
Ropivacaine	Naropin (Astra)	S-(−)-1-propyl-2',6'-pipecoloxylidide-Hcl monohydrate	8:1

Continued

TABLE 4-1
LOCAL ANESTHETICS—cont'd

DRUG	TOXICITY RATIO (PROCAINE = 1)	DOSAGE (%)	STABILITY	COMMENTS
Procaine	1:1	1-2 for infiltration and nerve block	Aqueous solutions are heat resistant, decomposed by bacteria	Hydrolyzed by liver and plasma esterase
Chloroprocaine	0.5:1	1-2 for infiltration and nerve block	Multiple autoclaving accelerates hydrolysis and impairs potency	Immediate onset of action; 2 hr duration with epinephrine
Lidocaine	0.5% 1:1 1% 1.4:1 2% 1.5:1	0.5-2 for infiltration and nerve block; topically 2-4	Aqueous solutions are thermostable; multiple autoclaving possible	Excellent penetrability; rate of onset twice as fast as procaine; 2 hr duration with epinephrine
	Less toxic than lidocaine	1-2 for infiltration and nerve block	Resistant to acid and alkaline hydrolysis; multiple autoclaving possible	Absence of vasodilator effects makes addition of a vasoconstrictor unnecessary
Mepivacaine	10:1	0.1 for infiltration and nerve block; topically 0.2	Crystals and solutions should not be autoclaved	Slow onset of anesthesia (5-10 min); 2 hr duration; for eye instillation
Tetracaine	2-4:1	0.5-1 for infiltration; 2 for nerve block; 5 topically	Crystals and solutions are thermostable	Recommended for epidural and topical anesthesia
Hexylcaine	15:1	Topically 0.1	Thermostable, but precipitation by alkalies	Slowly detoxified
Dibucaine	Greater margin of safety than lidocaine	0.25 for infiltration; 0.5 for nerve block; 0.75 for epidural block	Stable compound	Intermediate onset, lasting 4-6 hr
Bupivacaine	Greater margin of safety than bupivacaine	0.2 for infiltration; 0.5 for nerve block; 0.75 and 1.0 for epidural block	Stable compound	Intermediate onset, lasting 4-6 hr

   B. Procaine hydrochloride (Novocain)
      1. Prototype of all other local anesthetics
      2. Standard drug for comparison of anesthetic effects
      3. Hydrolyzed in plasma by pseudocholinesterase
   C. Chloroprocaine hydrochloride (Nesacaine)
      1. Minimal toxicity
      2. Good penetration
      3. Hydrolyzed by pseudocholinesterase
   D. Tetracaine hydrochloride (Pontocaine)
      1. 10 to 15 times more potent than procaine
      2. Relatively toxic
      3. Prolonged anesthetic effect
      4. Hydrolyzed by pseudocholinesterase

II. Amide-linked drugs
   A. Lidocaine hydrochloride (Xylocaine, lignocaine)
      1. Most stable drug in this group; not decomposed by boiling, acids, or alkali
      2. Superior penetration compared to procaine: effects evident in one-third the time; effects persist 1½ times longer; spread over a wider field
      3. Minimal tissue damage or irritation
      4. No allergy or hypersensitivity
      5. Sedative effects
      6. Antiarrhythmic
      7. Metabolized in the liver
   B. Mepivacaine hydrochloride (Carbocaine)
      1. Similar to lidocaine
      2. No irritation or tissue damage
      3. Metabolized in the liver
   C. Dibucaine hydrochloride (Nupercainal)
      1. 20 times more potent than procaine
      2. Anesthetic effect is three to five times longer
   D. Bupivacaine (Marcaine)
      1. Intermediate onset
      2. Decreased motor blocking potency
      3. Anesthetic effect is 4 to 6 hours
      4. Metabolized in the liver
   E. Ropivacaine (Naropin)
      1. Similar to bupivacaine
      2. Less cardiotoxic

TOPICAL ANESTHETICS

I. Commonly used topicals
    A. Butacaine (Butya sulphate)
    B. Tetracaine (Pontocaine)
    C. Piperocaine (Metycaine)
    D. Proparacaine (Ophthaine)
    E. Cetacaine (Benzocaine)
    F. EMLA Cream (lidocaine and prilocaine mixture)
II. Vascular effect: local anesthetic drugs are vasodilators, with the exception of cocaine (a vasoconstrictor) and lidocaine (minimal effect)
III. Toxicity dependent on:
    A. Rate of absorption
    B. Rate of detoxification

METHODS OF LOCAL ANESTHETIC APPLICATION

I. Surface anesthesia
    A. Sprayed or brushed on mucous membranes (mouth, nose)
    B. Dropped into the eye
    C. Infused into the urethra
    D. Injected subsynovially (synovial membranes)
    E. Injected intrapleurally
II. Infiltration anesthesia
    A. Diffuse infiltration of operative area
        1. Sensitive tissues: skin, nerve trunks, blood vessels, periosteum, synovial membranes, mucous membranes near orifices (mouth, nose, rectum, anus)
        2. Insensitive tissues: subcutaneous, fat, muscles, tendons, fascia, bone, cartilage, visceral peritoneum
    B. Techniques
        1. Bleb (very localized deposition of a small quantity)
        2. Tissue layer by tissue layer
    C. Uses
        1. Wound treatment
        2. Skin incision
            a. Surgical removal of superficial tumors
            b. Repositioning of fractured bones

III. Regional (perineural) anesthesia
  A. Linear block
  B. Field block: contraindications
    1. Fissures of bones
    2. Fractures of bones
  C. Epidural block
  D. Paravertebral block
IV. Intraarticular anesthesia
 V. Subsynovial anesthesia
VI. Intravenous regional anesthesia
VII. Refrigeration or hypothermic anesthesia

ANALGESIC ACTIVITY OF EPIDURALLY ADMINISTERED α_2-ADRENOCEPTOR AGONISTS, OPIOIDS, AND KETAMINE

α_2-Adrenoceptor agonists such as clonidine, xylazine, detomidine, romifidine, medetomidine, and dexmedetomidine are used for their sedative, analgesic, anxiolytic, anesthetic sparing, and hemodynamic stability properties; xylazine or detomidine injected epidurally in cattle and horses produce caudal (S3 to coccyx) localized analgesia with minimal impairment of motor function

  I. Site of action
  A. The site of action of α_2-adrenoceptor agonists in epidural analgesia is unknown
  B. The antinociceptive effects of epidurally and intrathecally (subarachnoid) administered α_2-adrenoceptor agonists are primarily the result of:
    1. Stimulation of α_2-adrenoceptors in the spinal cord; receptor binding results in release of norepinephrine, hyperpolarization of dorsal horn neurons, and inhibition of substance P (pain) release, thereby producing behavioral analgesia in animals
    2. Inhibition of impulse conduction in primary afferent nerve fibers; C-fibers (pain, reflex responses, and postsympathetic transmission) are blocked to a greater extent than A-fibers (somatic motor function and proprioception)
  C. The antinociceptive effects of epidurally and intrathecally (subarachnoid) administered α_2-adrenoceptor agonists

are independent of opiate receptor mechanisms; the α_2-agonists may provide effective alternatives in pain states that are resistant to opioids

D. The addition of xylazine to an epidural solution containing lidocaine prolongs the duration of analgesia

II. Receptors

A. α_2-adrenergic receptors are located on the dorsal horn of the spinal cord

B. The predominant α_2-adrenergic receptor in human cortex and the spinal cord in humans and rats is the α_2-A subtype

C. The density of α_2-adrenergic receptors in humans and rats is greater in the sacral cord than in the thoracolumbar cord

D. The density of α_2-adrenergic receptors in the spinal cord of domestic animals is unknown

III. Epidural xylazine

A. Xylazine is the most commonly used α_1-and α_2-agonist for epidural injection in cattle, horses, and pigs (Table 4-2)

1. Xylazine has a high affinity and selectivity for α_1- and α_2- receptors

2. The exact proportion of α_1 versus α_2-adrenoceptor—mediated analgesia and local anesthesia within the spinal cord has not been determined for domestic animals

3. Xylazine has local anesthetic properties that are independent of α-adrenergic stimulation

B. Clinical use of epidural xylazine

1. In cattle, xylazine (0.05 mg/kg expanded to a 5 ml volume with sterile saline) given in the epidural space at the first coccygeal intervertebral space produces anesthesia in the anal and perineal region for surgery and obstetric procedures (see Table 4-2)

2. Xylazine-induced caudal epidural anesthesia in cattle is associated with these side effects:

a. Marked sedation (head drop)

b. Mild ataxia

c. Bradycardia

d. Hypotension

e. Respiratory acidosis

    f. Hypoxemia

    g. Transient ruminal amotility

    h. Renal diuresis

3. The side effects in cattle are dose dependent and partially reversed by administration of tolazoline (Priscoline) (0.3 mg/kg IV)

4. In horses, xylazine (0.17 mg/kg) given in the epidural space at the first coccygeal intervertebral space produces anesthesia in the anal and perineal region for surgery and obstetric procedures, with minimal ataxia (Table 4-2)

5. In pigs, xylazine (2 mg/kg) given in the epidural space at the lumbosacral interspace produces bilateral surgical anesthesia of the trunk caudal to the umbilicus and analgesia and paralysis of rear limbs, with minimal cardiovascular depression (see Table 4-2)

    a. Smaller doses of epidural xylazine (<1 mg/kg) do not produce surgical anesthesia

    b. Larger doses of epidural xylazine (>3 mg/kg) induce weakness of rear limbs for 36 hours or longer

IV. Onset and duration of epidural analgesia

  A. Signs of analgesia develop within 20 to 30 minutes (compared to 5 to 10 minutes after epidural lidocaine)

  B. A mixture of xylazine and lidocaine can be used to shorten onset of analgesia to approximately 5 minutes and prolong analgesia to approximately 5 hours (see Table 4-2)

    1. Duration of analgesia is longer for the xylazine-lidocaine combination than for either drug used alone

    2. Approximate duration of analgesia after epidural drug administration is variable (see Table 4-2)

      a. 110 minutes after lidocaine

      b. 220 minutes after xylazine

      c. 330 minutes after xylazine-lidocaine combination

    3. Surgical and obstetric procedures can commence after injection without the need for additional anesthetic

V. Local anesthetic properties of xylazine

  A. Xylazine-induced epidural analgesia may be mediated by local spinal analgesic mechanisms because the systemic administration of α_2-, or α_1- and α_2-adrenoceptor antagonists does not abolish the analgesic effect

Text continued on p. 56

TABLE 4-2

XYLAZINE-, XYLAZINE/LIDOCAINE-, DETOMIDINE-, MORPHINE-, DETOMIDINE/MORPHINE-, AND KETAMINE-INDUCED ANALGESIA AFTER EPIDURAL ADMINISTRATION IN CATTLE, PONY, HORSE, PIG, AND LLAMA

SPECIES	AGONIST	CONCENTRATION OF DRUG (%)	DOSE (MG/KG)	VOLUME OF DILUENT (ML)
Cattle	Xylazine	2	0.05	5 ml of 0.9% NaCl
Pony	Xylazine	2	0.35	—
Horse	Xylazine	2	0.17	6 ml/450 kg with sterile water
	Xylazine	10	0.17	5 ml/450 kg with 2% lidocaine (0.22 mg/kg)
	Detomidine	1	0.06	10 ml/500 kg with sterile water
	Morphine	1.5	0.05	10 ml/450 kg with 0.9% NaCl
		0.1		
	Morphine	1.5	0.2	8 ml/450 kg with 0.9% NaCl
	+ Detomidine	1	0.03	
	Ketamine	1	2	10 ml/450 kg with 0.9% NaCl

Pig	Xylazine	10	2	5 ml of 0.9% NaCl
	Xylazine	10	1 in large sows >180 kg 2 in small pigs <50 kg	10 ml of 2% lidocaine
Llama	Detomidine	1	0.5	5 ml of 0.9% NaCl
	Xylazine	10	0.17	2 ml/150 kg of sterile water
	Xylazine	10	0.17	1.7 ml/150 kg with 2% lidocaine (0.22 mg/kg)

See Chapter 7 for epidural techniques in dogs and cats.

TABLE 4-2

XYLAZINE-, XYLAZINE/LIDOCAINE-, DETOMIDINE-, MORPHINE-, DETOMIDINE/MORPHINE-, AND KETAMINE-INDUCED ANALGESIA AFTER EPIDURAL ADMINISTRATION IN CATTLE, PONY, HORSE, PIG, AND LLAMA

SITE OF INJECTION	SPREAD OF ANALGESIA	ANALGESIA		SIDE EFFECTS
		ONSET (MIN)	DURATION (MIN)	
C_o-C_o2	S3 to coccyx	10	>120	Sedation, ataxia, cardiopulmonary depression, ruminal hypomotility, diuresis
C_o1-C_o2	S3 to coccyx	20-30	240	Mild ataxia
S5-C_o1	S3 to coccyx	30	200	—
S5-C_o1	S3 to coccyx	5	300	Mild ataxia
C_o1-C_o2	T14 to coccyx	10-15	130-150	Sedation, ataxia, cardiopulmonary depression, diuresis

Lumbosacral	Umbilicus to coccyx	5	>120	Sedation, immobilization
Lumbosacral	Umbilicus to coccyx	5-10	300-480	—
Lumbosacral	Umbilicus to coccyx	10	<30	Atipamazole (0.2 mg/kg IV) reverses sedation
C_o1-C_o2	S3 to coccyx	20	180	—
C_o1-C_o2	S3 to coccyx	<5	330	Mild sedation, occasional recumbency
C_o1-C_o2	Lumbosacral	20-480	480-780	Mild sedation, hypotension, occasional urticaria
L7-S1 (via catheter)	Entire pelvic limbs	60	>360	Marked sedation, mild ataxia, bradycardia, bradypnea
Midsacral (S2-S3), via catheter	Tail, perineum, upper pelvic limbs	5-15	80	Mild sedation, mild ataxia

    1. Atipamazole (0.2 mg/kg), a potent α_2-adrenoceptor antagonist, when injected IV, does not abolish the analgesic effect of epidurally administered xylazine in pigs

    2. Atipamazole (0.2 mg/kg), when injected IV, does not reverse xylazine-induced epidural immobilization in pigs

    3. Tolazoline (0.3 mg/kg), an α_1- and α_2-adrenoceptor antagonist, when injected IV, does not reverse xylazine-induced epidural analgesia in cattle

VI. Epidural detomidine

    A. In horses, detomidine (0.06 mg/kg expanded to a 10-ml volume with sterile saline) given in the epidural space at the first coccygeal intervertebral space produces variable analgesia. Analgesia may extend from the coccyx to the third sacral (S3) and coccyx to the fourteenth thoracic (T14) spinal cord segment (see Table 4-2)

        1. Detomidine-induced caudal epidural analgesia in horses is associated with side effects

            a. Marked sedation, head drop

            b. Bradycardia with second-degree, atrioventricular heart block

            c. Hypotension

            d. Hypercarbia

            e. Renal diuresis

        2. These side effects are dose dependent and can be partially antagonized by atipamazole (0.12 mg/kg IV)

VII. Restraint: movements of head, shoulder, and forelimbs are not suppressed by epidural analgesia/anesthesia and should be controlled by physical or chemical restraint

VIII. Toxicity: no detrimental histologic effects on the spinal cord of ponies, horses, and pigs have been noted after epidural administration of xylazine

  IX. Subarachnoid detomidine

    A. In horses, detomidine (0.03 mg/kg) expanded to a 3-ml volume with CSF given into the subarachnoid space at midsacral vertebrae (catheter technique) produces analgesia and side effects similar to that produced by epidural administration of detomidine (0.06 mg/kg)

        1. Most of the side effects, except bradypnea, are reversed by atipamazole (0.1 mg/kg IV)

CHAPTER FIVE

Local Anesthesia in Cattle, Sheep, Goats, and Pigs

"The pain of the mind is worse than pain of the body."

PUBLILIUS SYRUS

OVERVIEW

The most commonly used local anesthetic techniques in ruminants are surface (topical) anesthesia, infiltration anesthesia, nerve block (conduction) anesthesia, epidural anesthesia, and intravenous (IV) regional anesthesia. The standing position is optimal for surgery in ruminants because it reduces the problems associated with bloating, salivation, recumbency-related regurgitation, and nerve or muscle damage.

The most commonly used local anesthetic techniques in appropriately tranquilized pigs are infiltration anesthesia, lumbosacral epidural anesthesia, and intratesticular injection.

CATTLE: LOCAL ANESTHESIA FOR STANDING LAPAROTOMY

    I. There are four techniques for producing local anesthesia of the paralumbar fossa in ruminants:

        A. Infiltration anesthesia

        B. Proximal paravertebral anesthesia

        C. Distal paravertebral anesthesia

        D. Segmental dorsolumbar epidural anesthesia

II. Abdominal surgeries in which these anesthetic techniques may be used:
   A. Rumenotomy
   B. Cecotomy
   C. Correction of gastrointestinal displacement
   D. Intestinal obstruction
   E. Volvulus
   F. Cesarean section
   G. Ovariectomy
   H. Liver or kidney biopsy

III. Infiltration anesthesia
   A. Line block
      1. Area blocked: skin, muscle layers, and parietal peritoneum along the line of incision
      2. Needle: 18-gauge, 1½- to 3-inch
      3. Anesthetic: 50 ml of 2% lidocaine
      4. Method: make multiple subcutaneous injections of 0.5 to 1 ml of anesthetic, 1 to 2 cm apart; then infiltrate the muscle layers and parietal peritoneum through the desensitized skin
      5. Advantages
         a. Easiest technique
         b. Use of routinely sized needles (2.5-cm, 20-gauge or smaller for skin block; 7.5- to 10-cm, 18-gauge for infiltrating the muscle layers and peritoneum)
      6. Disadvantages
         a. Large volume of anesthetic
         b. Lack of muscle relaxation
         c. Incomplete block of deeper layers of the abdominal wall
         d. Formation of hematomas along the incision line
         e. Increased cost due to larger amounts of anesthetic use and time required
      7. Complications
         a. Potential toxicity if significant amount of anesthetic (i.e., 250 ml of 2% lidocaine hydrochloride solution given intraperitoneally to 450 kg cow) is injected into the peritoneal cavity in adult cattle
         b. Interference with healing

B. Inverted L block (Fig. 5-1)
   1. Area blocked: flank caudal and ventral to site of injection
   2. Site: a line along the caudal border of the last rib and along a line ventral to the lumbar transverse processes from the last rib to the fourth lumbar vertebra (inverted L)
   3. Needle: 18-gauge, 3-inch
   4. Anesthetic: up to 100 ml of 2% lidocaine, evenly distributed
   5. Method: inject drug into the tissues bordering the dorsocaudal aspect of the last rib and ventrolateral aspect

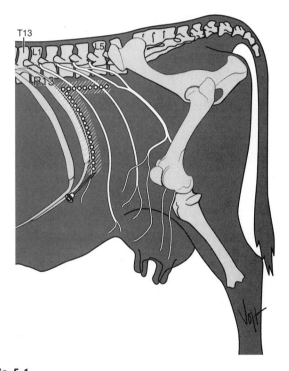

Fig. 5-1
Regional anesthesia of the cow's left flank using inverted L infiltration pattern.

of the lumbar transverse processes, creating a wall of anesthetic enclosing the incision site

6. Advantages
   a. Similar to line block
   b. Absence of anesthetic agent from the incision line minimizes edema, hematoma, and possible interference with healing
7. Disadvantages
   a. Large volume of anesthetic required
   b. Length of time required to infiltrate such a long line
   c. Incomplete block of the deep layers of the abdominal wall (particularly the peritoneum)
8. Complications: similar to line block

IV. Specific nerve anesthesia
   A. Proximal paravertebral anesthesia (Farquharson technique)
      1. Area blocked: flank of side on which technique is performed
      2. Nerves blocked: dorsal and ventral branches of T13, L1, and L2 and occasionally L3 (if L3 is blocked, the animal may become ataxic)
      3. Site: 2.5 to 5 cm from midline (Fig. 5-2); T13 immediately in front of transverse process of L1; L1 immediately in front of transverse process of L2; L2 immediately in front of transverse process of L3
      4. Needle: 14-gauge, ½-inch needle, creating passage for a 16- or 18-gauge, 4 ½-inch needle (up to 6 inches for bull)
      5. Anesthetic: 20 ml of 2% lidocaine at each site
      6. Method: palpate the lumbar transverse processes, starting from L5 and moving forward; L1 may be difficult to feel; measure 5 cm (2 inches) from midline; palpate the lumbar dorsal processes; injection site is at a 90-degree angle to the spaces between the dorsal processes; pass the needle vertically down until hitting the cranial edge of the transverse process, and proceed down through the intertransverse ligament; inject 15 ml of 2% lidocaine below the ligament to block the ventral branch of the nerve (there should be minimal resistance to injection); withdraw the needle sufficiently to inject 5 ml of 2% lidocaine above ligament, level

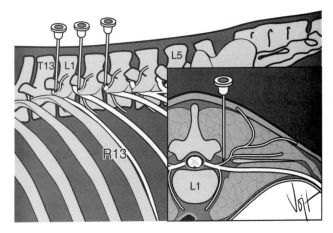

Fig. 5-2

Needle placement for proximal paravertebral nerve block in cattle. Left lateral aspect and cranial view of a transection of the first thoracolumbar vertebra at the location of the intervertebral foramen. *R13* is the last rib, *T13, L1,* and *L5* are the spinous processes of the last thoracic and the first and fifth lumbar vertebrae.

with dorsal surface of transverse process to block the dorsal branch (resistance to injection); if the first lumbar transverse process cannot be palpated, anesthetize the other nerves first, and then measure the distance between injection sites to find the site for blocking nerve T13

7. In sheep and goats, T13, L1, and L2 are desensitized similarly to the cattle method, but 2.5 to 3 cm off the midline and with less anesthetic (2 to 3 ml per site)

8. Advantages over local block
   a. Anesthesia of skin, musculature, and peritoneum
   b. No additional restraint required
   c. Large quantities of local anesthetic not required
   d. Shorter postsurgical convalescent period; incision site avoided

9. Disadvantages
   a. Procedure difficult in fat cattle and some beef cattle
   b. Arching of the spine due to paralysis of back muscles
   c. Anesthesia of abdominal viscera
   d. Bowing out toward the area of incision (after unilateral blockade), making the closure of the incision more difficult
10. Complications
    a. Possible penetration of the aorta
    b. Possible penetration of the thoracic longitudinal vein (posterior) or vena cava
    c. Loss of motor control of the pelvic limb due to caudal migration of drug (femoral nerve block)

B. Distal paravertebral anesthesia (Magda, Cakala, or Cornell technique)
   1. Area blocked: flank of side on which technique is performed
   2. Nerves blocked: dorsal and ventral rami of T13, L1, and L2
   3. Site: distal ends of lumbar transverse processes of L1, L2, and L4 (Fig. 5-3)
   4. Needle: 18-gauge, 3-inch
   5. Anesthetic: 10 to 20 ml of 2% lidocaine at each site
   6. Method: insert the needle ventral to the tips of the respective transverse process; inject anesthetic (up to 20 ml) in a fan-shaped infiltration pattern; withdraw the needle a short distance and reinsert it dorsal and caudal to the transverse process, and inject approximately 5 ml of the anesthetic
   7. Advantages of distal paravertebral nerve block over proximal paravertebral block
      a. Use of routinely sized needles
      b. Minimizes risk of penetrating a major blood vessel
      c. Lack of scoliosis
      d. Minimal ataxia or weakness in the pelvic limb
   8. Disadvantages
      a. Large volume of anesthetic
      b. Variations in efficacy, particularly if the nerves follow a variable anatomic pathway

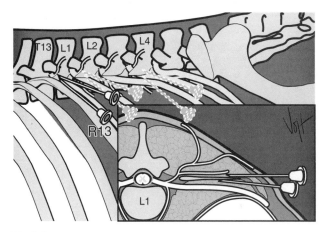

Fig. 5-3
Needle placement for distal paravertebral nerve blockades in cattle. Left lateral aspect and cranial view of a transection of the first lumbar vertebra at the location of the intervertebral foramen. *R13* is the last rib, and *T13, L1, L2,* and *L4* are the spinous processes of the last thoracic and first, second, and fourth lumbar vertebrae.

       9. Complications: none
  C. Segmental dorsolumbar epidural block (Fig. 5-4)
      1. Area blocked: flank on both sides
      2. Nerves blocked: T13 and anterior lumbar nerves, depending on the total dose administered
      3. Site: epidural space between L1 and L2 vertebrae
      4. Needle: spinal, preferably 18-gauge, 4½-inch
      5. Anesthetic: 8 ml of 2% lidocaine
      6. Method: to reach the epidural space, insert the spinal needle 8 to 12 cm ventral and cranial at an angle of 10 to 15 degrees from vertical; piercing of the interarcuate ligament is felt as slight resistance during the insertion process; no blood or cerebrospinal fluid (CSF) can be aspirated, and also no resistance to the injection of anesthetic results after correct needle placement

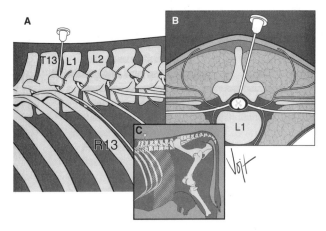

Fig. 5-4
Needle placement for segmental dorsolumbar epidural block. **A,** Left lateral aspect. **B,** Cranial view of a transection of the first lumbar vertebra at the location of the intervertebral foramen. **C,** *(inset)* Desensitized area of skin after segmental epidural anesthesia. *R13* is the last rib; and *T13, L1,* and *L2* are the spinous processes of the last thoracic and first and second lumbar vertebrae.

7. Advantages over proximal or distal paravertebral anesthesia
   a. Only one injection
   b. Small quantity of anesthetic
   c. Uniform anesthesia and relaxation of the skin, musculature, and peritoneum (begins 10 to 20 minutes after administration and continues for 45 to 120 minutes)
8. Disadvantages: difficult technique to perform
9. Complications
   a. Loss of motor control of the pelvic limbs due to overdose or subarachnoid injection
   b. Physiologic disturbance due to overdose or subarachnoid injection
   c. Potential for trauma to the spinal cord or venous sinuses

ANESTHESIA FOR OBSTETRIC PROCEDURES AND RELIEF OF RECTAL TENESMUS

I. Caudal epidural anesthesia and desensitization of the internal pudendal nerve are commonly used in ruminants for obstetric manipulations, caudal surgical procedures, and as an adjunct treatment for control of rectal tenesmus; these techniques are not effective in pigs

II. Cattle

    A. Low posterior or caudal epidural anesthesia (Fig. 5-5, *A*)

        1. Area blocked: anus, perineum, vulva, vagina

        2. Nerves blocked: coccygeal and posterior sacral nerves

        3. Site: first intercoccygeal space

        4. Needle: 18-gauge, 1½-inch (average dairy cow)

        5. Anesthetic: 5 to 6 ml of 2% lidocaine

        6. Method: locate the sacrococcygeal joint by moving the tail up and down; this joint moves very little and is located just anterior to the anal folds; the first intercoccygeal joint is easily located by its movement; it is much wider and is posterior to the anal folds; insert the

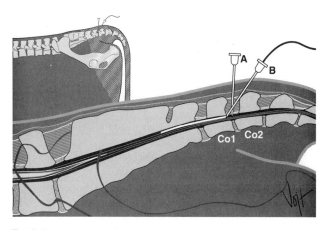

Fig. 5-5
Needle placement for **A,** caudal epidural anesthesia and **B,** continuous caudal epidural anesthesia in cattle. *Co1* is the first coccygeal vertebra, and *Co2* is the second coccygeal vertebra.

needle exactly at the midline of the first intercoccygeal space at a right angle to the skin surface; push the needle ventrally through the interarcuate ligament to the floor of the neural canal, which is at about 2 to 4 cm (¾ to 1½ inches); withdraw the needle slightly into epidural space and test by injecting 1 cc of air; no resistance should be felt

7. Advantages
   a. Minimal effect on cardiovascular and respiratory systems
   b. Little effect on organ systems
   c. Little problem with toxicity
   d. Good muscle relaxation
   e. Good postoperative analgesia
   f. Rapid recovery
   g. Relatively simple
   h. Inexpensive
8. Disadvantages
   a. Technically difficult if Co1-Co2 interspace is not identified
   b. Technically difficult if the sacrococcygeal interspace is ossified in older cows
9. Complications
   a. Rare
   b. Infection resulting in draining tracts or permanently paralyzed tail
   c. Possible ataxia and collapse due to overdose
   d. Hemorrhage due to puncture of a venous sinus

B. Continuous caudal epidural anesthesia (see Fig. 5-5, *B*)
   1. Indications: painful prolapse of the vagina and/or rectum that provokes severe continuous straining
   2. Nerves blocked: coccygeal and posterior sacral nerves
   3. Site: first intercoccygeal space
   4. Needle: 16- or 17-gauge, 2½-inch, thin-walled, Huberpoint directional needle or Hustead needle
   5. Catheter: 30-cm, medical-grade vinyl tubing (0.036 cm outside diameter) or a commercially available epidural catheter with gradual markings
   6. Anesthetic: 3 to 5 ml of 2% lidocaine

7. Method: identify the first intercoccygeal joint as previously described; desensitize the skin and needle tract; with stylet in place and bevel directed cranial, advance the spinal needle 5 to 8 cm approximately 45 degrees to vertical, until an abrupt reduction in resistance to needle passage is noted; remove the stylet from the needle, and inject 3 ml of 2% lidocaine with minimal resistance; the test dose ensures proper placement of the needle in the vertebral canal; place the catheter aseptically, introduce into the canal through the needle and advance it cranially approximately 3 cm beyond the tip of the needle (see Fig. 5-5, *B*); withdraw the needle, leaving the catheter in position; inject local anesthetic solution into the catheter at 3- to 5-hour intervals or as needed; place a catheter adapter on the free end of the catheter; secure the catheter at the entrance into the skin with adhesive tape sutured to the skin; place a protective sterile gauze over the free end of the catheter to allow the catheter to be used for many hours of infusion in the field
8. Advantages
    a. Similar to caudal epidural anesthesia
    b. Repeated administration of small fractional doses of local anesthesia
    c. No fibrosis of the extradural space from repeated standard epidural blocks
9. Disadvantages
    a. Similar to caudal epidural anesthesia
    b. Greater cost of equipment
    c. Acute tolerance to repeated injections
10. Complications
    a. Similar to caudal epidural anesthesia
    b. Kinking and curling of the catheter and occlusion of the tip with fibrin
C. Internal pudendal nerve block (Fig. 5-6)
    1. Indications
        a. Anesthesia and relaxation of the penis for examination
        b. Relief of tenesmus associated with vaginal and uterine prolapse

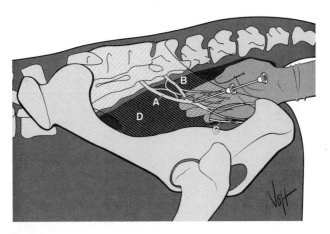

Fig. 5-6
Right hand and needle placement at the internal pudendal nerve on the medial side of the left pelvis. **A,** Internal pudendal nerve. **B,** Pelvic splanchnic
nerves. **C,** Pudendal artery. **D,** Sacrosciatic ligament.

2. Nerves blocked: internal pudendal (fibers of the ventral branches of S3 and S4), caudal rectal (fibers of the
   ventral branches of S4 and S5), and pelvic splanchnic
   nerves
3. Site: identified by rectal palpation
4. Needle: spinal, preferably 18-gauge, 3½-inch
5. Anesthetic: up to 25 ml of 2% lidocaine per side
6. Method: use rectal palpation to locate the lesser sciatic
   foramen, a soft, circumscribed depression in the
   sacrosciatic ligament; find the nerve a finger's width
   dorsal to the pudendal artery present in the fossa; pass
   the needle through the disinfected skin in the is-
   chiorectal fossa; deposit 15 ml of 2% lidocaine around
   the nerve; withdraw the needle 2 to 3 cm caudodorsally
   and inject another 10 ml of the anesthetic in the area of
   the pelvic splanchnic nerve; repeat the procedure on
   the opposite side of the pelvis
7. Advantages
   a. No loss of tail tone
   b. No sciatic nerve involvement

        c. Ballooning of the vagina may aid in retention of the vagina after it is repositioned in a cow with prolapse

    8. Disadvantages

        a. Technical difficulty and necessity of identifying the injection sites by rectal palpation

        b. Lack of cervical anesthesia

        c. Anesthesia duration of 3 to 6 hours

    9. Complications: injury to the bull's penis, which must be protected from injury by replacing it into the prepuce

III. Sheep and goats: low posterior or caudal, epidural anesthesia

    A. Similar to that used in cattle

    B. No more than 0.5 to 1 ml of 2% lidocaine per 50 kg of body weight injected at the first coccygeal interspace or sacrococcygeal (S4-Co1) space (Fig. 5-7); excellent for tail docking in lambs and intravaginal obstetric procedures

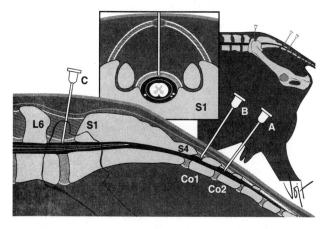

Fig. 5-7

Needle placement for caudal epidural anesthesia (**A** and **B**) and anterior epidural anesthesia (**C**) in the goat. **A,** Lateral aspect and cranial view of a transection to the first sacral vertebra. A needle is placed into **A,** the first intercoccygeal vertebral space; **B,** the sacrococcygeal space; and **C,** the lumbosacral space.

ANTERIOR EPIDURAL ANESTHESIA

I. Anterior epidural anesthesia can be used for all procedures caudal to the diaphragm; the lumbosacral space is commonly used in calves, sheep, and goats because the injection sites are usually palpable; this space is the only practical injection site for producing anterior anesthesia in pigs. The sacrococcygeal or first intercoccygeal space is the injection site of choice in adult cattle for producing anterior anesthesia, because the technique is relatively simple and avoids trauma to the spinal cord and meninges; proper techniques should provide anesthesia of the following areas:
   A. Perineal region
   B. Inguinal region
   C. Flank
   D. Abdominal wall caudal to the umbilicus

II. Increasing the dose of the anesthetic increases the area of blockade

III. Rapid epidural injections must be avoided to prevent consequences
   A. Discomfort to the patient
   B. Increased rate of vascular absorption, which can result in less drug for neural uptake; reduced neural uptake can result in the following:
      1. Reduced duration of action
      2. Higher incidence of incomplete anesthesia
      3. Only a slight increase in segmental spread

IV. The technique is contraindicated in animals with certain known conditions:
   A. Cardiovascular disease
   B. Bleeding disorders
   C. Shock or toxemic syndromes because of sympathetic block and resulting depression of blood pressure

V. The following complications may result from overdose or subarachnoid injection
   A. Transient loss of consciousness
   B. Flexor spasm
   C. Rapid muscular contractions
   D. Convulsions
   E. Respiratory paralysis

    F. Hypotension

    G. Hypothermia

VI. Small ruminants (sheep and goats)

    A. Landmarks and techniques for injection at the lumbosacral space are similar to those used in dogs (Fig. 5-7, *C*)

    B. Dose: 1 ml of 2% lidocaine per 10 lb of body weight

    C. Effect

        1. Onset of posterior paralysis occurs in 2 to 15 minutes

        2. Anesthesia generally reaches three fourths of the distance from pubis to umbilicus

        3. Duration of action is 1 to 2 hours

        4. Similar extent and duration of anesthesia can be achieved if only half the dose (0.5 ml/10 lb) is injected subarachnoidally (the space from which spinal fluid is aspirated into the syringe); true cerebrospinal fluid (CSF) anesthesia results with the onset of posterior paralysis within 1 to 3 minutes

        5. Gravity, not diffusion of drug in the CSF, determines the spread of anesthesia

        6. Morphine (0.05 mg/lb) diluted with saline to a volume of 0.06 ml/lb can be injected epidurally following orthopedic procedures to produce 6-hour analgesia and sedation with minimal cardiopulmonary complications

VII. Pigs

    A. Landmarks and techniques for injection at the lumbosacral space are similar to those used in dogs (Fig. 5-8)

    B. Dose when using 2% lidocaine:

STANDING CASTRATION	CESAREAN SECTION
4 ml/200 lb	10 ml/200 lb
6 ml/400 lb	15 ml/400 lb
8 ml/600 lb	20 ml/600 lb

    C. Effect

        1. Onset of anesthetic action generally occurs within 5 minutes

        2. Maximum effect is within 15 to 20 minutes

        3. Duration of action is 120 minutes

        4. Most pigs develop posterior paresis

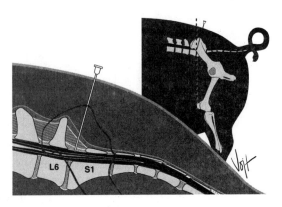

Fig. 5-8
Needle placement for epidural anesthesia in the pig. *L6* is the sixth lumbar vertebra, and *S1* is the first sacral vertebra.

LOCAL ANESTHESIA FOR DEHORNING

I. Cattle
  A. Area blocked: horn and base of the horn
  B. Nerves blocked: cornual branch of zygomaticotemporal (lacrimal) nerve, a portion of the ophthalmic division of the trigeminal nerve
  C. Site: temporal ridge, 2 cm from the base of horn (Fig. 5-9); needle penetration is from 1 cm (¼ inch) in small cattle to 2.5 cm (1 inch) in large bulls
  D. Needle: 18-gauge, 1- or 1½-inch
  E. Anesthetic: 5 to 10 ml of 2%
  F. Method: palpate the lateral temporal ridge of the frontal bone; the nerve is relatively superficial, 7 to 10 mm deep (¼ to ½ inch) on the upper third of the ridge, lying between the thin frontalis muscle and the temporal muscle, and can usually be palpated between these muscles; aspiration ensures that the needle point is not inadvertently intravascular; inject 2 to 3 cm in front of the horn
  G. Advantages
    1. Minimal systemic effects on the cardiopulmonary system
    2. Relatively simple procedure
  H. Disadvantages
    1. Cornual anesthesia does not result if the anesthetic is injected too deeply in the aponeurosis of the temporal muscle

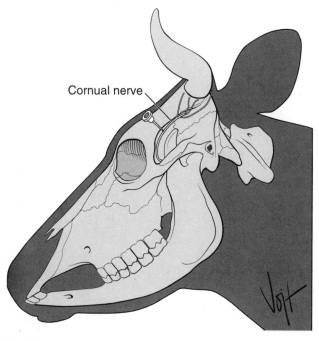

Cornual nerve

Fig. 5-9
Needle placement for desensitizing the cornual branch of the zygomaticotemporal nerve in the cow.

2. A second injection posterior to the horn may be required in adult cattle with well-developed horns
3. Anesthesia of a fractured horn involving the frontal bone or sinuses may require a Peterson eye block

I. Complications: none

II. Goats

A. Area blocked: horn and base of the horn

B. Nerves blocked: cornual branch of the zygomaticotemporal (lacrimal) nerve and cornual branch of the infratrochlear nerve

C. Site: halfway between lateral canthus of the eye and lateral base of the horn (lacrimal nerve) (Fig. 5-10, *A*) and halfway

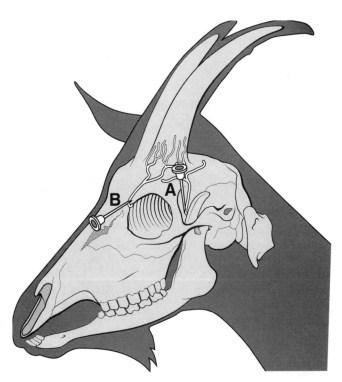

Fig. 5-10
Needle placement for desensitizing **A,** the cornual branch of the zygomaticotemporal (lacrimal) nerve; and **B,** the cornual branch of the infratrochlear nerve in the goat.

   between medial canthus of the eye and medial base of the
   horn (cornual branch of infratrochlear nerve) (Fig. 5-10, *B*)
D. Needle: 22-gauge, 1-inch
E. Anesthetic: 2 to 3 ml of 2% lidocaine at each site in the adult
   goat; no more than 0.5 ml of 2% lidocaine for ring block at
   the horn base in young kids 7 to 14 days of age
F. Method: to reach the cornual branch of the zygomaticotemporal nerve, insert the needle as close as possible to
   the caudal ridge of the supraorbital process and 1 to 1.5 cm

deep (see Fig. 5-10, *A*); to reach the cornual branch of the infratrochlear nerve, insert the needle dorsal and parallel to the dorsomedial margin of the orbit; inject the anesthetic in a line, since this nerve is frequently branched (see Fig. 5-10, *B*)

G. Advantages
1. Alleviation of pain during dehorning
2. Alleviation of pain during disbudding

H. Disadvantages
1. Sedation of the animal is required if the frontal sinus will be entered during horn removal
2. A total dose of 10 mg/kg (0.5 ml of 2% solution per kg or 1 ml of a 1% solution per kg) must not be exceeded to minimize adverse reactions

I. Complications: toxicity due to overdose of lidocaine and any of the following clinical signs:
1. Excitation
2. Lateral recumbency
3. Generalized tonic-clonic convulsions
4. Opisthotonus
5. Respiratory depression
6. Cardiac arrest

LOCAL ANESTHESIA FOR THE EYE

I. At present, topical and regional anesthetic techniques are used for surgery of the eye and its associated structures; paralysis of the eyelids (without analgesia) is accomplished by selectively desensitizing the auriculopalpebral branch of the facial nerve (producing akinesia); anesthesia of the eye and orbit and immobilization of the globe are commonly achieved by the Peterson technique (Fig. 5-11)

A. Area blocked: eye and orbit, orbicularis oculi muscle, *except* the eyelids

B. Nerves blocked: oculomotor, trochlear, and abducens nerves and the three branches of the trigeminal nerve (ophthalmic, maxillary, and mandibular)

C. Sites: the points at which these nerves emerge from the foramen orbitorotundum

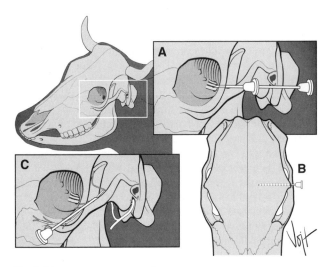

Fig. 5-11
Needle placement for Peterson eye block, with needle tip at the foramen orbitorotundum. **A,** Craniolateral aspect. **B,** Dorsal aspect. **C,** Needle placement for akinesia of the eyelids in the cow.

D. Needle: 14-gauge, 1-inch to serve as a cannula; 18-gauge, 4½-inch
E. Anesthetic: 7 to 15 ml of 2% lidocaine at the foramen orbitorotundum; 5 to 10 ml of 2% lidocaine for desensitizing the auriculopalpebral nerve
F. Method
1. Fully extend cow's head in a standing position with frontal and nasal bones parallel to the ground
2. Surgically prepare area posterior and ventral to the eye
3. Inject several milliliters of anesthetic with a small-gauge needle into the skin and subcutaneously into the notch formed by the zygomatic and temporal process of the malar bone (where the supraorbital process of the frontal bone meets the zygomatic arch) (see Fig. 5-11)
4. Place a 14-gauge, ½- or 1-inch needle (to serve as a cannula) through the skin as far anterior and ventral as possible in the notch

5. Direct a straight, 18-gauge, 4½-inch needle with no syringe attached (to feel the bony landmarks) through the cannula in a horizontal and slightly posterior direction, until it strikes the coronoid process of the mandible

6. Reposition the point of the needle anteriorly until it passes medially around this bone

7. Advance needle slightly posteriorly and somewhat ventrally until it strikes a solid bony plate, which is at a depth of between 3 and 4½ inches

8. Inject 15 ml of 2% lidocaine anterior to the foramen rotundum

9. Block the auriculopalpebral branch of the facial nerve (see Fig. 5-11, *C*)

   a. Fill a 10-ml syringe with local anesthetic, attach it to the needle, and partially withdraw the cannula

   b. Withdraw the needle until it almost leaves the skin, and direct it posteriorly for 2 to 3 inches lateral to the zygomatic arch while injecting lidocaine

   c. If the upper lid is involved in the surgical procedure, make a line of infiltration with local anesthetic subcutaneously about 1 inch from the margin of the lid

G. Advantages

   1. Technique is useful for enucleation of the eyeball and removal of tumors from the eye and eyelids

   2. Technique is quick, easy, safe, and effective if done properly

   3. Less edema and inflammation result than when the eyelids and the orbit are infiltrated

   4. Surgery of the cornea (removal of tumors and dermoids) can be done easily without retraction or fixation forceps if the eyeball is proptosed

   5. Peterson eye block is safer than retrobulbar injections of local anesthetic, which often lead to orbital hemorrhage, direct pressure on the globe, penetration of the globe, damage to the optic nerve, or injection into the optic nerve meninges

H. Disadvantages

   1. The cow's head is difficult to keep horizontal when the animal is in a chute or stanchion with the head tied to one side; this makes the landmarks difficult to locate

2. If the needle point strikes the pterygoid crest, the anesthetic drug will be deposited at the wrong site; therefore no anesthesia results following injection of the local anesthetic

3. In 50% of cases, incomplete anesthesia of the upper eyelid results because of sensory innervation from other nerves

4. Blinking is prevented for several hours

5. Sterile saline solution should be applied to the eye frequently during surgery to keep the cornea moist

6. Antibiotic eye ointments should be applied to the cornea after orbital replacement of the globe

7. Sunlight, dust, and wind in the eye must be avoided to prevent keratoconjunctivitis

8. The lids may be sutured together until motor activity of the lids returns

I. Complications

1. In procedures other than enucleation, keratitis may result from postoperative drying of the cornea because effective block prevents blinking for several hours

2. Penetration of the turbinates and injection with local anesthetic into the nasopharynx and optic nerve meninges can cause severe central nervous system toxicity, including certain clinical signs:

   a. Hyperexcitability
   b. Lateral recumbency
   c. Tonic-clonic convulsions
   d. Opisthotonus
   e. Respiratory arrest
   f. Cardiac arrest

LOCAL ANESTHESIA OF THE FOOT: THREE METHODS

I. Infiltrating the tissues around the limb with local anesthetic solution (ring block)

II. Desensitizing specific nerves (regional anesthesia)

III. Injecting local anesthetic solution into an accessible superficial vein in an extremity isolated from circulation by placing a tourniquet on an animal's leg (intravenous regional anesthesia)

   A. Area blocked: extremity distal to tourniquet

B. Veins used: *A,* Common dorsal metacarpal vein; *B,* radial vein; *C,* plantar metacarpal vein in the thoracic limb; *D,* cranial branch of the lateral saphenous vein, lateral plantar digital vein in the pelvic limb (see Fig. 5-12)

C. Needle: 18-gauge, 1 ½ inch

D. Anesthetic: 10 to 30 ml of 2% lidocaine in adult cattle; 3 to 10 ml lidocaine in small ruminants and pigs

E. Method: place rubber tourniquet proximal to the metatarsal or metacarpal region for foot surgery or at a more proximal position for surgery of the carpal or tarsal region; rapidly inject local anesthetic into the prominent vein, directing the needle either proximally or distally

F. Advantages
   1. No special skill or knowledge of anatomy of the limb is needed
   2. Only one injection is required, with little risk of introducing bacteria

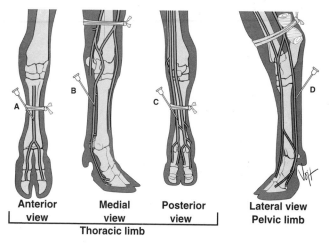

Anterior view | Medial view | Posterior view | Lateral view Pelvic limb

Thoracic limb

Fig. 5-12

Tourniquet and needle placement for intravenous regional anesthesia of the cow. In the thoracic limb, the needle tip is placed at **A,** the common dorsal metacarpal vein; **B** the radial vein; or **C,** the plantar metacarpal vein. In the pelvic limb, the needle tip is placed at **D,** the cranial branch of the lateral saphenous vein.

   3. Onset of anesthesia distal to the tourniquet is rapid (5 to 10 minutes); anesthesia occurs last in the interdigital region
   4. Recovery is rapid after removal of the tourniquet (5 to 10 minutes)
G. Disadvantages
   1. Inexplicable failure rate of 7%
   2. Occasional hematoma at the injection site
   3. Failure of anesthesia due to tourniquet slipping or extravascular injection
H. Complications: ischemic necrosis, severe lameness, and edema if the tourniquet is left in place longer than 2 hours

TEAT AND UDDER ANESTHESIA OF CATTLE

I. Techniques for surgical procedures on the forequarters and foreteats
   A. Paravertebral anesthesia of L1, L2, and L3 spinal nerves
   B. Segmental lumbar epidural anesthesia of L1, L2, and L3 spinal nerves
   C. Both techniques are difficult and often result in cows lying down
II. Techniques for surgical procedures of the caudal—most teats and escutcheon areas of the udder
   A. Desensitization of the perineal nerve in the standing cow
   B. High caudal epidural anesthesia in recumbent ruminants
   C. Lumbosacral epidural anesthesia in recumbent ruminants
III. Most surgical procedures on the teat (e.g., repair of a stenotic teat sphincter, repairs of teat fistulae and lacerations) are generally performed under local anesthesia
   A. Needle: 20- or 22-gauge, ½-inch or teat cannula
   B. Anesthetic: 6 to 10 ml of 2% lidocaine
   C. Methods
      1. Inverted V block: line infusion of the anesthetic using an inverted V pattern, which encloses the teat skin defect (Fig. 5-13, *A*)
      2. Ring block: local anesthetic infused into the skin and muscular tissue of base of the teat, after thorough cleaning of the external surface of the teat and quarter (Fig. 5-13, *B*)

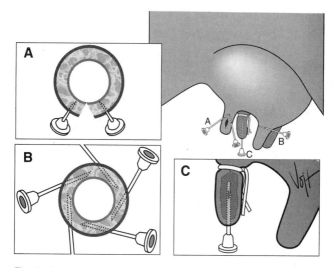

Fig. 5-13
Needle placement in the cow's teat. **A,** Inverted V block. **B,** Teat ring block.
C, Tourniquet and cannula placement for teat cistern infusion.

3. Teat infusion block
   a. Teat opening is cleaned
   b. Tourniquet is placed at the base of the teat
   c. 10 ml of 2% lidocaine is infused into the teat cistern
      (Fig. 5-13, *C*)
   d. Mucous membrane of the teat cistern is anesthetized
      within 5 minutes; the muscular and skin layers re-
      main sensitive; thereafter the remaining lidocaine is
      milked out, and the tourniquet is removed

CHAPTER SIX

Local Anesthesia in Horses

"A horse is dangerous at both ends and uncomfortable in
the middle."

IAN FLEMING

OVERVIEW

Many diagnostic and surgical procedures can be performed safely
and humanely on horses by coupling physical restraint and sedation
with surface (topical) anesthesia, infiltration anesthesia, nerve block
(regional) anesthesia, or epidural anesthesia. Peripheral nerve
blocks, intraarticular and intrabursal injections, and local infiltra-
tions (ring block) are used to diagnose equine lameness and to anesthetize surgical sites. Desensitization of the auriculopalpebral nerve
is most frequently used to prevent voluntary closure of the eyelids
during examination and treatment of the eye. Although regional
anesthesia of the head can be induced by various techniques, the
most frequently desensitized nerves are the supraorbital, infraorbital, and mandibular alveolar.

Caudal epidural anesthesia is used to facilitate surgery involving the tail, perineum, anus, rectum, vulva, vagina, and urethra
and for symptomatic relief of painful conditions during obstetric
manipulations.

Improper injection techniques contribute to inadequate anesthesia. Overdosing leads to more serious complications, including
ataxia of hind limbs, hind limb motor blockade, and recumbency.

REGIONAL ANESTHESIA OF THE HEAD
The Most Frequently Desensitized Nerves of the Head

I. Supraorbital (frontal)
II. Auriculopalpebral

III. Infraorbital
IV. Mandibular alveolar

ANESTHESIA OF THE UPPER EYELID AND FOREHEAD

   I. Area blocked: upper eyelid except medial and lateral canthi
  II. Nerve blocked: supraorbital (or frontal) nerve
 III. Site: supraorbital foramen (Fig. 6-1, *A*)
 IV. Needle: 22- to 25-gauge, 1-inch
  V. Anesthetic: 5 ml of 2% lidocaine
 VI. Method: palpate the supraorbital foramen about 5 to 7 cm above the medial canthus where it perforates the supraorbital process of the frontal bone; insert the needle into the foramen to a depth of 1.5 to 2 cm; inject 2 ml of lidocaine into the foramen; 1 ml as the needle is withdrawn and 2 ml subcutaneously over the foramen
VII. Use
    A. Desensitization of the upper eyelid
    B. Blockade of the palpebral motor supply derived from the auriculopalpebral nerve

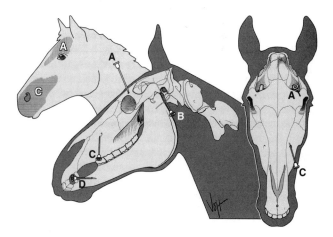

Fig. 6-1
Needle placement for nerve blocks on the head. **A,** Supraorbital (or frontal).
B, Auriculopalpebral. **C,** Infraorbital. **D,** Mandibular alveolar nerves.

AKINESIA OF THE EYELIDS

    I. Area blocked: paralysis of orbicularis oculi muscles; no desensitization

  II. Nerve blocked: auriculopalpebral nerve (Fig. 6-1, *B*)

 III. Site: caudal to posterior ramus of the mandible

  IV. Needle: 22- to 25-gauge, 1-inch

   V. Anesthetic: 5 ml of 2% lidocaine

  VI. Method: insert the needle into the depression caudal to the mandible at the ventral edge of the temporal part of the zygomatic arch; inject local anesthetic subfascially as the needle is withdrawn

 VII. Use: examination of the eye; successful blockade of the motor nerve supply prevents the horse from closing the eyelids

ANESTHESIA OF THE UPPER LIP AND NOSE

    I. Area blocked: upper lip and nostril, roof of nasal cavity, and related skin up to the infraorbital foramen

  II. Nerve blocked: infraorbital nerve

 III. Site: external opening of the infraorbital canal (Fig. 6-1, *C*)

  IV. Needle: 22- to 25-gauge, 1-inch

   V. Anesthetic: 5 ml of 2% lidocaine

  VI. Method: find the bony lip of the infraorbital foramen, about halfway along and 2.5 cm dorsal to a line connecting the nasomaxillary notch and the anterior end of the facial crest; push the flat levator labii superioris muscle, which runs over the foramen, upward with the fingertips and place the needle tip at the foramen opening

 VII. Use: simple lacerations in quiet or sedated horses

ANESTHESIA OF THE LOWER LIP

    I. Area blocked: lower lip, all parts of mandible rostral up to and including the third premolar tooth (PM3)

  II. Nerve blocked: mandibuloalveolar nerve

 III. Site: within mandibular canal (Fig. 6-1, *D*)

  IV. Needle: 20-gauge, 3-inch

   V. Anesthetic: 10 ml of 2% lidocaine

VI. Method: palpate the lateral border of the mental foramen as a ridge along the lateral aspect of the ramus in the middle of the interdental space; insert the needle into the mandibular canal as far as possible in a ventromedial direction; injection requires pressure, and fluid might partially drain back from the canal under the skin

VII. Use: simple lacerations in quiet or sedated horses

CAUDAL EPIDURAL ANESTHESIA

I. Area blocked: tail, perineum, anus, rectum, vulva, and vagina

II. Nerves blocked: caudal nerves and last three pairs of sacral nerves

III. Site: epidural space in the first intercoccygeal space (Co1-Co2) (Fig. 6-2)

IV. Needles: spinal with stylet (spinal: 18-gauge, 2- to 3-inch)

V. Anesthetic: 6 to 10 ml of 2% lidocaine; other drugs can be considered (e.g., xylazine, xylazine-lidocaine combination,

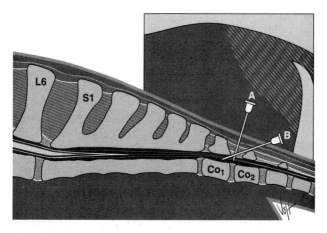

Fig. 6-2

Needle placement into **A** or **B,** caudal epidural space at the first intercoccygeal space (Co1-Co2). Stippled markings indicate desensitized subcutaneous area after caudal blockade.

detomidine, morphine, detomidine-morphine combination, and ketamine) (see Table 4-2)

VI. Method

    A. Use proper restraint, depending on the horse's temperament; clip, surgically scrub, and disinfect the injection site; make a skin wheal, and infiltrate the tissues down to the interarcuate ligament with 1 to 3 ml of 2% lidocaine to minimize movement during insertion of the spinal needle

    B. Method A (see Fig. 6-2, *A*): insert the spinal needle into the epidural space in the center of the first intercoccygeal space at a right angle to the general contour of the croup, and press the needle ventrally in a median plane until it strikes the floor of the vertebral canal; withdraw the needle approximately 0.5 cm

    C. Method B (see Fig. 6-2, *B*): insert the spinal needle about 1 inch posterior to the first intercoccygeal space and slide its point ventrocranially at an angle of about 30 degrees to the horizontal plane and to its full length into the vertebral canal

    D. Test with a syringe of air for resistance to the injection; alternatively, fill the needle hub with isotonic saline solution and manipulate slightly until the solution is aspirated from the needle by subatmospheric epidural pressure (hanging drop technique); inject local anesthetic; needle can be left in place with stylet reinserted; maximum blockade may require 10 to 30 minutes, and it is not advisable to redose during this time if surgery is to be done with the horse standing

VII. Use

    A. Anesthesia of pelvic viscera without loss of hind leg motor control during obstetric manipulations

    B. Anesthesia of genitalia without loss of hind leg motor control during obstetric manipulations

    C. For standing surgical procedures of viscera and genitalia

        1. Caslick operation (for pneumovagina)

        2. Rectovaginal fistula repair

        3. Prolapsed rectum repair

        4. Urethrostomy

     5. Tail amputation

     6. Tenesmus prevention

VIII. Common causes for inadequate anesthesia or incomplete block

  A. Improper injection technique

     1. Use of solutions of diminished potency

     2. Inadequate dispersal of anesthetic

  B. Inappropriate angulation of the spinal needle

     1. Needle point strikes the dorsal aspect of the vertebral arch

     2. Deviation of the needle from the midline

  C. Horses that have fibrous connective tissue from previous epidural injections, which limits diffusion of anesthetic agent

  D. Anatomic peculiarities

     1. Presence of septa within the epidural space

     2. Presence of patent intervertebral foramina

IX. Potential complications

  A. Trauma to coccygeal nerve(s)

  B. Infection of the neural canal

  C. Extensive cranial migration of local anesthetic solution causing the following:

     1. Ataxia

     2. Staggering

     3. Excitement

     4. Recumbency

REGIONAL ANESTHESIA OF THE LIMB

  I. Begin by blocking the most distal branches of the nerve trunks to most effectively localize potential sites of lameness. If lameness is not resolved, continue the examination by injecting local anesthetics more proximally, increasing the size of the desensitized area

 II. The palmar (volar) digital nerves of the forelimb or the plantar digital nerves of the hind limb branch dorsal to the fetlock at the level of the sesamoids, forming three digital nerves

  A. The anterior (or dorsal) digital nerve supplies sensory fibers to the anterior two thirds of the hoof

  B. The middle digital nerve (relatively unimportant)

C. The low palmar or plantar digital nerve, which is the most important clinically, supplies sensory fibers to the posterior third of the hoof, including portions, if not all, of the navicular area

PALMAR (VOLAR) OR PLANTAR DIGITAL NERVE BLOCK (Figs. 6-3, *A* and 6-4, *A*)

I. Area blocked: posterior third of the foot, including the navicular bursa
II. Nerves blocked: digital nerves
III. Site: palmar (volar)/plantar region of the pastern joint
IV. Needle: 20- to 25-gauge, 1-inch
V. Anesthetic: 2 ml of 2% lidocaine at each site
VI. Method: palpate the palmar (volar) or plantar nerve just palmar/plantar to the vein and artery, dorsal to the flexor tendon; insert the needle in the palmar/plantar region of the pastern joint, medially and/or laterally with the leg elevated or bearing weight
VII. Use: diagnosis of equine lameness

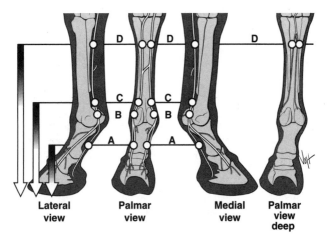

Fig. 6-3

Injection sites for nerve blocks on the left forelimb in the horse. **A,** Palmar (digital). **B,** Abaxial sesamoidean. **C,** Low palmar. **D,** High palmar metacarpal nerves.

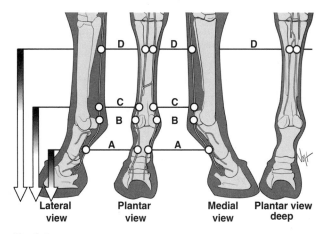

Fig. 6-4
Injection sites for nerve blocks on the left hind limb in the horse. **A,** Plantar digital. **B,** Abaxial sesamoidean. **C,** Low plantar. **D,** High plantar metatarsal nerves.

ABAXIAL (BASILAR) SESAMOIDEAN NERVE BLOCK
(Figs. 6-3, *B* and 6-4, *B*)

I. Area blocked: entire foot distal to the injection site, including the back of the pastern area and distal sesamoidean ligaments
II. Nerves blocked: anterior and posterior digital nerves
III. Site: palmar region of the fetlock joint over abaxial surface of proximal sesamoids
IV. Needle: 20- to 25-gauge, 1-inch
V. Anesthetic: 3 ml of 2% lidocaine at each site
VI. Method: palpate the digital nerve in the palmar region of the fetlock joint over the abaxial surface of proximal sesamoids, just palmar/plantar to the digital artery and vein; insert the needle subcutaneously at this site
VII. Use: diagnosis of equine lameness

PALMAR (VOLAR) OR PLANTAR NERVE BLOCK

I. The palmar (volar) or plantar nerves can be desensitized at either a low site (low palmar/volar or low plantar nerve block) or a high site (high palmar/volar or high plantar nerve block)

II. Midregion blocks (midmetacarpal or midmetatarsal) should be avoided because of the location of the anastomotic branch, which transverses downward from medial to lateral

LOW PALMAR (VOLAR) OR PLANTAR NERVE BLOCK
(Figs. 6-3, C and 6-4, C)

   I. Area blocked: almost all structures distal to the fetlock and fetlock joint, except for a small area dorsal to the fetlock joint supplied by sensory fibers of the ulnar (Fig. 6-5) and musculocutaneous nerves (Fig. 6-6)
   II. Nerves blocked: palmar or plantar nerves (medial/lateral: four-point block)
   III. Site: medially and laterally at the level of the distal enlargements of metacarpals II and IV and metatarsals II and IV (splints)
   IV. Needle: 20- to 25-gauge, 1-inch
   V. Anesthetic: 2 to 3 ml of 2% lidocaine at each site

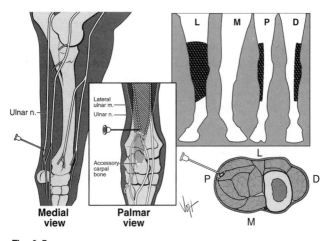

Fig. 6-5
Needle placement for ulnar nerve block: lateral, palmar, and cross-sectional views. Stippled markings indicate desensitized area (*L,* Lateral; *M,* medial; *P,* palmar; and *D,* dorsal views) after ulnar nerve block of the left forelimb.

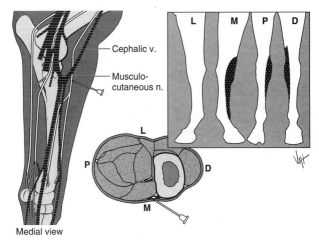

Medial view

Fig. 6-6

Needle placement for median nerve block: medial and cross-sectional views. Stippled markings indicate desensitized area (*L,* Lateral; *M,* medial; *P,* palmar; and *D,* dorsal views) after median nerve block of the left forelimb.

   VI. Method
   A. Desensitize the palmar nerves (medial/lateral) by injecting the anesthetic between the flexor tendon and suspensory ligament
   B. Desensitize the palmar metacarpal and metatarsal nerves (medial/lateral) by injecting the anesthetic between the suspensory ligament and the splint bone
   VII. Use: diagnosis of equine lameness

HIGH PALMAR (VOLAR) OR PLANTAR NERVE BLOCK
(Figs. 6-3, *D* and 6-4, *D*)

   I. Area blocked: palmar (volar) metacarpal or plantar metatarsal region and all of the digit distal to the fetlock
   II. Nerves blocked: palmar or plantar nerves (medial/lateral)
   III. Site: proximal quarter of the metacarpus or metatarsus proximal to the communicating branch of the medial and lateral palmar (volar) or plantar nerves
   IV. Needle: 22-gauge, 1½-inch

   V. Anesthetic: 2 to 3 ml of 2% lidocaine at each site

  VI. Method: desensitize the medial and lateral palmar (volar) and plantar nerves by injecting anesthetic subfascially into the groove between the suspensory ligament and the deep flexor tendon on both the medial and lateral sides

 VII. Use

     A. Diagnosis of equine lameness

     B. The ulnar, median, and musculocutaneous nerves must be desensitized to produce complete anesthesia of the forelimb from the carpus distally

ULNAR NERVE BLOCK (see Fig. 6-5)

    I. Area blocked: lateral, or dorsal and palmar skin areas

   II. Nerve blocked: ulnar nerve

  III. Site: 10 cm proximal to the accessory carpal bone

  IV. Needle: 22-gauge, 1-inch

   V. Anesthetic: 5 to 10 ml of 2% lidocaine

  VI. Method: the nerve is desensitized 1.5 cm deep beneath the fascia between the flexor carpi ulnaris and ulnaris lateralis muscle

 VII. Use: anesthesia of part of the forelimb

MEDIAN NERVE BLOCK (Fig. 6-7)

    I. Area blocked: lateral, medial, palmar, and dorsal skin areas

   II. Nerve blocked: median nerve

  III. Site: medial aspect of the forelimb 5 cm ventral to the elbow joint

  IV. Needle: 20- to 22-gauge, 1½-inch

   V. Anesthetic: 10 ml of 2% lidocaine

  VI. Method: the median nerve is desensitized between the posterior border of the radius and the muscular belly of the internal flexor carpi radialis

 VII. Use: anesthesia of part of the distal limb

MUSCULOCUTANEOUS NERVE BLOCK (see Fig. 6-6)

    I. Area blocked: medial, palmar, and dorsal skin areas

   II. Nerve blocked: cutaneous branch of the musculocutaneous nerve

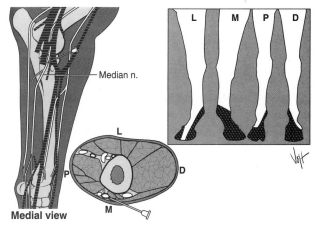

Fig. 6-7

Needle placement for musculocutaneous nerve block: medial and cross-sectional views. Stippled markings indicate desensitized area (*L,* Lateral; *M,* medial; *P,* palmar; and *D,* dorsal views) after musculocutaneous nerve block of the right forelimb.

III. Site: anteromedial aspect of the forelimb halfway between the elbow and carpus
IV. Needle: 22-gauge, 1-inch
V. Anesthetic: 10 ml of 2% lidocaine
VI. Method: the musculocutaneous nerve is desensitized subcutaneously, where it is easily palpated just cranial to the cephalic vein
VII. Use: anesthesia of part of the forelimb

INTRAARTICULAR INJECTIONS

I. General considerations
   A. Intraarticular injections require a surgical scrub to reduce the risk of introducing contaminants
   B. Use surgical gloves when performing complicated joint blocks

    C. Arthrocentesis implies aspiration of synovial fluid but is usually done to allow for instillation of diagnostic and therapeutic agents

        1. Local anesthetic

           a. Adequate amount of local anesthetic should be administered

           b. Enough time should be given for maximal effect and post-block examination

        2. Saline flushes

        3. Antibiotics

        4. Hyaluronic acid

        5. Antiinflammatory drugs

II. Common intraarticular and bursal injections at the most distal digit (Fig. 6-8)

    A. Podotrochlear (navicular) bursa

    B. Coffin joint

    C. Pastern joint

    D. Fetlock joint

    E. Distal flexor tendon sheath

INTRAARTICULAR PODOTROCHLEAR (NAVICULAR) BURSA BLOCK

    I. Site: podotrochlear (navicular) bursa (see Fig. 6-8, *A*)

    II. Needle: 18-gauge spinal needle, 2- to 3-inch

    III. Anesthetic: 2 to 5 ml of 2% lidocaine

    IV. Method: introduce the needle through the digital pad between the bulbs of the heel at the level of the coronary band until it strikes the bone along the midline while the limb is bearing weight; withdraw the needle until very little synovial fluid is aspirated, and then inject anesthetic

INTRAARTICULAR COFFIN BLOCK

    I. Site: interphalangeal (coffin) joint (P2-P3) (see Fig. 6-8, *B*)

    II. Needle: 18- to 20-gauge, 1½-inch

    III. Anesthetic: 5 to 10 ml of 2% lidocaine

    IV. Method: insert the needle 1.5 cm proximal to the coronet approximately 2 cm lateral to the vertical center of the pastern

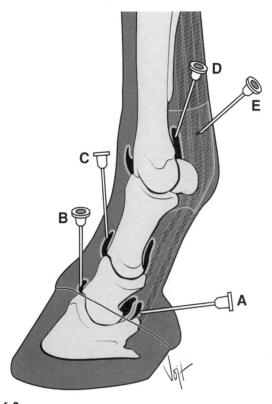

Fig. 6-8
Needle placement. **A,** Podotrochlear (navicular) bursa. **B,** Coffin joint. **C,** Pastern joint. **D,** Fetlock joint. **E,** Distal flexor tendon sheath.

and direct it obliquely ventral to the tendon toward the extensor process

INTRAARTICULAR PASTERN BLOCK

I. Site: interphalangeal (pastern) joint (P1-P2) (see Fig. 6-8, *C*)
II. Needle: 20- to 22-gauge, 1½-inch
III. Anesthetic: 5 to 8 ml of 2% lidocaine

IV. Method: insert the needle medially or laterally to the midline
on the palpable epicondyles of P2 for approximately 2.5 cm in
a vertical direction

INTRAARTICULAR FETLOCK BLOCK

   I. Site: metacarpophalangeal or metatarsophalangeal (fetlock)
joint (see Fig. 6-8, *D*)
  II. Needle: 20- to 22-gauge spinal needle, 1½-inch
 III. Anesthetic: 5 to 10 ml of 2% lidocaine
 IV. Method: insert the needle into the lateral pouch distal to the
splint bone and dorsal to the annular ligament of the fetlock to
a depth of approximately 0.5 to 1 cm

DIGITAL FLEXOR TENDON SHEATH BLOCK

   I. Site: digital flexor tendon sheath (see Fig. 6-8, *E*)
  II. Needle: 18- to 20-gauge, 1½-inch
 III. Anesthetic: 10 ml of 2% lidocaine
 IV. Method: insert the needle at the distal end of the splint ("but-
ton"), either medially or laterally, cranial to the deep and su-
perficial flexor tendons and caudal to the suspensory ligament

INTRAARTICULAR RADIOCARPAL BLOCK

   I. Site: radiocarpal (antebrachial carpal) joint (Fig. 6-9, *A*)
  II. Needle: 20-gauge, 1½-inch
 III. Anesthetic: 5 to 10 ml of 2% lidocaine
 IV. Method: with the carpus flexed, insert the needle between the
radiocarpal joint space on either side of the palpable extensor
carpi radialis tendon

INTRAARTICULAR INTERCARPAL BLOCK

   I. Site: intercarpal (middle carpal) joint (Fig. 6-9, *B*)
  II. Needle: 20-gauge, 1½-inch
 III. Anesthetic: 5 to 10 ml of 2% lidocaine
 IV. Method: with the carpus flexed, insert the needle between the
intercarpal joint space on either side of the palpable extensor
carpi radialis tendon

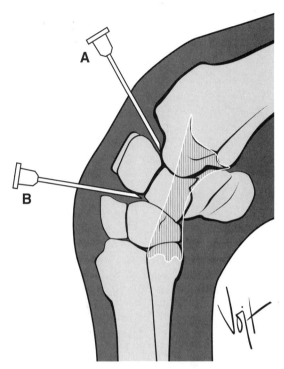

Fig. 6-9
Needle placement. **A,** Radial carpal joint spaces. **B,** Intercarpal joint spaces.

CUNEAN BURSA BLOCK

I. Site: cunean bursa on the medial aspect of the tarsus (Fig. 6-10, *A*)
II. Needle: 22-gauge, 1-inch
III. Anesthetic: at least 10 ml of 2% lidocaine
IV. Method: insert the needle approximately 1.5 cm distal to the cunean tendon (medial branch of the tibialis anterior muscle) and advance it between the cunean tendon and the tarsal bone to penetrate the bursa distally; at least 20 minutes are required for maximum anesthetic effect

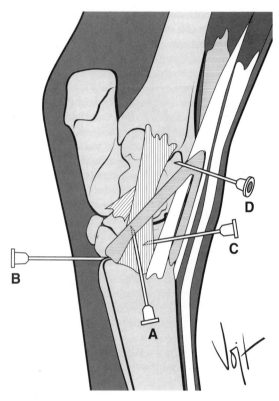

Fig. 6-10
Needle placement. **A,** Cunean bursa. **B,** The tarsometatarsal joint spaces. **C,** Intertarsal joint spaces. **D,** Tibiotarsal joint spaces.

INTRAARTICULAR TARSOMETATARSAL BLOCK

   I. Site: tarsometatarsal joint at the posterior lateral aspect of the hock over the lateral head of the splint (metatarsal IV) (Fig. 6-10, *B*)
   II. Needle: 22-gauge, 1-inch
   III. Anesthetic: 6 to 8 ml of 2% lidocaine
   IV. Method: the needle is most easily inserted into the tarsometatarsal joint on the posterior lateral aspect of the hock

proximal to the palpable lateral head of the splint; the bevel of
the needle must be turned away from the bone to allow injection of the anesthetic solution

INTRAARTICULAR INTERTARSAL BLOCK

  I. Site: distal intertarsal joint on the medial aspect of the tarsus
(Fig. 6-10, *C*)
  II. Needle: 22-gauge, 1-inch
 III. Anesthetic: 6 ml of 2% lidocaine
 IV. Method: insert the needle into the joint at a right angle to the
skin ventral to the cunean tendon; inject local anesthetic using
considerable pressure while turning the needle bevel

INTRAARTICULAR TIBIOTARSAL BLOCK

  I. Site: tibiotarsal (tarsocrural) joint at the craniomedial aspect of
the tibia (Fig. 6-10, *D*)
  II. Needle: 18-gauge, 1½-inch
 III. Anesthetic: 15 ml of 2% lidocaine
 IV. Method: the needle is easily inserted less than 2 cm deep into
the skin and superficial capsule, 2 to 3 cm ventral to the medial
malleolus of the tibia on either the medial or lateral side of the
saphenous vein; inject local anesthetic after synovial fluid is recovered on aspiration

CHAPTER SEVEN

Local Anesthesia in Dogs and Cats

"Think globally, act locally."
OLIVER WENDELL HOLMES, JR.

OVERVIEW

Local anesthetic techniques can be used in selected small animals to perform surgery, avoiding the depressant effects of general anesthesia. Local anesthesia is usually administered in combination with sedation or tranquilization to produce a cooperative patient. Local analgesic techniques can also be used to produce postoperative analgesia in surgical patients. Commonly used techniques in small animals include infiltration anesthesia, nerve blocks (e.g., selected nerve blocks about the head), brachial plexus block, intravenous (IV) regional anesthesia, and continuous epidural anesthesia. Epidural opioid or ketamine analgesia, intercostal nerve blocks, and interpleural analgesia can provide long-lasting postoperative pain relief.

REGIONAL ANESTHESIA OF THE HEAD (Fig. 7-1)

The following local anesthetic techniques, when combined with sedative administration and appropriate physical restraint, can be used to desensitize nerves of the head:

  I. Infraorbital
 II. Maxillary
III. Ophthalmic
 IV. Mental
  V. Mandibuloalveolar

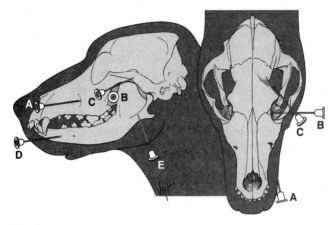

Fig. 7-1
Needle placement for nerve blocks on the head. **A,** Infraorbital. **B,** Maxillary. **C,** Ophthalmic. **D,** Mental. **E,** Mandibuloalveolar.

ANESTHESIA OF UPPER LIP AND NOSE

  I. Area blocked: upper lip and nose, roof of nasal cavity, and related skin ventral to the infraorbital foramen
 II. Nerve blocked: infraorbital
III. Site: point of emergence of the nerve from the infraorbital canal (see Fig. 7-1, *A*)
 IV. Needle: 22- to 25-gauge, 1-inch
  V. Anesthetic: 2 ml of 1% lidocaine
 VI. Method: insert the needle either intraorally or extraorally approximately 1 cm cranial to the bony lip of the infraorbital foramen; advance the needle to the infraorbital foramen, which can be felt between the dorsal border of the zygomatic process and the gum of the canine tooth

ANESTHESIA OF MAXILLA, UPPER TEETH, NOSE, AND UPPER LIP

  I. Area blocked: maxilla, upper teeth, nose, and upper lip
 II. Nerve blocked: maxillary

  III. Site: perpendicular portion of the palatine bone between the maxillary foramen and foramen rotundum (see Fig. 7-1, *B*)

  IV. Needle: 22- to 25-gauge, 1-inch

  V. Anesthetic: 2 ml of 1% lidocaine

  VI. Method: insert the needle through the skin at a 90-degree angle, in a medial direction, ventral to the border of the zygomatic process and approximately 0.5 cm caudal to the lateral canthus of the eye; advance the needle in close proximity to the pterygopalatine fossa; local anesthetic is administered where the maxillary nerve courses perpendicular to the palatine bone between the maxillary foramen and foramen rotundum

ANESTHESIA OF THE EYE

  I. Area blocked: eye, orbit, conjunctiva, eyelids, and forehead skin

  II. Nerves blocked: lacrimal, zygomatic, and ophthalmic (i.e., ophthalmic division of the trigeminal nerve)

  III. Site: at the orbital fissure (see Fig. 7-1, *C*)

  IV. Needle: 22- to 25-gauge, 1-inch

  V. Anesthetic: 2 ml of 1% lidocaine

  VI. Method: insert the needle ventral to the border of the zygomatic process at the lateral canthus of the eye; the needle point should be approximately 0.5 cm cranial to the anterior border of the vertical portion of the ramus of the mandible; advance the needle medial to the ramus of the mandible in a mediodorsal and somewhat caudal direction until it reaches the orbital fissure

ANESTHESIA OF THE LOWER LIP

  I. Area blocked: lower lip

  II. Nerve blocked: mental

  III. Site: rostral to the mental foramen (see Fig. 7-1, *D*)

  IV. Needle: 22- to 25-gauge, 1-inch

  V. Anesthetic: 2 ml of 1% lidocaine

  VI. Method: insert the needle over the mental nerve, rostral to the middle mental foramen at the level of the second premolar tooth

ANESTHESIA OF THE MANDIBLE

   I. Area blocked: cheek teeth, canine, incisors, skin, and mucosa of the chin and lower lip
  II. Nerve blocked: inferior alveolar branch of the mandibular nerve
 III. Site: point of entry of the nerve into the mandibular canal at the mandibular foramen (see Fig. 7-1, *E*)
  IV. Needle used: 22- to 25-gauge, 1-inch
   V. Anesthetic: 2 ml of 1% lidocaine
  VI. Method: insert the needle at the lower angle of the jaw approximately 1.5 cm rostral to the angular process; advance the needle 1.5 cm dorsally against the medial surface of the ramus of the mandible to the palpable lip of the mandibular foramen

ANESTHESIA OF THE FOOT

   I. Anesthesia of the foot may be induced by the following techniques:
   A. Infiltration of the tissues around the limb with local anesthetic solution (ring block)
   B. Infiltration of the brachial plexus by local anesthetic (brachial plexus block)
   C. IV injection of anesthetic into an accessible superficial vein in a distal extremity that is isolated from circulation by placing a tourniquet on the animal's leg (IV regional anesthesia)
   D. Injection of local anesthetic into the lumbosacral epidural space (anesthesia of the hind legs)
   E. Perineural infiltration of sensory nerves in the limbs

BRACHIAL PLEXUS BLOCK

   I. Area blocked: distal foot, up to the elbow region
  II. Nerves blocked: radial, median, ulnar, musculocutaneous, and axillary nerves
 III. Site: medial to the shoulder joint (Fig. 7-2)
  IV. Needle: 22-gauge, 3-inch
   V. Anesthetic: 10 to 15 ml of 2% lidocaine

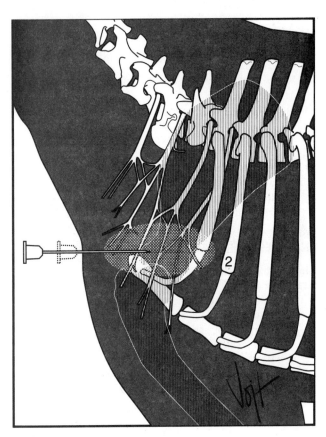

Fig. 7-2
Needle placement for brachial plexus block, lateral aspect of left thoracic limb in the dog. *2* represents the second rib.

VI. Method: insert the needle medial to the shoulder joint toward the costochondral junction and parallel to the vertebral column; inject the anesthetic slowly as the needle is withdrawn; anesthesia can be obtained within 20 minutes and for up to 2 hours

   VII. Advantages
     A. Relatively simple and safe to perform
     B. Produces selective anesthesia and relaxation of the limb distal to the elbow joint
VIII. Disadvantages
     A. Relatively long waiting period (15 to 30 minutes) required
     B. Occasional failure to obtain complete anesthesia, particularly in overweight dogs
   IX. Complications
     A. Toxic symptoms after intravascular administration of the local anesthetic
     B. Lack of anesthesia after inadvertent intravascular injection

INTRAVENOUS REGIONAL ANESTHESIA

    I. Area blocked: extremity distal to tourniquet
   II. Nerves blocked: nerve endings in peripheral tissues
  III. Site: any superficial vein distal to tourniquet
  IV. Needle: 22-gauge, 1½-inch
   V. Anesthetic: 2 to 3 ml of 1% lidocaine (without epinephrine)
  VI. Method: the limb is first desanguinated by wrapping it with an Esmarch bandage; a rubber tourniquet is placed around the forearm just proximal to the elbow for thoracic limb surgery or proximal to the hock for pelvic limb surgery; the tourniquet must be tight enough to overcome blood pressure; once the tourniquet is secured, the Esmarch bandage is unwrapped, and local anesthetic is injected with light pressure (BIER-block)
  VII. Advantages
     A. Safe and simple technique
     B. Lack of toxicity to organs if the occlusion of blood supply is limited to 2 hours
     C. Blood-free surgery site is ideal for taking biopsies and removing foreign bodies from the paws
VIII. Disadvantages: limited to 2 hours
   IX. Complications
     A. Shock can occur if tourniquet is left on more than 4 hours (reversible)

    B. Death can occur from sepsis and endotoxemia if tourniquet is left on more than 8 to 10 hours

LUMBOSACRAL EPIDURAL ANESTHESIA

I. Indications
- A. Animals that are severely depressed, are in shock, or require immediate surgery of the rear quarters
- B. Animals that are at high risk, are aged, or in which the use of other analgesic or anesthetic agents is contraindicated
- C. Opioids are used to provide analgesia after abdominal surgery or surgery of the rear limbs; paralysis is not produced

II. Specific procedures
- A. Surgery
    1. Tail amputation
    2. Anal sac therapy or perianal surgery
    3. Rear limb lacerations or fractures
    4. Urolithiasis therapy
    5. Abdominal surgery
    6. Cesarean section
    7. Obstetric manipulations
    8. Surgical procedures of the tail, perineum, vulva, vagina, rectum, and bladder
- B. Postoperative analgesia

III. Landmarks and anatomy (Fig. 7-3)
- A. Right and left cranial dorsal iliac wings of the ilium
- B. Spinous process of the seventh lumbar vertebra and the median sacral crest
- C. Important anatomic features
    1. Shape of lumbar and sacral spinous processes
    2. Interspinous ligament
    3. Ligamentum arcuatum (ligamentum flavum)
    4. Terminal portion of the dural sac
    5. Filum terminale
    6. Intervertebral disk
- D. The spinal cord usually ends at vertebral body L6 in dogs and S1 in cats; therefore the procedure is more hazardous when performed on cats

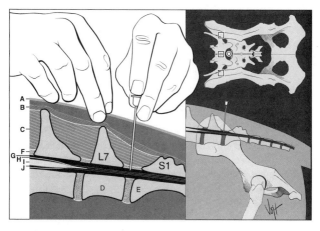

Fig. 7-3
Needle placement for lumbosacral epidural (between L7 and S1) anesthesia in the dog, lateral and dorsal aspects. *A,* Skin; *B,* supraspinous ligament; *C,* interspinous ligament; *D,* seventh lumbar vertebra; *E,* sacrum; *F,* interarcuate ligament (ligamentum flavum); *G,* epidural space; *H,* dura mater spinalis; *I,* spinal cord; *J,* subarachnoid space containing cerebrospinal fluid (CSF).

IV. Equipment
  A. 2- or 4-inch, 18- or 20-gauge short, beveled spinal needle with stylet (disposable needle preferred)
  B. One 2.5-ml and one 5-ml syringe
  C. A thin-walled, 18-gauge, 3-inch needle is used if a polyethylene catheter is to be placed for continuous epidural anesthesia
V. Procedure
  A. Perform a surgical scrub; this is a sterile procedure
  B. Place the spinal needle perpendicular to the skin surface at the midline of the lumbosacral space; this space can be palpated halfway between the dorsoiliac wings and just caudal to the dorsal spinous process of the seventh lumbar vertebra (see Fig. 7-3)
    1. Infiltration of the area with 2% lidocaine may facilitate placement of the spinal needle

      2. Push the spinal needle ventrally in a slight cranial or caudal angle as needed

  C. Resistance is usually encountered when the ligamentum flavum is reached; a distinct "pop" is usually felt when the needle is advanced through this ligament

  D. On penetrating the ligamentum flavum, the needle is in the epidural space

      1. Needle depth may vary from ½ to 1½ inches, depending on animal size

      2. Remove the stylet and examine the needle for blood or cerebrospinal fluid (CSF); if no blood or CSF is observed, the needle should be aspirated for blood or CSF

      3. Inject 1 to 2 ml of air to check for proper needle placement

         a. If subcutaneous crepitus is felt, the needle is incorrectly placed and should be repositioned

         b. No resistance should be felt to the injection of air or local anesthetic agent

VI. Doses

  A. The required dose varies depending on the desired effect

  B. 2% lidocaine or 0.75% bupivacaine is the agent of choice; inject 1 ml of local anesthetic for each 10 pounds of body weight; this will produce anesthesia as far cranial as L2; if anesthesia is required up to T5, the dose may be increased to 1 ml of local anesthetic per 7.5 pounds of body weight

      1. A test dose of 0.5 to 1 ml of 2% lidocaine produces almost immediate dilation of the external anal sphincter, followed by relaxation and ataxia of pelvic limbs within 3 to 5 minutes

      2. Small amounts of 1 : 200,000 epinephrine can be added to lidocaine to delay the rate of absorption, thus prolonging anesthetic action by 30 minutes (total of 2 hours)

  C. Bupivacaine with epinephrine (Marcaine) or ropivacaine (Naropin) produces 4- to 6-hour periods of anesthesia

VII. Continuous epidural anesthesia in dogs

  A. Procedure

      1. The procedure is similar to that previously described, except that a curved bevel spinal needle (Tuohy) is used, through which a catheter is passed (Fig. 7-4)

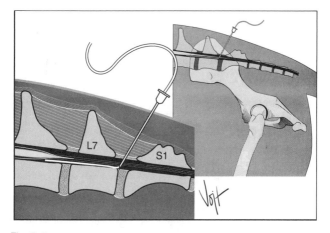

Fig. 7-4
Needle placement for continuous epidural anesthesia or opioid analagesia in
the dog, shown in the lateral aspect. *L7* and *S1* are the spinous processes of
the seventh lumbar and the first sacral vertebrae.

    2. The Tuohy needle is inserted into the epidural space
       with the needle bevel directed cranially
    3. Only ½ inch of catheter should be advanced into the
       epidural space
    4. Withdraw the needle, but leave the catheter in place
  B. Advantages
    1. Ability to tailor the duration of anesthesia to the length
       of operation
    2. Route for injecting epidural opioids during and after
       surgery (see epidural opioid analgesia)
  C. Disadvantages
    1. Technically difficult
    2. Potential for damage to the spinal cord, meninges, and
       nerves
    3. Risk of infection
    4. Catheter-related problems (e.g. kinks, displacement,
       clotting with fibrin)
VIII. Factors influencing cranial level of blockade
  A. Size of patient
  B. Conformation of patient

    C. Volume of drug injected

    D. Drug mass

    E. Rate of injection (volume × concentration)

    F. Direction of needle bevel

    G. Age of patient

    H. Obesity

    I. Intraabdominal pressure attributable to presence and size of abdominal mass (e.g., pregnancy)

       1. The volume of the epidural space in pregnant animals is decreased because of distention of epidural veins/engorgement

       2. The sensitivity of neural tissue to hormonal changes is increased

    J. Position of patient: gravity has a more definite role in the spread of subarachnoid anesthesia than in epidural anesthesia; however, with both techniques, a more rapid onset to maximal segmental anesthesia (unilateral anesthesia), a longer duration of anesthesia, and a more intensive motor blockade are achieved in the dependent side than in the upper side

IX. Proposed site of action after epidural injection (Table 7-1)

X. Possible complications

    A. Injection of local anesthetic into the vertebral sinuses

       1. Vomiting, tremors

       2. Decreased blood pressure caused by peripheral vasodilation

       3. Convulsions

       4. Paralysis

    B. Respiratory depression and paralysis in dogs and cats caused by drug overdose

       1. The drug must migrate to approximately C5 or C7 to produce complete respiratory paralysis from blockade of the phrenic nerves

       2. The cephalad spread of anesthesia after epidural or subarachnoid injection (of specifically prepared hyperbaric solution [e.g., "heavy nupercaine"] in 6% glucose) is limited in an animal that is kept in a sitting position

    C. Temperature may fall in small animals because they are unable to shiver; the patient's rear quarters should be kept

TABLE 7-1
PROPOSED SITE OF ACTION AFTER EPIDURAL INJECTION

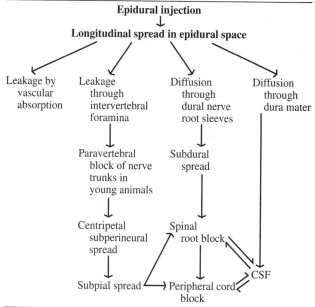

CSF, Cerebrospinal fluid.

warm by wrapping them in a towel or a heated water blanket

D. Administer a sedative or tranquilizer for patient cooperation

EPIDURAL OPIOID AND ALPHA₂-ADRENOCEPTOR ANALGESIA

I. Indications
   A. Intraoperative analgesia
   B. Postoperative analgesia
   C. Critical care patients
II. Site of opioid injection
   A. Lumbosacral epidural space (single-dose injection) (see Fig. 7-3)

    B. Anterior lumbar epidural space (catheter technique) (see Fig. 7-4)

III. Drugs

    A. Epidural morphine (0.1 mg/kg diluted in 0.13 to 0.26 ml/kg of 0.9% NaCl solution) produces pain relief 30 to 60 minutes after injection and for as long as 10 to 24 hours

    B. Epidural morphine (0.1 mg/kg) alone or combined with xylazine (0.02 mg/kg) or medetomidine (2-5 μg/kg) produces minimal cardiovascular changes in dogs anesthetized with 1.5 minimum alveolar concentration (MAC) of isoflurane

    C. Epidural morphine (0.1 mg/kg) with medetomidine (0.005 mg/kg) produces pain relief for at least 13 hours

    D. Epidural oxymorphone (0.05 to 0.1 mg/kg diluted in 0.26 ml/kg of 0.9% NaCl solution) produces pain relief 20 to 40 minutes after injection and for an approximate duration of 10 to 15 hours

    E. Epidural fentanyl (1 to 10 mg/kg diluted in 0.26 ml/kg of 0.9% NaCl solution) produces pain relief 15 to 20 minutes after administration, with analgesia lasting 3 to 5 hours

    F. Epidural fentanyl (0.1 mg/kg) with lidocaine (0.3 ml/kg, 2% solution + 1:200,000 epinephrine) produces scrotal anesthesia in 2 minutes after administration, with anesthesia lasting 2 to 2.5 hours

IV. Advantages

    A. Relief of somatic and visceral pain is more profound and prolonged with smaller doses than the analgesia produced by comparable parenterally administered (IM, IV) opioids

    B. No interference with sensory function

    C. No interference with motor function

    D. Minimal depression of the sympathetic nervous system

    E. Reversal of side effects by low-dose, IV infusion of opioid antagonists (e.g., naloxone)

V. Potential side effects (rare)

    A. Respiratory depression

    B. Urinary retention

    C. Delayed gastrointestinal motility

    D. Vomiting

    E. Pruritus

VI. Complications
   A. Respiratory depression after large doses (>1 mg/kg) of epidural morphine
   B. Catheter-related problems
      1. Catheter displacement
      2. Occlusion
      3. Infection

EPIDURAL KETAMINE ANALGESIA

I. Mechanism of action
   A. The precise mechanism of analgesic action after epidural or subarachnoid administration of ketamine has not been clearly defined
   B. Hypothetically, ketamine acts as an antagonist at the n-methyl-D-aspartate (NMDA) receptors preventing the development of neural changes involved in hyperesthesia
   C. NMDA receptors play an important role in spinal neural plasticity, such as central sensitization, wind-up, and hyperalgesia
II. Indication
   A. Preemptive (postoperative) analgesia when administered epidurally in the preoperative period
   B. Intraoperative analgesia lessens the cardiovascular depressant effects of inhalation anesthesia as a result of MAC-sparing effect
   C. Postoperative analgesia with minimal respiratory depression and cardiovascular changes (e.g., blood pressure, heart rate)
III. Method: ketamine (2 mg/kg) is diluted to a volume of 1 ml of sterile 0.9% NaCl/4.5 kg body weight and is injected into the lumbosacral epidural space
IV. Advantages
   A. Local anesthetic effects
   B. Alternative method to epidural opiate administration in dogs anesthetized with halothane or isoflurane
   C. Minimal changes in cardiovascular parameters, such as heart rate, blood pressure, central venous pressure, cardiac index, systemic and pulmonary vascular resistance, and

rate-pressured product in isoflurane-anesthetized dogs (MAC 1.2% to 1.6%)

V. Potential side effects

    A. Differences in the analgesic response to epidurally administered ketamine have been observed; attributable to anatomic differences, dose regimen, and inhalation anesthesia

INTRAARTICULAR BUPIVACAINE OR MORPHINE

  I. Indication: local analgesia for stifle surgery

  II. Method: an intra-articular injection of bupivacaine or morphine is given after surgical repair of ruptured cranial cruciate ligaments and before skin closure

    A. 0.5 ml of bupivacaine HCl (0.5%)/kg body weight or 0.1 mg morphine (preservative-free morphine, Duramorph, or Astramorph) diluted with 0.9% NaCl to a volume of 0.5 ml/kg

  III. Results

    A. Intra-articular bupivacaine and morphine provide postoperative analgesia without adverse reactions

    B. Intra-articular bupivacaine produces the greatest local anesthetic effect lasting up to 24 hours after administration, allowing dogs to recover completely while alert

    C. Intra-articular morphine provides some analgesia lasting at least 6 hours, but not to the extent of intra-articular bupivacaine

    D. Inflammation is needed for morphine to produce its antinociceptive effect; inflammation may cause activation of receptors already present within peripheral tissues

  IV. Advantages

    A. Local analgesia provides pain relief without the need for systemic administration of analgesic/sedative drugs allowing systemic functions to be undisturbed

    B. Local analgesia allows local inflammation to proceed while providing symptomatic relief of pain

  V. Potential side effects

    A. Limited effect of postoperative analgesia by intra-articular morphine as indicated by need for supplemental analgesia requirements postoperatively; attributable to low pain threshold (high cumulative pain score tests)

INTERCOSTAL NERVE BLOCKS

I. Indications
   A. Relief of pain during thoracotomy
   B. Analgesia after thoracotomy
   C. Pleural drainage
   D. Rib fractures

II. Nerves blocked: intercostals both cranial and caudal to the incision or injury site because of overlap of nerve supply

III. Site: intercostal spaces (R3 to R6) near the intercostal foramen (Fig. 7-5)

IV. Needle: 22- to 25-gauge, 1-inch

V. Anesthetic: 0.25 to 1 ml of 0.25% or 0.5% bupivacaine, or 0.2% or 0.5% ropivacaine/site, with or without epinephrine 1:200,000
   A. Small dog: 0.25 ml/site
   B. Medium dog: 0.5 ml/site
   C. Large dog: 1 ml/site

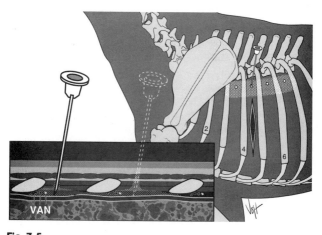

Fig. 7-5
Needle placement for intercostal nerve blocks in the dog, shown in the lateral aspect and the sagittal section. *2, 4, 6* are the second, fourth, and sixth rib; *VAN* is the intercostal vein, artery, and nerve.

VI. Method: insert the needle through the skin at a 90-degree angle caudal to the rib (R3 to R6) near the intervertebral foramen; inject small volumes and/or diluted anesthetic solutions into a minimum of two adjacent intercostal spaces, both cranial and caudal to the incision or injury site because of overlap of nerve supply; the total dosage should not exceed 3 mg/kg because the technique produces high blood concentrations of the anesthetic

VII. Advantages

    A. Selective intercostal nerve block is easily performed because of the proximity of each nerve to its adjacent rib

    B. The intercostal nerves can be visualized beneath the pleura during thoracotomy

    C. The technique provides consistent analgesia for 3 to 6 hours without respiratory depression

VIII. Complications

    A. Pneumothorax after faulty technique

    B. Impaired blood-gas exchange (hypercarbia, hypoxemia) in dogs with pulmonary diseases

INTRAPLEURAL REGIONAL ANALGESIA

I. Indications

    A. Relief of pain originating from the following conditions:

        1. Thoracotomy

        2. Rib fractures

        3. Mastectomy

        4. Chronic pancreatitis

        5. Cholocystectomy

        6. Renal surgery

        7. Abdominal cancer

        8. Metastasis of the chest wall, pleura, and mediastinum

II. Nerves blocked: mechanisms of pain relief are not fully understood

    A. Retrograde diffusion of local anesthetic through the parietal pleura, causing intercostal nerve block

    B. Desensitization of the thoracic sympathetic chain and splanchnic nerves

III. Site: place a catheter into the pleural space either percutaneously or before closure of a thoracotomy (Fig. 7-6).

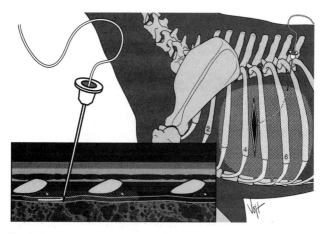

Fig. 7-6
Needle and catheter placement for intrapleural regional analgesia in the dog, shown in the left lateral aspect and the sagittal section. *2, 4, 6* are the second, fourth, and sixth rib.

IV. Equipment: 17-gauge, 2-inch, Huber-point (Tuohy) needle; medical grade silastic tubing, 5 to 10 cm, 2-mm inside diameter; sterile sets for single, continuous interpleural analgesia are available

V. Anesthetic: approximately 1 to 2 mg of 0.25% bupivacaine/kg or 0.2% ropivacaine/kg (0.5%, with or without 1 : 200,000 epinephrine)

VI. Method: in a well-sedated dog, desensitize the skin, subcutaneous tissue, periosteum, and parietal pleura over the caudal border of the rib with 1 to 2 ml of 2% lidocaine, using a 22-gauge, 1-inch needle; then use the Huber-point needle to place the catheter with minimal resistance into the subatmospheric pleural space, 3 to 4 cm beyond the needle tip (see Fig. 7-6); withdraw the needle over the catheter and leave the catheter in place; catheter placement in the open chest is accomplished by inserting the Tuohy needle through the skin at least two intercostal spaces caudal to the incision and passing the catheter through the needle subpleurally under direct vision; inject local anesthetic over 1 to 2 minutes following

negative aspiration of air or blood through the catheter; then
clear the catheter with 2 ml of physiologic saline solution

VII. Advantages

  A. The procedure is simple to perform

  B. One needlestick is needed in contrast to multiple intercostal nerve blocks

  C. Post thoracotomy pain relief lasts longer (3 to 12 hours)
than analgesia produced by subcutaneous morphine (0.5
mg/kg) or selective intercostal nerve blocks with bupivacaine (0.5 ml of 0.5% bupivacaine per site)

  D. Long-term use (over several weeks) of an interpleural
catheter is possible

VIII. Complications

  A. Infection

  B. Phrenic nerve paralysis or paresis; paradoxic respiration
with negative intraabdominal pressure

  C. Tachyphylaxis to local anesthetic

  D. High anesthetic blood concentration

  E. Systemic toxicity after excessive doses of the local anesthetic (>3 mg bupivacaine/kg)

  F. Catheter-related complications (e.g., pneumothorax)

  G. Minimal pain relief

    1. Misplaced catheter

    2. Excessive bleeding into the pleural space

    3. Pleural effusion

CHAPTER EIGHT

Acupuncture Analgesia

"Medicine is not only a science, but also the art of letting our
own individuality interact with the individuality
of the patient."

ALBERT SCHWEITZER

OVERVIEW

Acupuncture can be used to induce pain relief (hypalgesia) in clinical disorders and as a complementary method of pain control during surgical procedures in well-restrained, large and small animal patients. Acupuncture analgesia is best achieved by electrostimulation through acupuncture needles in acupuncture points. Many acupuncture points can be used to induce electroacupuncture analgesia (EAA) in animals. It is not known which point combination is best for a particular operation. Generally, the area of analgesia is related to the site of electrostimulation. The major advantages of EAA are good analgesia in high-risk patients without producing CNS and respiratory depression, bradycardia, and hypotension commonly observed after the use of sedatives, opioids, and general anesthetics; excellent postoperative pain relief; fast postoperative recovery of appetite and gut and bladder function; and fast postoperative wound healing with minimal infection. The major disadvantages are the need for very good restraint; a long induction period (mean time is 20 minutes) with variable degrees of analgesia; maintenance of sensations to touch, pressure, and traction; poor relaxation of abdominal muscles attributable to "ballooning" of viscera; nausea and/or vomiting attributable to prolonged manipulation of viscera and organs or traction on mesentery; and maintenance of reflexes to sight, sound, and fear in conscious animals.

119

TYPES OF OPERATIONS POTENTIALLY PERFORMED UNDER EAA

I. Dog
   A. Cesarean section with no depressive effects on the fetus
   B. Ovariohysterectomy, including toxic pyometra
   C. Abdominal laparotomy
   D. Gastric and intestinal surgery
   E. Nephrectomy
   F. Splenectomy
   G. Umbilical hernioplasty
   H. Removal of mammary and skin tumors
   I. Ear cropping
   J. Craniotomy
   K. Open reduction and repair of long bone fractures
II. Horses, cattle, sheep, pigs
   A. Castration
   B. Orchidopexy
   C. Reposition of prolapsed uterus
   D. Surgery of anal and vaginal region
   E. Relief of dystocia
   F. Surgery on esophagus and rumen
   G. Repair of navel and umbilical hernia
   H. Surgery on the bladder and urethra
   I. Orthopedic surgery (bones and joints)

Equipment

I. Acupuncture needles
   A. Human acupuncture needles: 29 to 34 gauge
   B. Veterinary acupuncture needles: 22 to 26 gauge for large animals; 26 to 30 gauge for small animals
   C. The needles are inserted at acupuncture points to the correct depth, taped or sutured firmly in position, and connected in pairs to the output socket of an acupuncture electrostimulator
   D. Each pair of electrodes should be on the same side of the spinal cord. To prevent cardiac fibrillation, any one pair of leads must not cross the spine between the cervical and thoracic vertebrae

    E. The leads may be alternated between needles if more nee-
       dles are used than can be stimulated simultaneously

II. Acupuncture electrostimulators

    A. There are many electrostimulators on the market today. They
       are manufactured in China, Japan, the United States, Canada,
       Europe, and Australia

    B. There is little standardization of equipment. The equipment
       is expected to have the following characteristics:

       1. Strength
       2. Portability
       3. Battery-operated
       4. Outputs for at least six to eight electrodes
       5. Delivers a bipolar waveform $(+)$ and $(-)$ at each elec-
          trode to prevent electrolytic injury from prolonged use of
          monopolar waveform
       6. Delivers a square or spike wave form biphasic

    C. A hand-held unit (Pointer Plus, M.E.D. Servi-Systems,
       Canada Ltd.) to locate and stimulate acupuncture and trig-
       ger points, using 10 Hz, 1 to 25 volts, and 1 to 50 milliamps,
       is shown in Fig. 8-1

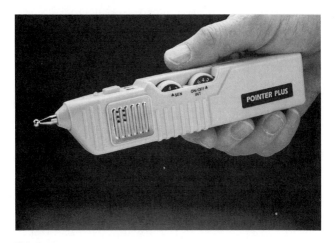

Fig. 8-1
Pointer Plus, a handheld unit for locating and stimulating acupuncture points.

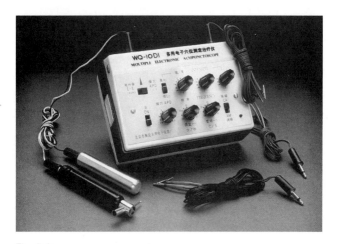

Fig. 8-2
Electronic acupunctoscope for locating and stimulating acupuncture points percutaneously.

D. A multiple electronic acupunctoscope (WQ10C, M.E.D. Servi-Systems, Canada Ltd.) is shown in Fig. 8-2. It possesses the following characteristics:
1. It reflects the latest in research and clinical practice in China
2. It detects acupuncture and auricular points
3. It stimulates three pairs of acupuncture needles for acupuncture analgesia and therapy
4. It generates three different wave forms to minimize facilitation
5. The frequency can be varied between 1 and 1000 Hz
6. It has a constant amplitude and amplitude modulation switch
7. It operates on 9-volt batteries

RESTRAINT

I. Technique in small animals
A. Small animals are generally operated on in lateral, dorsal, or ventral recumbency

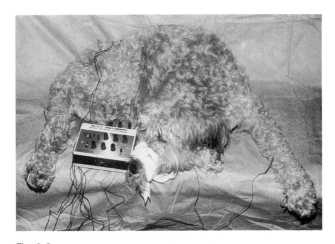

Fig. 8-3
Sedated and restrained dog during electroacupuncture stimulation.

  B. Dogs are given a sedative/analgesic and small doses of general anesthetics
  C. The animal's elbows and hocks are tied with bandages and secured to the operation table
  D. A tape bandage may be tied around the dog's jaws to prevent biting (Fig. 8-3)
  E. The owner or an attendant should comfort and speak to the dog from time to time during surgery
II. Technique in large animals
  A. Electroacupuncture may be performed in horses and cattle restrained in the standing position or in dorsal, lateral, or ventral recumbency
  B. For a standing animal, usual methods for restraint (stock, chute, cattle crate) as applied for surgery under local anesthesia may be used
  C. Nervous animals may be given a sedative/analgesic intravenously
  D. Recumbency may be induced with a short-acting, intravenous anesthetic
  E. Recumbent animals should be securely restrained with ropes
  F. The operator should keep noise and movement to a minimum

SELECTION OF ACUPUNCTURE POINTS

I. General statements
  A. Point combinations for induction of hypalgesia sufficient for surgery vary with the operative site and the preference and experience of the surgeon
  B. Points are generally chosen based on the channel (meridian) theory of human acupuncture
  C. Acupuncture points in animals have the same name and code as in humans and are transposed from human acupuncture anatomy
  D. Channels have a superficial course (from the first to the last point on the channel), a deep course (going to the organ of the channel), and a collateral course (linking to interior and exterior parts of the body). This may explain why a Liver point is used for operations of the eye, a Heart point for operation of the tongue, and a Kidney point for operation of the ear and bone.

II. Acupuncture point selection in the dog. In general, the following points bilateral of the spine are chosen:
  A. For surgery in all areas: Bl 23 +/or SP 6; Ll 11 + Japanese point In Ko Ten; ST 36 + Japanese point Bo Ko Ku
  B. For surgery on the head, neck, thorax, and front limb: PC 6 + TH 5
  C. For surgery on the abdomen and hind limbs: SP 6 + ST 36 and paraincisional for ovariohysterectomy
  D. For surgery on high-risk dogs: Ll 4 + Ll 11 + SP 6 + ST 36
  E. For back surgery: BL 23 + BL 40 + BL 60 + ST 36 + GB 34

III. Anatomical location of acupuncture points in dogs
  A. Fig. 8-4 illustrates the location of the various acupuncture points for dogs
  B. The International Veterinary Acupuncture Society (IVAS) describes the abbreviation and location of these points as follows:
    1. Ll 4 (large intestine point 4): between the first and second metacarpal bones, approximately in the middle of the second metacarpal bone on the radial side
    2. Ll 11 (large intestine point 11): at the end of the lateral cubital crease, halfway between the biceps tendon and

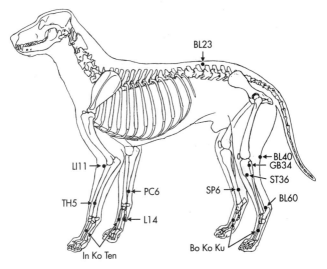

Fig. 8-4
Location of various acupuncture points to induce analgesia in dogs.

the lateral epicondyle of the humerus, with the elbow flexed

3. PC 6 (pericard point 6): at two ribs-width above the transverse crease of the carpus between the tendons of the flexor digitorum superficialis and flexor carpi radialis

4. TH 5 (tripple Heater point 5): at two ribs-width above the carpus, on the cranial aspect of the interosseous space between the radius and ulna

5. In Ko Ten: between metacarpal bones 2 and 3

6. BL 23 (bladder point 23): at one- to two ribs-width lateral to the caudal border of the spinous process of the second lumbar vertebra

7. ST 36 (stomach point 36): at one finger-width from the anterior crest of the tibia, in the belly of the medial tibialis cranialis

8. GB 34 (gallbladder point 34): in the depression anterior and distal to the head of the fibula

9. BL 40 (bladder point 40): in the center of the popliteal crease
10. SP 6 (spleen point 6): at three ribs-width directly above the tip of the medial malleolus, on the posterior border of the tibia
11. BL 60 (bladder point 60): in the depression, between the lateral malleolus and tendon calcaneus, level with the tip of the lateral malleolus
12. Bo Ko Ku: between metatarsal bones 2 and 3

C. The needle penetrates completely from TH 5 to PC 6 between the radius and ulna of both limbs

D. The needle may penetrate completely through the limb at ST 36 and SP 6 of both hind limbs

IV. Acupuncture point selection in horses (Fig. 8-5, *A, B*) and cattle (Fig. 8-6)

A. For abdominal surgery: LU 1 (lung point 1) + TH 8 (tripple heater point 8)

1. Technique: one needle is inserted in LU 1 (caudal to the shoulder in the second intercostal space) for a depth of 3 to 5 cm (positive pole). A second needle is inserted at TH 8 (approximately one hand-width ventral to the elbow joint, on the lateral side) and is advanced ventromedially caudal to the radius/ulna to reach PC 4.5, subcutaneously dorsal to the "chestnut" (negative pole). A third needle is inserted at small intestine point 10 (SI 10, approximately on the caudal border of the deltoids and between the long and lateral heads of the triceps brachii). A fourth needle is inserted in the center depression between the bulbs of the heel on the forelimb

B. For abdominal, vaginal, and hind limb surgery: Bai Hui (main point) + Wei Gan (secondary point) + San Tai (tertiary point) + Tian Ping (minor point) + added points on or near the spinal nerves supplying the surgical site

1. Technique: one needle is inserted in acupuncture point Bai Hui (GV 3a point) at the dorsal midline of the lumbosacral space, 3 to 5 cm deep. A second needle is inserted in Wei Gan (at the dorsal midline of the second coccygeal intervertebral space), 1 to 1.5 cm deep. A third needle is inserted in San Tai (at the dorsal midline

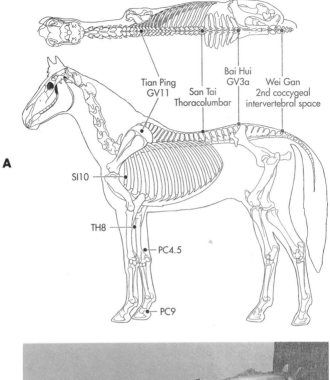

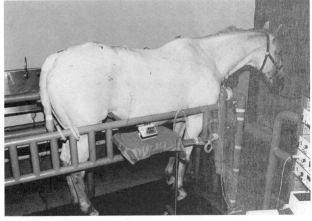

Fig. 8-5
A, Location of various acupuncture points to induce analgesia in horses. **B,** Percutaneous electrical nerve stimulation of various acupuncture points in a 560-kg Thoroughbred mare, which is well sedated (detomidine 5 mg IM) and physically restrained.

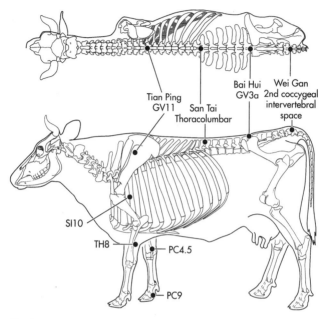

Fig. 8-6
Location of various acupuncture points to induce analgesia in cattle.

of the thoracolumbar intervertebral space), 2 to 4 cm deep. A fourth needle is inserted at Tian Ping (at the dorsal midline of the fourth or fifth thoracic intervertebral space, GV 11 point) and advanced cranioventrally 6 to 8 cm

V. Acupuncture point selection in pigs
   A. The Akita Veterinary Acupuncture Research Unit in Japan tested many point combinations in pigs, including LU 1 and TH 8 penetrating to PC 4.5
   B. The most effective points for producing hypalgesia are located in the midline of the thoracolumbar space (point Tian Ping) and lumbosacral spaces (Bai Hui) penetrating almost to the dura mater spinalis

NEEDLE PLACEMENT

I. The needles are inserted deeply into the acupuncture points
   A. The points are palpated at precise anatomical landmarks
   B. Point finders (Fig. 8-1 and Fig. 8-2) are helpful in localizing acupuncture points
II. The needles are taped or sutured in position to prevent dislodgment

ELECTROACUPUNCTURE (EA) STIMULATION

I. Voltage, current, frequency
   A. The power controls of the stimulator are set at zero
   B. The pairs of needles are attached to each circuit of the electrostimulator with alligator clips
   C. The power switch is turned on and the electrical stimulation frequency is set at 2 to 15 Hz
   D. The output voltage is increased slowly until the needles begin to twitch in time with the frequency of the stimulator at 2 to 15 Hz
   E. At higher frequencies (more than 15 Hz), the muscle goes into local spasm, and the needle vibration is not obvious
   F. The output voltage from each control is first increased to maximum tolerance of anesthesia mode, dense-disperse wave form
   G. The output is then reduced to a level the animal can tolerate without obvious discomfort or pain (e.g., restlessness, struggling, vocalization)
II. Onset and duration of hypalgesia
   A. Induction time for hypalgesia ranges from 10 to 40 minutes; 20 minutes is the duration most commonly reported
   B. The surgery site is tested for analgesia by grasping the skin with toothed forceps or clamps or pricking the skin with needles or pins every 5 minutes after the onset of electrical stimulation
   C. The EA stimulation is continued during the entire surgery
   D. Inadequate or excessive EA stimulus produces little or no analgesia

ADVANTAGES OF EAA

I. EAA can induce hypalgesia sufficient for surgery
   A. It can be used in "balanced anesthesia" to greatly reduce the dose of sedatives/analgesic and anesthetic drugs
   B. It is advantageous in Cesarean sections because it has no depressive effects on the fetus
   C. It is suitable for animals that are in shock, debilitated, or toxic
II. EAA is suitable for prolonged surgery (up to 10 hours)
   A. Autonomic functions remain stable
III. When compared to general anesthesia:
   A. The technique is relatively simple and inexpensive
   B. There is less hemorrhage
   C. Postoperative recovery of appetite as well as gastrointestinal and bladder function are faster
   D. Postoperative healing is faster; attributable to no chemical interference with wound healing
   E. Postoperative infection is less
   F. Postoperative pain is reduced

DISADVANTAGES OF EAA

I. An induction period of 10 to 40 minutes (average is 20 minutes) is necessary
II. To facilitate surgery, sedatives and anesthetics are needed in 50% to 95% of cases
III. Intrathoracic surgery cannot be performed
IV. Physical restraint is necessary
   A. The amount of restraint needed depends on the skill of the surgeon and tolerance of the patient
V. Muscle relaxation may be inadequate
   A. Poor relaxation of abdominal muscles can cause "ballooning" of viscera
VI. All sensory inputs except pain are present
   A. Manipulation of viscera and organs or traction of mesentery can induce nausea, vomiting, and shock
VII. Certain body regions are more sensitive to pain than others
   A. The skin, serosa (peritoneum, pleura), periosteum, and nerves are very sensitive

    B. Incision of such organs requires the frequency and output voltage to be increased to counteract the pain

    C. The success rate for intestinal surgery is higher than for limb surgery

VIII. Pain thresholds vary among species

    A. Cattle and sheep are the most tolerant, followed by dogs, pigs, and horses

  IX. Temperaments vary among species

    A. Nervous animals may be tolerant but are easily frightened and difficult to restrain, even with good analgesia

MECHANISMS OF ACUPUNCTURE ANALGESIA

  I. The mechanisms of acupuncture analgesia have been reviewed in the medical literature.*

  II. Modern theories attribute the effects of EAA to:

    A. Inhibition of ascending (sensory) pain signals at the peripheral, spinal ("pain inhibition gates"), and central level

    B. Activation of descending brain-based pain inhibition mechanism, especially the midbrain and hypothalamus

 III. Sensory nervous system components involved in pain sensation include A-delta and C fibers

    A. Acupuncture points are cutaneous areas with high concentrations of nerves (particularly A-delta fibers), mast cells, capillaries, and venules and lower electrical resistance than surrounding areas

    B. Acupuncture stimuli are transmitted to the spinal cord by peripheral nerves

    C. A-delta fibers are 10 times thicker, transmit impulses 10 times faster, have a lower threshold, and are associated with milder pain sensation than C fibers

    D. The "gate" theory suggests that A-delta fibers carry non-painful sensations rapidly to the spinal cord where inhibitory neurons are stimulated and prevent slower pain impulses from reaching higher pain centers of conscious perception

---

*Kho H-G, Robertson EN: The mechanisms of acupuncture analgesia: review and update, *Am J Acupunct* 25 (4):261-281, 1997.

   IV. Neurotransmitters involved in acupuncture therapy and pain inhibition include:
      A. Endorphins (beta-endorphin, enkephalins, dynorphin)
      B. Serotonin
      C. Norepinephrine
      D. Acetylcholine
   V. Other neurotransmitters that potentiate acupuncture analgesia include:
      A. Parasympathomimetics
      B. Substance P
      C. Histamine
      D. Cyclic guanosine monophosphate (cGMP)
   VI. Frequency of stimulation affects fibers and neurotransmitters involved in pain perception response
      A. <5 Hz: A-delta fibers and enkephalin
      B. >100 Hz: C fibers and dynorphin
      C. >200 Hz: analgesia via serotonin and norepinephrine
   VII. Duration of stimulation may change the mechanism of analgesia from opiate to nonopiate
      A. Segmental acupuncture analgesia usually occurs rapidly
      B. Generalized opiate effects take 20 to 40 minutes
   VIII. Intensity of stimulation (voltage) traditionally is increased until muscle fasciculation is seen at 1 to 5 Hz. This produces the following conditions:
      A. General analgesia with prolonged induction
      B. Prolonged analgesia after cessation of stimulation
      C. Endorphin-mediated analgesia
      D. Analgesia that is reversible by naloxone
   IX. High frequency/low intensity stimulation results in local segmental analgesia, which is irreversible by naloxone

ACUPUNCTURE SUPPLIES

M.E.D. Servi-Systems Canada Ltd.
8 Sweetnam Drive
Stittsville, Ontario
Canada K2S 1G2
1 (613) 836-3004
1-800-267-6868 (Canada and United States)
www.medserv.ca

OMS Medical Supplies
1950 Washington Street
Braintree, MA 02184
1-800-323-1839 (orders)
(781) 331-3370 (information)
www.osmsmedical.com

LHASA Medical, Inc.
539 Accord Station
Accord, MA 02018-0539
1-800-722-8775 (orders)
(781) 335-6484 (information)
(781) 335-6296 (fax)
www.lhasamedical.com

PROFESSIONAL ORGANIZATIONS

The International Veterinary Acupuncture Society (IVAS)
PO Box 1478
Longmont, CO 80502
(303) 682-1167
(303) 682-1168 (fax)
lvasoffice@aol.com (e-mail)

American Academy of Veterinary Acupuncture (AAVA)
PO Box 419
Hygiene, CO 80533-0419
(303) 722-6726
(303) 772-6726 (fax)
aavaoffice@aol.com (e-mail)

CHAPTER NINE

Specific Intravenous Anesthetic Drugs

"To sleep: perchance to dream"
WILLIAM SHAKESPEARE

OVERVIEW

Intravenous and intramuscular anesthetic drugs can be used to induce chemical restraint and general anesthesia. Proper use of preanesthetic medication (tranquilizers, sedatives, analgesics) is imperative if anesthetic drugs are to produce the desired effect and if side effects are to be avoided. Injectable anesthetic drugs are often more convenient and economical than inhalation anesthetic drugs. Their principal disadvantage is that once administered, they cannot be controlled and are not immediately eliminated. Several injectable drugs (thiopental, methohexital, propofol, etomidate) have a very short duration of action.

GENERAL CONSIDERATIONS

I. Increasing degrees of central nervous system (CNS) depression can be produced, from drowsiness and mild sedation to anesthesia and coma

II. Factors that determine rate of onset and amount of depression
   A. Type of anesthetic drug used
   B. Dose
   C. Rate of drug administration when administered intravenously (IV)
   D. Route of administration (intravenous, intramuscular [IM], intraperitoneal [IP])

     E. Animal's level of consciousness (excited versus depressed) when the drug is administered

     F. Acid-base and electrolyte balance; acidosis enhances barbiturate anesthesia

     G. Animal's cardiac output

     H. Drug tolerance (age, breed)

     I. Interactions with other drugs

III. Most injectable anesthetic drugs produce unconsciousness by depressing the cerebral cortex

     A. Many are used to control convulsions (barbiturates; propofol)

     B. Barbiturates increase the threshold of spinal reflexes and can be used clinically for the treatment of strychnine poisoning

IV. Routes of administration

     A. Most injectable drugs are administered intravenously; ketamine and tiletamine-zolazepam can be administered intramuscularly

     B. Sodium salts of barbiturates can be injected in a solution of up to 10%, guaifenesin in a solution of up to 10%, and chloral hydrate in a solution of up to 7%

     C. Because of the extreme alkalinity of barbiturate solutions, subcutaneous injection results in necrosis and sloughing; thiobarbiturates are not injected intramuscularly or subcutaneously

V. Dose should be calculated on the basis of lean body mass (body weight minus fat)

BARBITURATE ANESTHESIA

   I. Barbiturates are categorized according to their duration of action

     A. Long: 8 to 12 hours

     B. Intermediate: 2 to 6 hours

     C. Short: 45 to 90 minutes

     D. Ultrashort: 5 to 15 minutes

II. Official names

DRUG	APPROPRIATE DURATION OF ACTION
Phenobarbital sodium	Long
Pentobarbital sodium	Short (Table 9-1)
Thiopental sodium	Ultrashort
Methohexital	Ultrashort

III. General anesthetic actions of barbiturates
   A. Effects on the CNS
   1. CNS depression ranging from drowsiness and mild sedation to coma results from interaction with the CNS inhibitor/gamma aminobutyric acid A ($GABA_A$) receptors
   2. Response to barbiturate anesthesia
      a. Pentobarbital sodium and ultrashort-acting barbiturates decrease cerebral blood flow (CBF), cerebral metabolic rate of oxygen ($CMRO_2$), and neuronal activity of the brain (e.g., dogs); the $CBF/CMRO_2$ ratio is unchanged or increased; there are minimal changes in CSF pressure if ventilation is normal
      b. Anesthetic concentrations of barbiturates depress arterial blood pressure (BP) and intracranial pressure and increase cerebral perfusion pressure
      c. Barbiturates are used to produce a general anesthesia (short-acting) or to induce a patient to surgical anesthesia (ultrashort-acting)
      d. Barbiturates are universally poor analgesics at subhypnotic dosages
   B. Organ system effects and responses
   1. Effects on the respiratory system
      a. Barbiturates are respiratory depressants
         (1) They depress respiratory centers in the medulla and the areas of the brain responsible for the characteristic rhythmic pattern of respiratory movement (apneustic and pneumotaxic centers)
         (2) The degree of respiratory depression is related to the dose and rate of drug administration
      b. Coughing, sneezing, hiccoughing, and laryngospasm occur frequently; these effects are caused by exces-

TABLE 9-1

INTRAVENOUS (MG/LB) DRUGS COMMONLY USED TO PRODUCE ANESTHESIA OF SHORT DURATION

	AGENT	HORSE	DOG	CAT	PIG	COW	GOAT
1	Thiopental	3-5	4-6	4-6	4-6	2-5	2-5
2	Etomidate		0.5-2	0.5-2	0.5-2		
3	Propofol	4-6	2-6	2-6	2-6		
4	Guaifenesin	30-60	20-40		20-40	30-60	30-60
5	Chloral hydrate		—	—	6-9 g/100 lb	6-10 g/100 lb	6-10 g/100 lb
6	Chloral hydrate (7% solution)	10 ml/100 lb*	—	—	20-30 ml/100 lb	20-30 ml/100 lb	20-30 ml/100 lb
7	Chloropent	10 ml/100 lb	—	—	—	10 ml/100 lb	10 ml/100 lb
	Thiopental	2-4	—	—	—	2-4	2-4
8	Ketamine		—	1-3	1-3		1-3
9	Telazol		2-5	1-5	2-5	2-5	1-5
10	Guaifenesin	20-40	15-40	—	15-40	20-40	15-40
	Thiopental	2-4	2-4	—	2-4	2-4	—

TABLE 9-1

INTRAVENOUS (MG/LB) DRUGS COMMONLY USED TO PRODUCE ANESTHESIA OF SHORT DURATION—cont'd

	AGENT	HORSE	DOG	CAT	PIG	COW	GOAT
11	Guaifenesin	20-40	15-40	—	—	20-40	20-40
	Ketamine	0.5-0.7	0.5	—	—	0.3-0.5	0.3-0.5
12	Acepromazine	—	0.1	0.2	0.2	—	—
	Ketamine	—	5.0	1-3	1-3	—	—
13	Xylazine†	0.5	0.3	0.3	—	0.04	0.02
	Ketamine	0.5-1	3	1-3	—	1-3	1-3
14	Xylazine	0.5	0.2	0.3	0.3	0.05	0.04
	Telazol	0.5-1	3	1-3	1-3	1-3	1-3
15	Diazepam‡		0.15	0.2	0.1	0.1	
	Ketamine		2-3	2-3	2-3	2-3	
16	Xylazine, guaifenesin, ketamine	(500 ml 5% guaifenesin + 500 mg ketamine + 25 mg xylazine [ruminants]; 500 ml 5% guaifenesin + 500 mg ketamine + 500 mg xylazine [horses]); approximately 3-5 ml/min to effect					

*Sedative dose.
†Detomidine, 1-5 µg/lb intravenously, can be used in xylazine drug combinations.
‡Midazolam, 0.1-0.3 mg/lb intravenously, can be used in diazepam drug combinations.

sive salivary secretion and are minimized by pre-anesthetic medication (atropine, glycopyrrolate)

  (1) Laryngospasm is a common complication of barbiturate anesthesia in dogs and cats

  (2) A short period of apnea frequently occurs after IV bolus administration of barbiturates

c. When respiratory arrest occurs, attention should be directed toward establishing an airway and ventilating the patient; respiratory stimulants (doxapram) may be necessary if the animal does not begin to ventilate spontaneously

2. Effects on the cardiovascular system

  a. Barbiturates produce significant cardiovascular depression when administered rapidly as a bolus or in extremely large doses

  b. Cardiac arrhythmias may occur

    (1) Thiobarbiturates sensitize the heart to epinephrine and induce autonomic imbalance; arrhythmias, particularly ventricular extrasystoles and ventricular bigeminy, can occur after thiopental administration

    (2) Thiobarbiturates increase both parasympathetic and sympathetic tone; this may lead to atrial or ventricular arrhythmias; sinus bradycardia; or first-, second-, or third-degree heart block and cardiac arrest

  c. Barbiturates may cause a transient drop in BP; if the patient is already in a state of surgical anesthesia, small doses of a barbiturate may cause dramatic decreases in cardiac contractility and arterial BP

    (1) Barbiturates should be administered slowly and in reduced dosages to sick, debilitated, or depressed animals

    (2) Concentrations greater than 2.5% are toxic to tissues and may injure the capillary musculature, causing capillary dilation and thrombophlebitis

    (3) Induction doses of thiobarbiturates may prompt an initial increase in BP caused by tachycardia and an increase in peripheral vascular resistance caused by increases in sympathetic tone

3. Actions on the gastrointestinal (GI) tract
    a. Depress intestinal motility; thiobarbiturates may depress GI tract motility initially, then increase both tone and motility
    b. Diarrhea and intestinal stasis are generally not observed at recommended doses
4. Kidney and liver
    a. No direct effect on the kidney has been observed, unless a large dose is given, in which case a decrease in renal blood flow occurs; systemic hypotension may cause a cessation in urine production
    b. Single administrations at therapeutic doses have no effect on liver function; large doses of barbiturates may cause injury in patients with liver damage
5. Effects on the uterus and fetus
    a. The short-acting barbiturate, pentobarbital, is contraindicated in near-term animals
    b. Barbiturates readily diffuse across the placenta into the fetal circulation; thiopental reaches mixed fetal cord blood within 45 seconds
    c. Doses of barbiturates that do not produce anesthesia in the mother can completely inhibit fetal respiratory movements

IV. Absorption, elimination, and excretion
A. Absorption
    1. IV administration
        a. Adequate provisions should be available to support respiration and circulation
        b. Short-acting barbiturates (pentobarbital) require approximately 5 to 10 minutes to produce maximal CNS effect
        c. Ultrashort-acting barbiturates (thiopental, methohexital) reach maximal effect within 30 seconds of administration
    2. Barbiturates are absorbed from the GI tract after oral administration
B. Elimination
    1. Redistribution: ultrashort-acting barbiturates (thiopental, methohexital) rely on redistribution to lean body tissues (muscle) for their duration of action (Fig. 9-1)

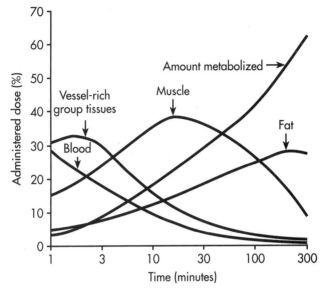

Fig. 9-1
Distribution of thiopental to various tissues. Note that the accumulation of drug in the muscle tissue corresponds to the approximate duration of thiopental anesthesia.

a. Emergence from sleep depends on a shift of the drug from the brain to lean body tissues
b. Concentrations in muscle and skin peak in about 15 to 30 minutes after thiobarbiturate injection
c. Concentrations in fat peak in several hours
d. Repeated doses have a cumulative effect
e. Extremely thin, heavily muscled animals (e.g., greyhounds, whippets) demonstrate prolonged recoveries (3 to 5 hours) from thiopental anesthesia
f. Obesity delays drug elimination because of the high lipid solubility of barbiturates
g. "Acute tolerance" (minimal effect with a usual dose) is rarely observed following the administration of thiobarbiturates in horses and dogs; the mechanism

is unknown but is probably related to the patient's level of excitement and the distribution of cardiac output; if this occurs, alternative anesthetic techniques should be used

2. Barbiturates are eliminated by oxidative activity of hepatic enzymes and by renal excretion
3. The amount of active (nonionized, nonprotein-bound) drug is increased by acidosis; alkalinazation of the urine hastens drug elimination

C. Excretion
   1. Hepatic metabolism
      a. Barbiturates are metabolized by both hepatic and extrahepatic mechanisms; metabolites are eliminated by the kidneys and appear in the urine
      b. Liver disease may prolong the duration of drug action; avoid using short-acting barbiturates in the presence of liver disease
      c. Hypothermia and depressed cardiovascular function may prolong hepatic metabolism of barbiturates

V. Dosage and administration of specific barbiturate drugs
   A. Pentobarbital sodium (Nembutal)
      1. IV anesthetic dose varies from 3 to 13 mg/lb of body weight, depending on type and amount of preanesthetic medication; when administered as the only source of anesthesia, approximately half the anticipated dose should be injected rapidly; the rest should be administered in small increments until the desired effect is reached
      2. May be used in combination with other anesthetics (inhalants) to produce surgical anesthesia
      3. Preanesthetic drugs decrease the dose of barbiturates required to produce anesthesia
      4. Atropine sulfate or glycopyrrolate decrease salivary secretions, the potential for laryngospasm, and vagal activity
      5. The anesthetic duration can be prolonged by administration of 50% glucose intravenously; this is known as the *glucose effect*
      6. Complete recovery occurs in 8 to 24 hours
      7. The minimum lethal dose in dogs is 23 mg/lb IV

      8. Overdose is treated by cardiopulmonary support, respiratory stimulants, fluid therapy, alkalinizing solutions (Na^+ $HCO3^-$), and diuresis

      9. Oral administration is neither safe nor practical for dogs or cats

B. Thiopental sodium (Pentothal)

    1. Administer intravenously in small increments to produce anesthesia (3 to 8 mg/lb)

    2. Use in 2% to 10% solutions

      a. Solution should be discarded after being stored for 3 days at room temperature; precipitated solutions should not be used

      b. More concentrated solutions cause severe tissue damage (pH $\approx$ 13) if accidentally administered subcutaneously

      c. Subcutaneous injection causes necrosis of tissue; tissue necrosis may be minimized by infiltrating the area with saline; pain can be minimized by injecting 2% lidocaine

    3. Dose for induction and intubation is 4 to 6 mg/lb of body weight; solutions of up to 10% are used in horses; repeated doses are cumulative, resulting in prolonged recovery from anesthesia

    4. Dose is based on lean body weight (body weight minus fat)

    5. Anesthesia usually occurs in 20 to 60 seconds

    6. Ventricular arrhythmias (ventricular bigeminy) may occur following induction of anesthesia

    7. Apnea is more common following rapid IV injections; ventilation should be supported early in anesthesia

    8. Recovery occurs in 10 to 30 minutes, but the animal may remain depressed for many hours depending on the dose; repeated doses are cumulative

    9. Overdose is best treated with O_2, controlled ventilation, fluids, alkalinizing solutions, and diuretics

C. Methohexital (Brevane)

    1. Similar to thiopental, except it is not cumulative (it is rapidly metabolized)

    2. 3 to 7 mg/lb provides light anesthesia in small animals

3. Recommended in sight hounds (e.g., greyhounds, whippets, borzois) because of its short duration effect
4. Duration is 5 to 10 minutes
5. Respiratory depression and apnea are common
6. Induction and recovery may be accompanied by pronounced involuntary excitement and convulsions (delirium); CNS effects can be prevented by diazepam (0.1 mg/lb)
7. Not routinely used in large animals

NONBARBITURATE ANESTHETIC DRUGS

I. Etomidate (Amidate)
   A. A rapid-acting, ultrashort, nonbarbiturate, noncumulative IV anesthetic
   B. General anesthetic actions
      1. Produces hypnosis (sleep), minimal analgesia at subhypnotic doses; as with barbiturates, interacts with CNS $GABA_A$ receptors
      2. Produces depression of the reticular formation of the brain stem
      3. Enhances monosynaptic reflex activity, which may result in myoclonal activity
      4. Decreases CBF and $CMRO_2$; increases ratio of CBF to $CMRO_2$
   C. Organ system effects
      1. Respiratory system
         a. Brief periods of apnea may occur immediately after IV injection
         b. Tidal volume and respiratory rate are minimally affected during anesthetic maintenance; respiratory rate may increase
      2. Cardiovascular system
         a. Produces little change in heart rate, arterial BP, and cardiac output when administered at induction dosages
         b. Cardiac contractility is mildly depressed
         c. Does not sensitize the myocardium to catecholamine-induced cardiac arrhythmias
         d. Does not produce histamine release

    3. GI system
       a. Nausea and vomiting are occasionally observed during induction and following anesthesia; these effects can be inhibited by proper preanesthetic medication
       b. GI motility is minimally affected
    4. Endocrine system
       a. An antiglucocorticoid and mineralocorticoid effect is produced; adrenocorticotropic hormone stimulation tests and glucose tolerance tests may be invalid
       b. Adrenocorticoid function is suppressed for 2 to 3 hours in dogs after a single IV administration of etomidate
    5. Crosses the placenta, but effects are minimal because of the rapid clearance

D. Fate and elimination
    1. Rapidly distributed to the brain, heart, spleen, lungs, liver, and intestines
    2. Anesthetic duration of action depends on drug redistribution and capacity; limited ester hydrolysis by the liver
    3. Noncumulative

E. Other
    1. Produces good muscle relaxation during anesthesia; involuntary muscle movements and myoclonic reactions occur during induction and recovery
    2. Does not trigger malignant hyperthermia in susceptible pigs but predisposes them to a more rapid onset of malignant hyperthermia if triggered by other drugs
    3. Pain may occur during IV injection
    4. Decreases intraocular pressure

F. Clinical uses
    1. Induction agent for general anesthesia
    2. Short-term (5 to 10 minutes) anesthesia in dogs and cats; produces excessive muscle rigidity and seizures in horses and cattle

G. Dosages
    1. 0.25 to 1.5 mg/lb IV in dogs and cats
    2. The best results are obtained after sedating the animal with diazepam, xylazine, or acepromazine

II. Propofol

A. A rapid-acting, ultrashort, nonbarbiturate, and relatively noncumulative IV anesthetic

B. General anesthetic actions
1. Produces sedation-hypnosis similar to that induced by thiopental and methohexital. Like barbiturates interact with CNS $GABA_A$ receptors
2. Produces dose-dependent depression of the cerebral cortex and CNS polysynaptic reflexes; may enhance the effects of nondepolarizing neuromuscular blocking drugs
3. Produces minimal analgesia at subhypnotic doses
4. Anesthetic doses decrease CBF and $CMRO_2$; the $CBF/CMRO_2$ ratio is unchanged or minimally increased
5. Possesses anticonvulsant properties similar to barbiturates

C. Chemistry
1. An alkylphenol poorly soluble in water
2. Solubilized in a lecithin-containing emulsion (10% soybean oil and 1.2% egg lecithin) called *Intralipid*

D. Organ system effects
1. Respiratory system
   a. Similar to thiopental
   b. Dose-dependent respiratory depression and initial periods of apnea
2. Cardiovascular system
   a. Produces little change in heart rate
   b. Dose-dependent decreases in arterial BP caused by decreases in cardiac output and systemic vascular resistance
   c. Minimal but dose-dependent negative inotropic effect at anesthetic doses
3. Other organ systems: effects of propofol on the liver, kidney, and GI system are secondary to changes in arterial BP and organ blood flow
4. Crosses the placenta and can induce fetal depression, which is dose dependent

E. Fate and elimination
1. Termination of anesthetic effects and short duration of action are due to redistribution from well-perfused (vessel-rich) tissues such as the brain to muscle and fat
2. Relatively rapid biotransformation by the liver compared to thiobarbiturates

       3. Rapid clearing from the body by hepatic and extrahepatic metabolism compared to thiobarbiturates

       4. Noncumulative

  F. Other

       1. Produces good to excellent muscle relaxation

       2. May elicit pain on induction to anesthesia

       3. Rapid recovery; little or no "hangover" effect

  G. Clinical uses

       1. From induction to general anesthesia

       2. Maintenance of general anesthesia when combined with opioid analgesics or other sedative-analgesic drugs

  H. Dosages

       1. 1 to 3 mg/lb intravenously in dogs and cats for induction

       2. 0.2 to 0.4 mg/lb/min IV infusion in dogs and cats for anesthetic maintenance; usually used with diazepam and oxymorphone or fentanyl for added muscle relaxation and analgesia; medetomidine is an excellent adjunct to propofol anesthesia

III. Chloral hydrate

  A. Chloral hydrate is no longer sold as an anesthetic for veterinary use but is occasionally purchased as crystals and solubilized in water for IV administration as a sedative, hypnotic, or for euthanasia in horses; administered IV or orally to cattle

  B. General anesthetic actions

       1. Drug is sedative-hypnotic, depressing the cerebral cortex, resulting in hyporeflexia

       2. CNS depression believed to result from trichloroethanol; CBF is decreased or unchanged; $CMRO_2$ is decreased

       3. Subanesthetic doses depress motor and sensory nerves and produce mild sedation

       4. Anesthetic doses produce deep sleep lasting for several hours; recovery is prolonged (6 to 24 hours)

       5. Drug is a poor analgesic at subhypnotic doses; excitement or delirium are precipitated by painful stimulation

  C. Chemistry

       1. Physical properties: colorless, translucent crystals that volatilize when exposed to air

    2. Chemical properties
      a. Readily soluble in both water and oil
      b. Largely reduced to trichloroethanol in the body
      c. Bitter, caustic taste; irritating to the skin and mucous membranes

D. Organ system effects
    1. Respiratory system
      a. Sedative doses minimally depress both respiratory rate and tidal volume
      b. Anesthetic doses markedly affect ventilation by depression of the respiratory centers; death is usually caused by progressive respiratory center depression
    2. Cardiovascular system
      a. Anesthetic doses produce depression of the myocardium (decreased contractility)
      b. Chloral hydrate potentiates vagal (parasympathetic) activity, causing bradycardia, P-R interval prolongation, and sinus arrest or atrioventricular block
      c. Supraventricular arrhythmias and a transient period of atrial fibrillation have been observed after chloral hydrate anesthesia in horses
    3. GI system
      a. GI secretions and motility are increased because of the parasympathomimetic effect; diarrhea may occur following anesthesia
      b. Nausea and vomiting, salivation, and defecation may occur when chloral hydrate is given orally
    4. Liver and kidney: effects on these systems appear to be secondary to parasympathetic and cardiovascular effects
    5. Uterus and fetus: chloral hydrate readily crosses the placenta

E. Absorption, fate, and excretion
    1. May be administered orally, rectally, intravenously, or intraperitoneally; very irritating if given perivascularly, intramuscularly, or intraperitoneally
    2. A small amount is excreted unchanged in the urine; the majority is reduced to trichloroethanol, a less potent hypnotic, and then conjugated with glucuronic acid, after which it is excreted in the urine

        3. Recovery is often prolonged and characterized by a "hangover" effect

  F. Clinical uses

      1. Chloral hydrate is frequently used as a sedative and adjunct to surgical anesthesia in horses and cattle; the dosage for anesthesia is variable (100 to 300 mg/lb)

      2. Casting harnesses or hobbles are generally necessary

      3. Drug is generally used in combination with pentobarbital and magnesium sulfate

      4. Pharmaceutical companies no longer supply chloral hydrate for veterinary use, but it can be obtained from chemical companies (Sigma, Aldrich)

  G. Dosage

      1. Sedation: 1 to 3 g/100 lb IV

      2. Anesthesia: 6 to 10 g/100 lb IV

IV. Guaifenesin (glyceryl guaiacolate)

  A. Chemistry

      1. Physical properties: a white, finely granular powder that is soluble in water

      2. Chemical properties

         a. A decongestant and antitussive also noted for its centrally acting muscle relaxant properties

         b. Very similar to mephenesin chemically; mephenesin is an aromatic glycerol ether

  B. General anesthetic actions

      1. Blocks impulse transmission at the internuncial neurons of the spinal cord and brain stem; guaifenesin is a centrally acting muscle relaxant

      2. Produces relaxation of skeletal muscles but produces minimal effects on the function of the diaphragm at relaxant dosages

      3. Relaxes laryngeal and pharyngeal muscles, thus potentiating intubation of the trachea

      4. Compatible with preanesthetic and anesthetic agents

      5. Produces excitement-free induction and recovery from anesthesia

      6. In excessive doses, produces paradoxic increases in muscle rigidity

C. Organ system effects
   1. Respiratory system
      a. Little, if any, effect at relaxant dosages
      b. Ventilatory rate may increase initially; tidal volume decreases
      c. Excessive doses produce an apneustic pattern of breathing
   2. Cardiovascular system
      a. Initial mild decrease in BP, which returns to normal
      b. Myocardial contractile force and cardiac rate are relatively unchanged
   3. GI system: increases GI motility
   4. Uterus and fetus: guaifenesin crosses the placental barrier but has minimal effects on the fetus
D. Absorption, fate, and excretion: excreted in the urine after conjugation in the liver to a glucuronide
E. Clinical uses
   1. Used for restraint and muscle relaxation in horses and cattle
   2. Used for short anesthetic procedures of up to 30 to 60 minutes
   3. Used as a 5%, 10%, or 15% solution; high concentrations (>6%) may cause hemolysis and hemoglobinuria in cattle; solutions greater than 15% cause hives and hemolysis
   4. Often made by mixing 50 g of guaifenesin with 50 g of dextrose and 1 L warm sterile water (5% solution)
   5. Compatible with other IV and inhalation anesthetic drugs
F. Dosage
   1. The dose varies from 15 to 50 mg/lb
   2. Guaifenesin may be administered to effect with the following agents:
      a. 2 g thiopental
      b. 2.5 g pentobarbital
      c. 500 mg ketamine; 500 ml of 5% guaifenesin; 20 to 50 mg xylazine for ruminants and up to 500 mg xylazine for horses has been administered to effect to produce total IV anesthesia (TIVA)

    3. The margin of safety (guaifenesin alone) is three times the therapeutic dose (approximately 150 mg/lb IV)
    4. Excessive doses cause muscle rigidity and an apneustic pattern of breathing

DISSOCIOGENIC ANESTHETIC DRUGS

Dissociative anesthetics include the arylcyclohexylamines: ketamine, tiletamine, and phencyclidine

  I. Anesthesia is characterized by profound amnesia, analgesia, and catalepsy

    A. Oral, ocular, and swallowing reflexes remain intact, and muscle tone generally increases

    B. Large doses can produce convulsions, which can be controlled with small doses of pentobarbital, thiopental, propofol, or diazepam

  II. Psychosomatic effects such as hallucinations, confusion, agitation, and fear have occurred in humans and seem to occur in animals when large doses are administered

 III. Muscle rigidity is minimized by the prior administration of tranquilizers, sedatives, or benzodiazepines (diazepam, midazolam)

  IV. Effects are partially reversed by adrenergic and cholinergic blockade

  V. Specific drugs

    A. Ketamine HCl is the most commonly used dissociative anesthetic in veterinary practice. Telazol (tiletamine-zolazepam drug combination) is used as an alternative and in aggressive animals

      1. Used for restraint, anesthetic induction, and minor surgical procedures

      2. Palpebral, conjunctival, corneal, and swallowing reflexes persist; nystagmus is common

    B. Telazol, a 1:1 drug combination of zolazepam (a benzodiazepine) and tiletamine, is a dissociogenic drug combination for use in all animal species; it is very useful in aggressive dogs or cats and exotic animals

  VI. Salivation and lacrimation are common and may become copious

VII. Tremors, oculogyria, tonic spasticity, and convulsions occur when excessive doses are administered

VIII. Muscle relaxation is poor; for best results, ketamine and other arylcyclohexylamines should be used with drugs that produce muscle relaxation

IX. Animals are hyperresponsive and ataxic during recovery (a result of emergence delirium)

X. Analgesia is selective, with the best results obtained in superficial pain models; visceral pain is not abolished

XI. System effects and responses

    A. Central nervous system

        1. Produces dissociative anesthesia characteristics by poor muscle relaxation and catalepsy; inhibits N-methyl-d-aspartate (NMDA), resulting in analgesia

        2. Ketamine increases CBF and causes no change or an increase in $CMRO_2$; the $CBF/CMRO_2$ ratio increases; arterial BP and intracranial pressure increase; cerebral perfusion pressure decreases

    B. Respiratory system

        1. Apneustic pattern of breathing; respiratory rate may be increased; arterial Po_2 generally falls after IV administration

        2. Possible increases in Pco_2 and decreases in arterial pH caused by the irregular pattern of breathing

    C. Cardiovascular system

        1. Increased heart rate

        2. Increased BP

        3. Decreased cardiac contractility; increase in heart rate and decrease in cardiac contractility, may induce pulmonary edema or acute heart failure in animals with preexisting cardiac disease

        4. Ketamine and other cyclohexamines minimally sensitize the heart to catecholamine-induced arrhythmias

    D. Kidney and liver

        1. Ketamine HCl is metabolized by the liver and excreted by the kidneys

        2. Ketamine should be used with caution in animals with hepatic or renal disease; ketamine can be used in cats with urethral obstruction, provided renal disease is ab-

sent or not severe and the obstruction has been eliminated

XII. Dose

    A. Ketamine

        1. Cat: 2 to 15 mg/lb intramuscularly or subcutaneously; 0.5 to 5 mg/lb intravenously; doses as small as 1 to 3 mg *total* are administered intravenously to sick animals and cats with urethral obstruction

        2. Dog: xylazine 0.1 to 0.3 mg/lb intravenously and ketamine 3 to 5 mg/lb intravenously; diazepam 0.1 mg/lb intravenously and ketamine 2.5 mg/lb intravenously; 1 ml diazepam plus 1 ml ketamine administered 1 ml/20 lbs intravenously

        3. Pigs: 2 to 5 mg/lb ketamine plus 1 mg/lb xylazine administered intramuscularly produces short-term anesthesia in pigs

    B. Telazol

        1. Dogs, cats, cattle, sheep, goats: 2 to 8 mg/lb intramuscularly

        2. Horses: xylazine 0.5 mg/lb followed by 0.25 to 0.5 mg/lb Telazol, intravenously

        3. Pigs: Telazol-ketamine-xylazine (TKX); add 4 ml ketamine and 1 ml of 100 mg/ml xylazine to a 5-ml bottle of Telazol; administer 1 ml per 60 to 80 lbs intramuscularly

CHAPTER TEN

Inhalation Anesthesia

"O sleep! O gentle sleep! Nature's soft nurse, how have I
frightened thee, That thou no more will weigh my eyelids
down and steep my senses in forgetfulness?"

WILLIAM SHAKESPEARE

OVERVIEW

Inhalational anesthetic drugs are used to produce general anesthesia. They are suitable for use in all species, including reptiles, birds, and zoo animals. Their safe use requires knowledge of their pharmacologic effects and physical and chemical properties. Anesthetic doses produce unconsciousness (hypnosis), hyporeflexia, and analgesia. Inhalation anesthetics provide optimal control of anesthesia, rapid induction and recovery from anesthesia, and relatively few adverse side effects. This chapter outlines the basic principles of inhalation anesthesia and its use.

GENERAL CONSIDERATIONS

I. Inhalation anesthetic drugs are vapors or gases that are breathed directly into the respiratory system

II. To produce anesthesia, they must be absorbed from the alveoli into the bloodstream and carried by the blood to the brain

III. Inhalation anesthetics are primarily eliminated by the lungs

IV. Because the uptake and elimination of inhalation anesthetics are relatively rapid, the depth of anesthesia can be controlled effectively, but constant patient monitoring is required

PROPERTIES OF A DESIRABLE GENERAL ANESTHETIC

I. Nonirritating and free from disagreeable odors
II. Easily controlled, producing rapid induction and rapid recovery from anesthesia
III. Produces adequate muscular relaxation
IV. Produces adequate analgesia
V. Should not promote bleeding
VI. Minimal to no side effects
VII. Nontoxic to the patient and to humans
VIII. Not flammable or explosive (stable during storage)
IX. Compatible with other drugs
X. Easy to deliver

FACTORS CONTROLLING THE BRAIN CONCENTRATIONS OF VOLATILE ANESTHETIC (Table 10-1)

I. Factors governing the delivery of a suitable concentration of inhalation anesthetic
  A. Physical and chemical properties of the agent
    1. Vapor pressure of the agent governs the volatility of inhalation anesthesia
    2. Boiling points (other than nitrous oxide and desflurane) are higher than room temperature (70° F or 27° C)
  B. Anesthetic system
    1. The concentration of anesthetic delivered to the patient is primarily determined by the type of anesthetic circuit, fresh gas flow rate, type of vaporizer, and vaporizer temperature
    2. Frequent inspection and maintenance of inhalation anesthetic equipment is necessary to prevent malfunctions caused by factors such as leaks and sticky one-way valves
II. Factors responsible for the delivery of inhalation anesthetic to the lungs and alveoli
  A. The partial pressure of inhalation anesthetic in the brain depends on the alveolar partial pressure of anesthetic; the alveolar partial pressure of the anesthetic is the result of the inspired concentration and the alveolar ventilation

TABLE 10-1

BOILING POINTS, VAPOR PRESSURES, AND VAPORIZATION OF INHALATION AGENTS

DRUG	BOILING POINT (°C)	VAPOR PRESSURE AT 20° C (mm Hg)	MAXIMUM CONCENTRATION OF VAPOR DELIVERED BY SATURATION VAPORIZER AT 20° C (%)	USEFUL RANGES OF CONCENTRATION (AGENT USED ALONE)	
				INDUCTION (%)	MAINTENANCE (%)
Volatile anesthetics					
Ether	36	443	58	10-40	3-12
Desflurane	23.5	664	87.4	8-15	5-9
Sevoflurane	59	160	22	4-5	2-3.5
Isoflurane	48	252	33	2-6	1-3
Halothane	50	243	32	1-4*	0.5-2
Enflurane	57	180	24	3-7	1-3
Methoxyflurane	105	24	3	Up to 3	0.25-1
Anesthetic gas					
Nitrous oxide†	−89	39,500 0 (50 atm).			

*Up to 10% may be used in induction of large animals.
†Nitrous oxide is a gas at room temperature.

B. Inspired concentration
 1. Concentration effect: the greater the inspired concentration administered (vaporizer setting), the more rapid the rate of rise of alveolar concentration
 2. Second gas effect
  a. Theoretically suggests that a 50% to 80% inspired concentration of nitrous oxide initially augments the inflow and rate of uptake of the second gas (e.g., halothane, isoflurane) in the inspired mixture; it is not a clinically valid concept
C. Alveolar ventilation
 1. Generally, the greater the ventilation (tidal volume), the more rapid the approach of the alveolar gas concentration to the inspired gas concentration*
 2. Limited by lung volume; the larger the functional residual capacity, the longer it takes to wash in a new inhalant
 3. Factors affecting ventilation
  a. Breathing rate
  b. Tidal volume
  c. Increased dead space (anatomic and physiologic) during anesthesia decreases effective alveolar ventilation; tidal volume (V_T) = dead space volume (V_D) + alveolar ventilation (V_A): $V_T = V_D + V_A$
  d. Effective alveolar ventilation requires a patent airway
III. Factors responsible for uptake of anesthetic from the lungs
 A. Solubility: describes how much of a substance can be dissolved in a gas, liquid, or solid (e.g., fat); the solubility of inhalation anesthetics is usually expressed as a partition coefficient; how an anesthetic is distributed between two phases (e.g., between blood and gas, between tissue and blood); Ostwald's partition coefficient

---

*See Eger EI, editor: *Anesthetic uptake and action,* Baltimore, 1974, Williams & Wilkins.

expresses the solubility of an inhalant anesthetic between blood and gas

AGENT	BLOOD-GAS PARTITION COEFFICIENT (OSTWALD'S COEFFICIENT)
Diethyl ether	15.2
Methoxyflurane	13
Halothane	2.36
Enflurane	1.91
Isoflurane	1.41
Sevoflurane	0.69
Nitrous oxide	0.49
Desflurane	0.42

A gas with a blood-gas partition coefficient of 2 has *one* volume in the alveoli per *two* volumes in the blood at equilibrium

1. Anesthetic blood-gas partition coeffcent and drug potency determine the rapidity of onset of anesthetic effect
2. The greater the blood-gas partition coefficient, the greater the solubility of anesthetic in the blood; therefore the tension of anesthetic in arterial blood rises slowly for drugs that are highly soluble in blood (high blood-gas coefficients); onset of the clinical effect is contingent on the tension of anesthetic developed in the blood; very soluble drugs, such as methoxyflurane, have long induction and recovery periods because large amounts of anesthetic must be taken into the blood before the tension or partial pressure of the anesthetic rises sufficiently to produce anesthesia; clinically, slow induction may be overcome by raising the inspired concentration to values exceeding those necessary to maintain anesthesia
3. The lower the blood-gas partition coefficient, the less soluble the drug is in the blood (only small quantities are carried in the blood; thus both alveolar concentration and tension will rise rapidly) and the more rapidly the tension or partial pressure of the drug increases in the blood; less soluble drugs such as nitrous oxide, isoflurane, and sevoflurane have relatively short induction and short recovery periods

    4. Generally, drugs with high blood-gas partition coefficients exhibit long induction and recovery times; drugs with low blood-gas partition coefficients exhibit short induction and recovery times

B. Cardiac output: blood carries anesthetic drug away from the lungs; the greater the cardiac output, the slower the rate of rise of alveolar concentration and tension in the lung; excited, stressed animals have a slower rate of induction; animals with depressed cardiac output may be induced to anesthesia very rapidly

C. Alveolar-venous anesthetic tension difference: during induction, tissues remove nearly all the anesthetic brought to them because of the high tissue solubility of most inhalant anesthetics; venous blood returning to the lungs contains little anesthetic; as time passes, increasing tissue saturation raises the venous blood concentration; less anesthetic is taken up in the lungs; anesthetic uptake by the lung is a changing but continuous process

D. Shunts
    1. Right-to-left intracardiac or intrapulmonary shunts (e.g., Fallot's tetralogy) delay induction; this effect is more important for poorly soluble agents (nitrous oxide)
    2. Left-to-right shunts may speed the rate of induction, particularly if cardiac output is low

E. Pathologic changes in alveoli: if the alveolar membranes are affected by disease resulting in exudate, transudate, emphysema, or pulmonary fibrosis, diffusion may be impaired, and the uptake of the inhaled anesthetic is thus reduced

IV. Factors governing brain and tissue uptake of anesthetic

A. Same as those determining uptake from the lungs
    1. Solubility (blood versus tissue)
    2. Tissue blood flow
    3. Arterial blood to tissue anesthetic tension difference

B. The uptake by tissue is dependent on anesthetic concentration, blood flow, and tissue capillary density; tissues can be divided into four groups according to blood supply
    1. Vessel-rich group (VRG): 75% of cardiac output (e.g., brain, heart, intestines, liver, kidneys, spleen)
    2. Vessel-moderate group, or muscle group (MG): 15% to 20% of cardiac output (e.g., muscle, skin)

      3. Neutral fat group (FG): 5% of cardiac output (e.g., adipose tissue)

      4. Vessel-poor group (VPG): 1% to 2% of cardiac output (e.g., bone, tendons, cartilage)

C. Tissue-blood partition coefficients vary far less than blood-gas coefficients (except for fat)

      1. Lowest is approximately 1 (nitrous oxide in lung tissue)

      2. Highest is approximately 4 (halothane in muscle tissue)

D. Important considerations

      1. Equilibration of an anesthetic drug in the VRG is complete in 5 to 20 minutes; this is approximately how long it will take for anesthesia to become deep enough to do surgery, providing the anesthetic concentration (vaporizer setting) is appropriate

      2. Equilibration in the MG may take 1½ to 4 hours

      3. Because of a higher blood flow, arterial-tissue partial-pressure difference, and therefore uptake, decrease far more rapidly in VRG than in MG

      4. Solubility of an inhalation drug in VRG and MG may affect recovery time

      5. The fat group occupies 10% to 30% body mass and receives about 5% of the cardiac output; the FG has a higher tissue solubility for inhalation anesthetics than most other tissues and thus has a greater and more prolonged capacity to absorb anesthetic; because of its low blood flow, the FG has little effect on induction of anesthesia; the FG may affect recovery time after prolonged anesthetic periods (3 hours or longer)

AGENTS	FAT-BLOOD PARTITION COEFFICIENT
Diethyl ether	4.2
Methoxyflurane	61
Halothane	65
Enflurane	37
Isoflurane	48
Sevoflurane	65
Nitrous oxide	2.3
Desflurane	27.2

      6. VPG tissues have very little effect on short duration anesthesia

7. Rubber solubility: methoxyflurane is freely absorbed into rubber components of the anesthetic system; during recovery, they equilibrate back into the anesthetic circuitry

8. Methoxyflurane, halothane, isoflurane, and desflurane are stable in moist soda lime; sevoflurane produces a potentially toxic substance called *Compound A* when it comes in contact with moist soda lime; the concentrations of Compound A measured in circle-systems are five to ten times lower than those reported to produce toxic effects

ELIMINATION OF INHALATION ANESTHETICS

I. By the lung

A. Inhalation anesthetics are excreted largely unchanged by the lungs

B. The same factors that affect the rate of anesthetic uptake are important in anesthetic elimination

1. Pulmonary ventilation
2. Blood flow
3. Solubility of inhalation in blood and tissue

C. As anesthetic gas washes out of the lungs, the arterial blood tension falls, followed by the tension in tissues; because of the high blood flow to the brain, the anesthetic tension falls rapidly and accounts for the rapid awakening from anesthesia with insoluble agents such as sevoflurane and desflurane; decreases in anesthetic drug concentration from other tissues are progressively slower and dependent on blood flow

II. Other routes through which small quantities of inhalation anesthetic agent may be excreted are skin, milk, mucous membrane, and urine

III. Biotransformation

A. Anesthetic gases are metabolized in the body to variable degrees

BIOTRANSFORMATION OF INHALATION ANESTHETICS TO METABOLITES

AGENT	% RECOVERED AS METABOLITE
Diethyl ether	50.0
Methoxyflurane	50.0
Halothane	20.0
Enflurane	3.0
Isoflurane	3.0
Sevoflurane	3.0-5.0
Nitrous oxide	0.0
Desflurane	0.0

B. Metabolism is generally by hepatic microsomal enzyme systems; various intermediate metabolites are formed; these may be responsible for certain toxic effects or aftereffects
  1. Approximately 20% inspired halothane is metabolized, compared to 50% methoxyflurane; approximately 2.5% enflurane and 0.25% isoflurane are metabolized; less than 1% of desflurane is metabolized
  2. Toxic metabolites are primarily inorganic fluoride and bromide ions

IV. Diffusion hypoxia may occur at the end of anesthesia and is discussed in the nitrous oxide section in Chapter 11; briefly, the rapid elimination of N_2O from the blood into the alveoli results in the dilution of alveolar O_2 by N_2O and hypoxemia if ventilation is not maintained

POTENCY OF INHALATION ANESTHETICS

I. Anesthetic potency can be expressed in several ways; one way to compare inhalant anesthetic potency is to measure the minimum alveolar concentration (MAC) of the inhalation anesthetic at surgical anesthesia (Table 10-2); MAC is generally defined as the minimum alveolar concentration of an anesthetic (1 atm) that produces no response in 50% of patients exposed to a painful stimulus

A. MAC is generally measured as the end-tidal concentration of anesthetic

B. MAC values are not vaporizer settings

TABLE 10-2
MINIMAL ALVEOLAR CONCENTRATIONS OF INHALATION ANESTHETICS IN VARIOUS SPECIES

	HUMAN	DOG	CAT	HORSE
Diethyl ether	1.92	3.04	2.1	—
Methoxyflurane	0.16	0.29	0.23	0.22
Halothane	0.76	0.87	1.19	0.88
Enflurane	1.68	2.06	2.4	2.12
Isoflurane	1.2	1.3	1.63	1.31
Sevoflurane	1.93	2.34	2.58	2.34
Desflurane	6.99	7.20	9.80	7.23
Nitrous oxide	101.1	188-200	150	190

    C. MAC values are used to compare the potency of anesthetics

  II. MAC values vary among species and are affected by the following factors:

    A. Age: older patients require less inhalation anesthetic

    B. Temperature: hypothermia reduces MAC

    C. Administration of other CNS depressant drugs

    D. Disease:

        1. Hyperthyroidism or hypothyroidism

        2. Hypovolemia, anemia

        3. Septicemia

        4. Extreme acid-base imbalances

    E. Pregnancy

 III. Studies using dogs suggest the following:

    A. 1 MAC produces light anesthesia

    B. 1.5 MAC produces moderate surgical anesthesia

    C. 2 MAC produces deep anesthesia

CHAPTER ELEVEN

Pharmacology of Inhalation Anesthetic Drugs

"Sleep is pain's easiest salve, and doth fulfill all offices of death, except to kill."

JOHN DONNE

OVERVIEW

Inhalation anesthetic drugs are pharmacologically active chemicals that cause unconsciousness, various degrees of muscle relaxation and analgesia, and changes in organ system function. Their administration requires familiarity with a variety of equipment (e.g., vaporizers, flow meters, pressure valves) needed to vaporize the anesthetic liquid and the anesthetic circuits used to accurately deliver the anesthetic to the patient. Theoretically, the depth of inhalation anesthesia is easily controlled compared to injectable anesthesia. This chapter outlines the pharmacologic properties and the interactions of inhalation anesthetic drugs.

GENERAL CONSIDERATIONS

I. The factors that influence the ability of an inhalation anesthetic to produce general anesthesia are discussed in Chapter 10 and include tissue membrane effects and physiochemical properties (Table 11-1)

   A. Factors that influence anesthetic uptake and delivery to the brain include:
   1. Alveolar ventilation
   2. Blood-gas partition coefficient
   3. Cardiac output (brain blood flow)

    4. Alveolar to mixed, venous anesthetic, partial pressure difference

II. Ventilation-perfusion abnormalities and hypoventilation hinder the rate of anesthetic uptake and the rate of induction to anesthesia

III. Left-to-right intracardiac shunts may slow the rate of induction to anesthesia

IV. Hypothermia decreases the need for anesthesia

V. The metabolites of inhalation anesthetics can be toxic

VI. Familiarity with an anesthetic drug is the key to its safe and effective use

NITROUS OXIDE

I. General anesthetic properties (see Table 11-1)

    A. A gas at room temperature, but readily compressible at 30 to 50 atm (750 psi) to a colorless liquid; returns to gaseous state when released from the cylinder into atmospheric pressure

    B. Nonflammable, but supports combustion by decomposing into nitrogen and oxygen

II. Effect on systems

    A. Nervous system

        1. Mild analgesic and anesthetic action produced by cerebrocortical depression

        2. Dangerous in excessive concentrations (more than 70% total gas flow) because it interferes with patient oxygenation

    B. Respiratory system

        1. Nonirritating to the respiratory tract

        2. Does not depress cough reflex

        3. Causes only minimal respiratory depression; respiratory rate may increase

    C. Cardiovascular system

        1. Few side effects occur except in the presence of hypoxia

        2. Heart rate, cardiac output, and arterial blood pressure (BP) remain relatively unchanged

        3. Tachycardia may develop

        4. N_2O does not sensitize the myocardium to catecholamines

TABLE 11-1
SUMMARY OF PHYSIOCHEMICAL PROPERTIES
OF INHALATION AGENTS

PROPERTIES	ETHER	NITROUS OXIDE	HALOTHANE
Chemical formula	$(C_2H_5)_2O$	N_2O	$\begin{matrix} F & Br \\ \mid & \mid \\ F-C-C-H \\ \mid & \mid \\ F & Cl \end{matrix}$
Molecular weight	74	44	197.4
Boiling point (at 760 mm Hg)	36.5° C	−89° C	50° C
Specific gravity (g/ml)	0.72	1.53	1.87
Vapor pressure (mm Hg at 20° C)	443	39,500	243
Odor	Pungent, unpleasant	Pleasant	Sweet, pleasant
Preservative	Necessary	None	Necessary (thymol)
Stability			
To metal	May react	Nonreactive	May react
To alkali	Stable (traces of aldehydes)	Stable	Slight decomposition
Explosiveness	Explosive (in air or oxygen)	None	None
Presentation at room temperature	Colorless liquid	Colorless gas (liquid under pressure)	Colorless liquid

MAC, minimum alveolar concentration (see Table 10-2).

TABLE 11-1
SUMMARY OF PHYSIOCHEMICAL PROPERTIES OF INHALATION AGENTS—cont'd

METHOXY-FLURANE	EN-FLURANE	ISO-FLURANE	SEVO-FLURANE	DES-FLURANE
$\begin{array}{ccc} Cl & F & H \\ \mid & \mid & \mid \\ H-C-C-o-C-H \\ \mid & \mid & \mid \\ Cl & F & H \end{array}$	$\begin{array}{ccc} Cl & F & F \\ \mid & \mid & \mid \\ H-C-C-o-C-H \\ \mid & \mid & \mid \\ F & F & F \end{array}$	$\begin{array}{ccc} F & Cl & H \\ \mid & \mid & \mid \\ F-C-C-o-C-H \\ \mid & \mid & \mid \\ F & H & F \end{array}$	$\begin{array}{ccc} F & H & F \\ \mid & \mid & \mid \\ H-C-o-C-C-F \\ \mid & \mid & \mid \\ H & CF_3 & F \end{array}$	$\begin{array}{ccc} F & F & H \\ \mid & \mid & \mid \\ F-C-C-o-C-K \\ \mid & \mid & \mid \\ F & H & F \end{array}$
165	185	185	200	168
105° C	57° C	49° C	59° C	23.5° C
1.41	1.52	1.52	1.52	1.47
24	180	252	160	664
Fruity, pleasant	Pleasant	Pungent	Pleasant	Pungent
Necessary (butylated hydroxytoluene)	None	None	None	None
May react	Non-reactive	Non-reactive	Stable	Non-reactive
Stable	Stable	Stable	Decomposes	Stable
None	None	None	None	None
Colorless liquid	Colorless liquid	Colorless liquid	Colorless liquid	Colorless liquid

  D. Other organ systems
     1. Ileus may occur secondary to gas accumulation within the gastrointestinal tract
     2. The kidney and liver are not significantly affected
  E. Muscular system
     1. Does not cause muscle relaxation
     2. Does not potentiate muscle relaxants
  F. Uterus and fetus
     1. Passes placental barrier
     2. May cause fetal hypoxemia
III. Absorption, fate, and excretion
  A. Readily crosses alveolar membranes because of relatively large inspired concentrations (40% to 75%)
  B. May accelerate the uptake of inhalation anesthetics (second gas) into the blood (second-gas effect); the enhanced uptake of the second gas (e.g., isoflurane) is caused by an N_2O-dependent increase in alveolar ventilation
  C. Diffuses into closed air cavities (Fig. 11-1): N_2O is 30 times more soluble in blood than nitrogen; when N_2O is given in high concentrations (over 50%), it diffuses into air-containing cavities faster than nitrogen diffuses out; if the cavity is closed (e.g., pneumothorax, obstructed bowel,

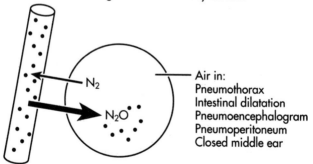

Effect of anesthetic agents on air and gases in closed body cavities

Air in:
Pneumothorax
Intestinal dilatation
Pneumoencephalogram
Pneumoperitoneum
Closed middle ear

Fig. 11-1
Distribution of N_2O from blood to air-containing cavities.

air embolism, blocked paranasal sinuses) and N_2O administered, then either the volume or pressure inside the cavity increases; volume or pressure increases until the alveolar nitrous oxide ratio is in equilibrium with the closed cavity; the relative volume increase can be calculated using this formula:

$M = 100/100\text{-}FiN_2O$; M = magnitude of volume change; FiN_2O = fraction of inspired N_2O; Example: If a patient is exposed to 50% N_2O, FiN_2O = 50%; $M = 100/100\text{-}50$ = 2; volume increases by a factor of 2

    D. Has no value as an O_2 source nor does it form any chemical combinations in the body; carried in simple solution

    E. Eliminated through the lungs rapidly and completely in minutes

    F. Diffusion hypoxia is a result of the low blood-gas partition coefficient (0.49); rapid diffusion of nitrous oxide into the alveoli at the end of anesthesia dilutes the oxygen in the alveoli; alveolar oxygen tension may be drastically reduced, especially if the patient is breathing room air; hypoxia is prevented by administering high oxygen flow rates for at least 5 to 10 minutes after discontinuing N_2O

    G. Recovery is fast and devoid of unpleasant sequelae

    H. Circumstantial evidence suggests some biotransformation; bone marrow depression may occur after prolonged exposure; N_2O may be teratogenic, especially in females after prolonged exposure in the first trimester of pregnancy

IV. Clinical use

    A. Used as an analgesic adjunct in veterinary anesthesia

    B. Adds to the effect of other inhalation anesthetics; therefore, less inhalant anesthetic is needed to produce general anesthesia

    C. Often used to supplement narcotic or inhalation anesthesia

    D. A minimum of 30% O_2 must be used to prevent hypoxia

    E. The ratio of N_2O to O_2 delivered by the anesthetic machine must be continually monitored; no more than 70% N_2O should be used

    F. The administration of N_2O is contraindicated during low flow or closed system anesthesia

V. Dosages
  A. Up to 70% F_iN_2O
  B. Maintenance concentrations are usually 50% or 66% (N_2O:$O_2 = 1:1$ or $2:1$)
  C. If the patient becomes cyanotic or the cardiopulmonary status deteriorates while receiving nitrous oxide, it should be discontinued
  D. N_2O is not potent enough in most animal species to make administration of less than 40% worthwhile

DIETHYL ETHER (ETHER)

I. Ether was once a frequently used inhalation anesthetic; it is now occasionally used in laboratory animals and to make tape sticky
II. Ether is highly flammable and explosive
III. Ether is an ideal anesthetic in some respects because it maintains respiration and minimally depresses cardiac output
IV. Ether may cause salivation, nausea, and vomiting during induction and recovery
V. The signs and stages of ether anesthesia (Table 11-2), as developed by Guedel, can be loosely applied to most inhalant anesthetics
  A. Stage I: analgesia (from the beginning of induction to the loss of consciousness)
    1. Disorientation, with normal reflexes or hyperreflexia, is the most common feature
    2. Fear and subsequent release of epinephrine with increased heart rate and rapid respirations may occur
    3. Excessive salivation may occur
  B. Stage II: delirium or excitement, which represents the period of early loss of consciousness
    1. Potential hazards of stage II include struggling, physical injury, and the consequences of increased sympathetic tone
    2. Voluntary centers in the brain become depressed; the patient becomes unaware of its surroundings and its actions
    3. During light anesthesia, the patient reacts to any sort of external stimuli with exaggerated reflex struggling

TABLE 11-2
STAGES OF ETHER ANESTHESIA

STAGE OF ANESTHESIA	RESPIRATION	PUPILS	EYE MOVEMENT	ABOLITION OF REFLEXES	SOMATIC MUSCLES	PULSE RATE AND BLOOD PRESSURE (BP)
Analgesia	Regular	Normal	Voluntary	All present	Normal tone	Rapid pulse; elevated BP
Delirium	Irregular	Dilated	Involuntary (nystagmus)	All present	Excited movement	Rapid pulse; elevated BP
Surgical						
Plane I	Increased depth, rate	Constricted	Involuntary; fixed	Conjunctival; pharyngeal; cutaneous	Slight relaxation	Normal pulse; normal BP
Plane II	Regular rate, depth	Normal		Laryngeal; corneal; peritoneal	Moderate relaxation	Normal pulse; normal BP
Plane III	Decreased rate, depth	Slightly dilated			Marked relaxation	Rapid, normal, or slow fall in BP
Plane IV	Abdominal breathing	Moderately dilated				Slow, weak pulse; then no pulse; fall in BP to zero

The classical stages described by A.E. Guedel.

    4. Respirations are generally irregular in depth and rate, and breath holding may occur

    5. The eyelids are widely open, and the pupil is dilated because of sympathetic stimulation

    6. Reflex vomiting may occur unless food has been withheld for 6 or more hours before anesthesia; defecation and urination may occur

    7. The duration of stage II can be decreased by temporarily administering higher inhalant anesthetic concentrations and inhalant drugs that have a low blood-gas solubility coefficient (e.g., isoflurane versus methoxyflurane)

C. Stage III

    1. Plane I: marked by the appearance of more regular respiration

       a. CO_2 retention during the preceding stages may double tidal volume for the first few minutes

       b. Preanesthetic medication directly affects the rate and volume of respiration throughout anesthesia

       c. Responses to pain, although depressed, are still present

       d. Cardiovascular function is only minimally affected

    2. Plane II: respiratory rate may be increased or decreased and respiratory volume (tidal volume) is decreased; cardiovascular function is mildly depressed

    3. Plane III: loss of intercostal muscle activity

       a. Respiratory depression is significant

       b. Cardiovascular function is noticeably depressed, dependent on the specific characteristics of the anesthetic drug used

       c. The level of anesthesia is potentially dangerous

    4. Plane IV: complete paralysis of intercostal muscles

       a. Cessation of all respiratory effort and dilation of the pupils

       b. Cardiovascular function is generally impaired, producing decreased cardiac contractility and vasodilation leading to hypotension

D. Stage IV: respiratory arrest followed by circulatory collapse; death ensues within 1 to 5 minutes

METHOXYFLURANE (METOFANE, PENTHRANE)

I. General anesthetic properties (see Table 11-1): the vapor pressure of methoxyflurane is low; the highest concentrations that can be produced at room temperature by a draw-over vaporizer are between 2.5% and 3%

II. Effects on organ systems
   A. Nervous system
      1. Dose-dependent CNS depression
      2. Potent CNS depressor
      3. Excitement (delirium) may occur during mask induction (not recommended)
      4. Good muscle relaxation and analgesia
      5. Most potent inhalation anesthetic (minimum alveolar concentration [MAC] = 0.29)
   B. Respiratory system
      1. Produces more respiratory depression than halothane
      2. Ventilation may need to be assisted to prevent hypercarbia
      3. Nonirritating to the respiratory tract
   C. Cardiovascular system
      1. Decreases cardiac contractile force (negative inotrope)
      2. May cause changes in heart rate (bradycardia) and rhythm
      3. Sensitizes the heart to catecholamines, but less so than halothane
   D. Gastrointestinal system: decreases smooth muscle tone and motility
   E. Renal system
      1. Acute renal failure (inorganic fluoride, a metabolite) has been reported after methoxyflurane anesthesia in obese patients, those with renal disease, those given concurrent nephrotoxic drugs (tetracyclines, aminoglycosides), or those undergoing extensive surgical procedures
      2. Acute methoxyflurane administration has not produced renal failure in animals, except when administered with other nephrotoxic drugs (e.g., aminoglycosides, tetracyclines)

   F. Muscular system
      1. Excellent muscle relaxation and analgesia at relatively
         low inspired concentrations
      2. Muscle relaxation is due to drug effects on the CNS
         (spinal cord) rather than the neuromuscular junction
   G. Uterus and fetus
      1. Rapidly crosses the placental barrier
      2. Does not significantly affect motility and tone
III. Absorption, fate, and excretion
   A. Absorbed and eliminated by the lung
   B. Up to 50% absorbed methoxyflurane may be metabolized
      by the liver; metabolites include inorganic fluoride
   C. Metabolites are excreted by the kidney
IV. Clinical use
   A. Good, potent muscle relaxation is produced; therefore, low
      concentrations of methoxyflurane can be used clinically for
      many minor surgical procedures
   B. Recovery is prolonged in laboratory animals because of the
      relatively high blood-gas partition coefficient (13)
   C. Analgesia may continue into the recovery period
   D. Accurate concentrations can be delivered by precise, heat-
      compensated, calibrated vaporizer; however, simple draw-
      over wick vaporizers can be used
   E. If nitrous oxide is used, the required amount of methoxyflu-
      rane is reduced
V. Dosages
   A. Maintenance: 0.2% to 1%

HALOTHANE (FLUOTHANE)

I. General anesthetic properties (see Table 11-1)
   A. Nervous system
      1. Depresses the central nervous system (CNS)
      2. Depresses body temperature regulating centers, result-
         ing in hypothermia
      3. Rarely causes hyperpyrexia and malignant hyperther-
         mia in humans, pigs, horses, dogs, and cats; this has been
         linked to a genetic defect in humans, pigs, and dogs
      4. The stages of anesthesia are not exactly the same as those
         for ether; pupils may be constricted at all stages, respi-

      ration may be shallow but rapid, and the abdominal muscles are relaxed only at deeper planes of anesthesia; the arterial BP may provide the best information about the depth of halothane anesthesia

    5. Increases cerebral blood flow

II. Effects on organ systems

   A. Respiratory system

     1. Respirations are depressed at all levels of halothane anesthesia

     2. Tidal volume is decreased

     3. Minute volume is smaller than in the conscious state, but breathing is usually adequate

     4. Increased breathing in response to hypercarbia does not occur during deeper anesthesia, and ventilation becomes inadequate

     5. Respiratory depression is pronounced in ruminants

     6. Tachypnea may occur; the mechanism is uncertain

   B. Cardiovascular system

     1. Hypotension is related to the depth of anesthesia

     2. Directly depresses vascular smooth muscle causing vasodilation (e.g., in cerebral, skeletal muscle, and peripheral tissues) and decreasing total peripheral resistance

     3. Directly depresses the myocardium, decreasing cardiac output, stroke volume, and cardiac contractility

     4. Decreases efferent sympathetic nervous system activity

     5. Cardiac rate is less affected but is usually decreased at deeper planes of anesthesia

     6. May cause sinus bradycardia and cardiac arrhythmias

     7. Sensitizes the heart to catecholamines, occasionally producing cardiac arrhythmias

   C. Gastrointestinal system

     1. Decreases intestinal tract motility, tone, and peristaltic activity

     2. Liver: a number of studies on humans have related halothane to jaundice and fatal postanesthetic liver necrosis; biotransformation of halothane to hepatotoxic metabolites may produce hypersensitivity in a small number of individuals; the effect is believed to be related to halothane administration in conjunction with tissue hypoxia

    D. Renal system: no nephrotoxic effects have been reported other than those resulting from hypotension

    E. Muscular system

       1. Relaxation is only moderate during light anesthesia

       2. Skeletal muscle relaxants may be needed if pronounced muscle relaxation is required

       3. Halothane potentiates the action of nondepolarizing muscle relaxants

       4. Malignant hyperthermia can occur

    F. Uterus and fetus

       1. Decreases uterine tone; may decrease uterine involution postpartum

       2. Readily crosses the placental barrier

III. Absorption, fate, and excretion

    A. Absorption takes place rapidly in the lungs

    B. As much as 20% to 40% inspired halothane is metabolized by liver microsomes; trifluoroacetic acid, bromide, and chloride radicals are produced and excreted in the urine for many hours to days

    C. Metabolites may persist for many days in the liver

    D. The major portion of administered halothane is excreted unchanged by the lungs

IV. Clinical uses

    A. Halothane is one of the most useful anesthetics, because it is nonflammable, potent, nonirritating, controllable, and relatively nontoxic

    B. Can be used in all species

    C. Accurate concentrations of halothane can be delivered from precision, thermostable or thermocompensated, calibrated vaporizers; draw-over, in-the-circle vaporizers have been used once the wick is removed

    D. Decomposes slowly when exposed to light; stored in dark bottles with thymol added as a preservative; thymol is potentially tissue toxic

    E. Can be used in rebreathing and nonrebreathing techniques

    F. Used in in-the-circle, draw-over vaporizers during "low-flow" techniques (see Chapter 14)

V. Dosage

    A. 2% to 4% at induction; careful monitoring is important to avoid overdosage

B. Because of the second-gas effect, induction time may be decreased if nitrous oxide is given simultaneously

C. Concurrent use of nitrous oxide reduces the amount of halothane required

D. Maintenance: 0.5% to 1.5% in small animals; 1% to 2% in large animals

ISOFLURANE (FORANE, AERRANE)

I. General anesthetic properties (see Table 11-1)
  A. An isomer of enflurane and exceptionally stable
  B. Produces comparatively rapid induction and recovery from anesthesia
  C. Can be used in all species

II. Effects on organ systems
  A. Nervous system
    1. Generalized CNS depression
    2. Cerebral blood flow is not increased if ventilation is maintained
    3. Burst suppression on the EEG is observed in moderate to deep surgical anesthesia
  B. Respiratory system
    1. Respiratory depression is similar to methoxyflurane; respiratory patterns may be different
    2. Tidal volume increases initially with depth of anesthesia; respiratory rate decreases
    3. $Paco_2$ concentration increases with time, although surgical stimulation increases respiration and thus prevents a large rise in $Paco_2$
  C. Cardiovascular system
    1. Cardiac depression is less than with halothane or methoxyflurane
    2. Cardiac contractility is depressed less than halothane at concentrations producing surgical anesthesia, but cardiac output is maintained
    3. Progressive vasodilation occurs with increasing depth of anesthesia, increasing muscle and skin blood flow
    4. Hypotensive: mean arterial BP and peripheral vascular resistance decrease with depth of anesthesia
    5. Isoflurane does not sensitize the heart to catecholamine-induced arrhythmias

    D. Gastrointestinal system
       1. Smooth muscle tone and motility are decreased
       2. No hepatotoxicity reported (metabolism is very low)
    E. Renal system: no changes in renal function reported; very little metabolism to trifluoroacetic acid
    F. Muscular system
       1. Produces excellent muscle relaxation
       2. Potentiates nondepolarizing muscle relaxants
       3. Can cause malignant hyperthermia in swine
    G. Uterus and fetus
       1. Rapidly crosses the placenta
       2. Reduces uterine tone
       3. Safety in pregnancy not evaluated

III. Absorption, fate, and excretion
    A. Absorbed and eliminated by the alveoli
    B. Primarily excreted unchanged by the lungs
    C. Very little biodegradation; approximately 0.25% is metabolized to inorganic fluoride (trifluoroacetic acid)

IV. Clinical use
    A. Produces fast, smooth induction and recovery in all species tested
    B. Rapid recovery may predispose some animals to emergence delirium
    C. Calibrated vaporizer is used to deliver accurate concentrations
    D. Can be used in in-the-circle, draw-over vaporizers during "low-flow" (closed system) techniques (see Chapter 14)
    E. Can be used with nitrous oxide
    F. Can be used for mask induction
    G. Is classified as a respiratory depressant

  V. Dosages
    A. Induction: 2.5% to 4.5% is usually necessary
    B. Induction is facilitated by the use of intravenous anesthesia or nitrous oxide
    C. Maintenance: 1% to 3%

ENFLURANE (ETHRANE)

I. General anesthetic properties (see Table 11-1)
    A. Similar to isoflurane

    B. Low blood-gas partition coefficient (1.9)
    C. Stable in moist soda lime
    D. Rarely used in clinical veterinary medicine

SEVOFLURANE (ULTANE)

  I. General anesthetic properties (see Table 11-1)
    A. Low blood-gas partition coefficient (0.6 to 0.7)
      1. Rapid, smooth induction; rapid recovery
      2. MAC of approximately 2.4%
    B. Nonpungent
    C. Relatively stable in moist soda lime
  II. Effects on organ systems
    A. Similar to isoflurane
    B. Depresses CNS; no convulsive activity
    C. Produces good muscle relaxation and analgesia
    D. Dose-dependent cardiorespiratory depression
      1. Respiratory depression similar to isoflurane
      2. Cardiovascular effects similar to, but more desirable than, isoflurane (slower heart rate, less myocardial depression)
    E. Does not sensitize the heart to catecholamine-induced cardiac arrhythmias
    F. Rapidly crosses the placenta, producing fetal depression
    G. Used in precision vaporizers
    H. Maintenance: 3.0% to 4.0%

DESFLURANE (SUPRANE)

  I. General anesthetic properties (see Table 11-1)
    A. Identical in structure to isoflurane, except that fluorine is substituted for chlorine
    B. Extremely low blood-gas partition coefficient (0.42); extremely rapid induction and recovery
    C. Less potent than other halogenated agents; MAC is approximately 7.2%
    D. Pungent; produces airway irritation, provoking coughing or breath holding
    E. Requires a special, electrically heated vaporizer
    F. Stable in moist soda lime
    G. Expensive

II. Effects on organ systems

   A. Similar to isoflurane

   B. Nervous system

      1. Similar to isoflurane

      2. Dose-dependent CNS depression

      3. Good muscle relaxation; enhances nondepolarizing neuromuscular blocking drugs

   C. Respiratory system

      1. Causes dose-dependent respiratory depression; decreases the breathing response to increases in $Paco_2$

      2. Pungent odor irritates the airway; induction to anesthesia may be difficult unless preceded by a preanesthetic drug

   D. Cardiovascular system

      1. Qualitatively and quantitatively similar to isoflurane

      2. Can cause sympathetic activation "storm" in some patients

   E. Gastrointestinal system: decreases smooth muscle tone and motility

   F. Renal system: does not affect renal function

   G. Muscular system

      1. Produces good muscle relaxation

      2. Can cause malignant hyperthermia in swine

   H. Uterus and fetus

      1. Crosses the placental barrier; causes fetal depression

      2. Allows rapid recovery (fetus) from anesthesia because of low blood-gas partition coefficient (0.42)

III. Absorption, fate, excretion

   A. Absorbed and eliminated by the lung

   B. Resists degradation by the liver; produces even less inorganic fluoride than isoflurane

   C. Has shown no hepatotoxicity or nephrotoxicity

IV. Clinical use

   A. Induction and recovery from anesthesia is about twice as fast as with isoflurane because of the extremely low blood-gas partition coefficient (0.42), despite comparatively low potency (MAC ~ 7.2%)

   B. Produces good muscle relaxation and analgesia

   C. Pungent odor makes mask induction difficult unless appropriate preanesthetics are used

    D. Recovery may be so rapid that resedation is needed to avoid emergence delirium

V. Dosages

    A. Mask induction: 10% to 15% concentration

    B. Anesthetic maintenance: 6% to 9% concentrations

    C. Preanesthetic use, N_2O, and adjuncts to anesthesia (fentanyl) can reduce MAC

CHAPTER TWELVE

Neuromuscular Blocking Drugs

"Don't fight forces; use them."

R. BUCKMINSTER FULLER

OVERVIEW

Neuromuscular blocking drugs (NMBDs), commonly referred to as *peripheral "muscle relaxants,"* as opposed to centrally acting muscle relaxants, interfere with or block neuromuscular transmission and are useful adjuncts to general anesthesia. Neuromuscular blocking drugs do *not* provide analgesia, sedation, amnesia, or hypnosis. Breathing ceases, which necessitates controlled ventilation and constant patient monitoring.

GENERAL CONSIDERATIONS

I. The primary pharmacologic effect of peripheral neuromuscular blocking drugs is to produce skeletal muscle (SM) relaxation

II. NMBDs are potentiated by many intravenous (IV) and inhalation anesthetic drugs

III. Other clinically useful drugs (some antibiotics) and some toxins can cause SM weakness or paralysis

IV. Potential mechanisms of SM relaxation

   A. NMBDs interfere with cholinergic (nicotine) neuromuscular transmission in the peripheral somatic nervous system

   B. Some NMBDs enhance the activity of endogenous inhibitory mechanisms in the central nervous system, which normally modulate SM tone

   V. NMBDs are used adjunctively during anesthesia to produce controlled, transient muscle weakness

  VI. NMBDs produce muscle relaxation but do not produce analgesia or a hypnotic effect

 VII. NMBDs can produce respiratory paralysis, which necessitates mechanical or manual support of ventilation

VIII. Hypothermia is an important secondary effect of prolonged SM relaxation in small animals

  IX. NMBDs are positively charged (ionized) and therefore do not pass the blood-brain barrier or cross the placenta in significant amounts

   X. Various electrical stimulators and stimulation protocols can be used to determine the degree of neuromuscular blockade

NORMAL NEUROMUSCULAR FUNCTION

  I. Acetylcholine (ACh) is released in small amounts even in resting muscles

    A. Random ACh release causes mini-endplate potentials at the postsynaptic muscle membrane, which are insufficient to evoke muscle contraction

 II. Action potential (AP)-dependent ACh release

    A. APs cause large depolarization in nerve terminals of α-motor neurons

    B. Depolarization in the presence of extracellular Ca^{++} causes simultaneous fusion of many ACh-containing vesicles with the terminal nerve membrane (Fig. 12-1)

    C. Release of ACh packets evokes a large endplate potential, leading to muscle contraction

III. Combination of ACh with postjunctional nicotine receptors (Nm receptors)

    A. Receptors on the muscle endplates are nicotinic, type IV cholinergic (Nm) receptors

    B. Strength of muscle contraction is proportional to the number of receptors activated by ACh

IV. Hydrolysis of ACh, reuptake of choline, synthesis and packing of ACh

    A. The duration of ACh activity at any cholinergic synapse is limited by the action of acetylcholinesterase (ACh esterase); ACh is metabolized to acetic acid plus choline at the synaptic cleft

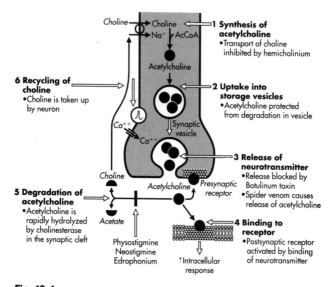

Fig. 12-1
Release of acetylcholine from neurons at the neuromuscular junction.

B. Choline produced by hydrolysis of ACh is taken up by the nerve terminals and resynthesized into ACh; choline + acetyl CoA ↔ ACh (choline acetyl transferase) at the nerve terminal membrane

C. ACh is packaged into vesicles or stored freely in the cytoplasm of the nerve terminals

MECHANISMS OF SKELETAL MUSCLE RELAXATION EVOKED BY INTERFERENCE WITH NORMAL PERIPHERAL NEUROMUSCULAR FUNCTION

I. At presynaptic sites
   A. Inhibition of ACh synthesis (e.g., hemicholinium blocks choline uptake)
   B. Inhibition of ACh release
      1. Calcium deficiency, Mg^{++} increases
      2. Procaine

      3. Tetracyclines and aminoglycoside antibiotics

      4. Some β-blockers

      5. Botulinum toxin

II. At postsynaptic sites

  A. Persistent depolarization with an agonist that has a longer duration of action than ACh (e.g., succinylcholine chloride)

  B. Competitive block of ACh receptors causing *nondepolarizing* blockade (e.g., curare, pancuronium)

TYPES OF NEUROMUSCULAR BLOCKS

  I. Phase I block: depolarizing block (succinylcholine)

 II. Phase II block: nondepolarizing block (pancuronium)

III. Mixed block: any combination of I and II

IV. Dual block: excessive amounts of depolarizing agents producing phase II block

  V. Nonacetylcholine block (procaine, botulinum, decreased Ca^{++}, increased Mg^{++}, increased K^+, decreased K^+)

SEQUENCE OF MUSCLE RELAXATION

  I. Oculomotor m. → palpebral m. → facial m. → tongue and pharynx → jaw and tail → limbs → pelvic m. → caudal abdominal m. → cranial abdominal m. → intercostal m. → larynx → diaphragm

  A. The sequence of motor blockade is highly variable in clinical patients

  B. Motor activity to the limbs may appear to return (twitching, jerking) before the diaphragm is fully functional

 II. Intercostal and diaphragmatic muscles are thought to be affected last

III. Recovery is generally in the reverse order of paralysis

IV. It is possible but difficult to titrate the specific neuromuscular blocking drug to paralyze the muscles of the eye while maintaining diaphragmatic function

TABLE 12-1

DOSE OF NEUROMUSCULAR BLOCKING ANESTHETICS WITH SIDE EFFECTS AND CONTRADICTIONS

AGENT	SPECIES	DOSE IV (mg/lb)	DURATION OF ACTION (min)	SIDE EFFECTS	CONTRAINDICATIONS
Succinylcholine chloride	Dog	0.1	1-10	Little cardiovascular effect; muscarinic effect-bradycardia; nicotinic effect-hypertension, increased intraocular pressure; hyperpyrexia	Organophosphate anthelmintics, chronic liver disease, malnutrition, high-K, glaucoma, penetrating eye injury
	Cat	0.5	2-3		
	Pig	0.5			
	Horse	0.04	1-10		
Pancuronium bromide	Dog	0.02	15-20	Negligible	Liver or kidney disease
	Cat				
	Pig	0.05			
Vecuronium	Dog	0.006-0.1	10-15	Negligible	
	Cat	0.05-0.1	10-15	Negligible	
Atracurium	Dog	0.05-0.1			
	Horse	0.01-0.03	15-20	Negligible	

SPECIFIC NEUROMUSCULAR BLOCKING DRUGS
(Tables 12-1, 12-2)

I. Depolarizing drugs act like ACh
   A. Succinylcholine chloride (Sucostrin, Anectine, Quillicine, Suxamethonium)
   B. Decamethonium bromide (Syncurine)
II. Nondepolarizing drugs; competitive blocking drugs
   A. D-Tubocurarine chloride (curare, Metubine)
   B. Gallamine triethiodide (Flaxedil)
   C. Pancuronium bromide (Pavulon)
   D. Vecuronium bromide (Norcuron)
   E. Atracurium besylate (Tracrium)
   F. Mivacurium chloride (Mivacron)
   G. Doxacurium chloride (Nuromax)
   H. Pipecuronium (Arduran)

CLINICAL DIFFERENTIATION BETWEEN DEPOLARIZING AND NONDEPOLARIZING DRUGS

I. Depolarizing
   A. First: transient muscle fasciculations caused by asynchronous depolarization
   B. Second: paralysis caused by prolonged depolarization of the motor endplate
   C. Paralysis is not reversed by anticholinesterase drugs

TABLE 12-2
AUTONOMIC EFFECTS OF NEUROMUSCULAR BLOCKING DRUGS

DRUG	AUTONOMIC GANGLIA	CARDIAC MUSCARINIC RECEPTORS	HISTAMINE RELEASE
Succinylcholine	Stimulated	Stimulated	Slight
Pancuronium	None	Blocked weakly	None
Atracurium	None	None	Slight
Vecuronium	None	None	None
Mivacurium	None	None	Slight
Doxacurium	None	None	None
Pipecuronium	None	None	None

    D. Paralysis is terminated by metabolism of the NMBD by pseudocholinesterase

  II. Nondepolarizing

    A. No muscle fasciculation occurs before muscle paralysis, and there is no depolarization of motor endplate; the animal gradually relaxes or "fades"

    B. Effects can be partially reversed by anticholinesterase drugs (see Fig. 12-1)

      1. Neostigmine

      2. Pyridostigmine

      3. Edrophonium

  III. Onset of effect

    A. Rapid (less than 1 minute): succinylcholine

    B. Medium (1 to 2 minutes): mivacurium, atracurium, vecuronium

    C. Slow (3 to 5 minutes): doxacurium, pancuronium

  IV. Duration of effect

    A. Ultra-short (1 to 3 minutes): succinylcholine

    B. Short (5 to 10 minutes): mivacurium, atracurium

    C. Intermediate (10 to 20 minutes): vecuronium

    D. Long (20 to 40 minutes): doxacurium, pancuronium, pipecuronium

  V. Speed of antagonism by anticholinesterases

    A. Rapid (less than 1 minute): mivacurium

    B. Medium (1 to 2 minutes): atracurium, vecuronium

    C. Slow (3 to 5 minutes): doxacurium, pancuronium

  VI. Metabolism

    A. Hoffman elimination: atracurium

    B. Plasma cholinesterase: succinylcholine, mivacurium

    C. Liver: vecuronium, pancuronium, pipecuronium, atracurium

DEPOLARIZING BLOCKING DRUGS

  I. Mechanism of action

    A. Persistent depolarization alone may result in neuromuscular block because of Na^+ inactivation, which prevents electrical impulse generation

    B. Dual block: prolonged exposure of ACh membrane receptors to large doses of depolarizing drugs (ACh, succinylcholine, C-10) reduces the ability of these drugs to cause conductance changes; the reason for this is uncertain

II. Indications

    A. Diagnostic or surgical procedures requiring a short duration of muscle relaxation

    B. Facilitation of endotracheal intubation in humans and primates

    C. Cesarean sections

    D. Fracture reductions

III. Contraindications with depolarizing drugs

    A. Disease states causing prolonged NMBD activity

        1. Liver disease: pseudocholinesterase is produced in the liver

        2. Chronic anemia: acetylcholinesterase is associated with red blood cell membranes

        3. Chronic malnutrition

        4. Organophosphates (anthelmintics): enzyme activity is inhibited

    B. Other conditions

        1. High serum K^+ levels

            a. Burns, muscle trauma, renal failure

            b. Depolarizing blockade can cause potassium release from muscles

        2. Ophthalmologic conditions

            a. Glaucoma, penetrating eye wounds

            b. Depolarizing blockade can transiently increase intraocular pressure

IV. Specific depolarizing drugs: succinylcholine, decamethonium (see Table 12-2)

    A. Succinylcholine: adverse effects

        1. Muscle soreness: reason unknown; probably related to muscle fasciculations and K^+ release before paralysis

        2. Histamine release

        3. Cardiovascular effects

            a. Potential for bradycardia

            b. The more common response is tachycardia and hypertension caused by sympathetic stimulation

        4. Hyperkalemia: caused by increased efflux of K^+ from endplate region of skeletal muscle

        5. Some patients have a deficiency of plasma cholinesterase; in these patients, neuromuscular block may be prolonged

6. Genetic anomaly in which plasma cholinesterase is replaced by an atypical cholinesterase may prolong drug effects; differentiation is possible with dibucaine, which inhibits normal plasma cholinesterase 80% and atypical cholinesterase, only 20%

7. Malignant hyperpyrexia: manifested by a severe, rapid rise in temperature, which may be accompanied by significant muscle rigidity
    a. Usually occurs when using succinylcholine and halothane together
    b. Treat with 100% O_2, rapid cooling, sodium bicarbonate to control acidosis, and dantrolene sodium (1 to 2 mg/lb)
    c. A genetic disease of pigs and humans

B. Decamethonium (Syncurine)
   1. Basically identical to succinylcholine except for the following characteristics:
       a. Does not release histamine
       b. Is not metabolized by plasma cholinesterase, thereby prolonging the duration of action
       c. Does not undergo metabolism; excreted by the kidney unchanged; not used for renal disease

NONDEPOLARIZING BLOCKING DRUGS (SEE SPECIFIC NMBDs)

I. Mechanism of action
   A. Competitive blocking drugs: compete with ACh for postsynaptic receptors, thereby reducing the depolarization caused by ACh

II. Indications
   A. Same as depolarizing drugs
   B. High-risk cases as part of a balanced anesthetic technique with narcotics, inhalation, or other analgesic drugs
   C. Ocular surgery
   D. Control of ventilation at any time

III. Specific nondepolarizing drugs (see Table 12-2)
   A. Pancuronium (Pavulon)
      1. No histamine release or ganglionic block; no catecholamine release or inhibition

    2. Effects are enhanced by inhalation anesthetics

    3. Major portion is excreted unchanged in urine

    4. Tachycardia is occasionally seen following administration

B. Atracurium (Tracrium)

    1. Developed as a rapid-onset and duration-competitive NMBD; can be administered by infusion

    2. pH and temperature-dependent degradation (Hoffman elimination); a potential benefit is that biologically mediated metabolism and elimination by the liver and kidneys are not needed

    3. Some histamine release at high dosages

    4. Occasionally decreases heart rate and arterial blood pressure (BP)

C. Vecuronium (Norcuron)

    1. Developed in an attempt to produce a competitive NMBD with short onset and duration and to eliminate the tachycardia seen occasionally with pancuronium

    2. Eliminated in bile (40%) and through the kidneys (15%)—a potential advantage in patients with compromised renal function

    3. Minimal cardiovascular effects; no histamine release; no ganglionic block

D. Mivacurium

    1. Slight histamine release

    2. Rapid clearance by plasma cholinesterase

    3. Occasional decrease in arterial BP

E. Doxacurium

    1. No histamine release

    2. Low clearance eliminated by the kidney

    3. Minimal cardiovascular effects

F. Pipecuronium

    1. No histamine release

    2. Low clearance eliminated by the kidney

    3. Minimal cardiovascular effects

G. Tubocurarine

    1. Infrequently used in veterinary medicine

    2. Used to poison the tips of arrows

H. Gallamine

    1. Infrequently used

    2. Causes tachycardia and occasionally hypertension

FACTORS THAT MAY INFLUENCE NEUROMUSCULAR BLOCKADE (Table 12-3)

I. Temperature

    A. Hyperthermia antagonizes competitive blockade but enhances and prolongs depolarizing blockade

    B. Hypothermia prolongs nondepolarizing neuromuscular blocking drugs

II. Acid-base balance

    A. Respiratory acidosis augments nondepolarizing neuromuscular blockade

    B. Inadequate reversal of nondepolarizing drugs causes depressed ventilation and respiratory acidosis, which enhances the blockade (a vicious cycle)

III. Fluid and electrolyte imbalance

    A. Hypokalemia and hypocalcemia potentiate nondepolarizing drugs

    B. Dehydration increases the plasma concentration of a normal dose of a nondepolarizing drug, augmenting its effect

    C. High Mg blood levels enhance both depolarizing and nondepolarizing neuromuscular blocking drugs

TABLE 12-3
FACTORS ALTERING INTENSITY OF DEGREE AND DURATION OF MUSCLE RELAXATION

FACTOR	DEPOLARIZING AGENT	NONDEPOLARIZING AGENT
Tranquilizers	↑	↑
Volatile anesthetic agents	↑	↑
Decreased body temperature	↑	↑
Decreased cardiac output/kg body weight	↓	↓ (Gallamine)
Increased age	↑	↑
Antibiotics		
Streptomycin	↑	↑
Neomycin	↑	↑
Kanamycin	↑	↑
Organophosphates	↑	—

↑, Increase; ↓, decrease; —, no effect.

IV. Other drugs

    A. The following antibiotics potentiate nondepolarizing drugs: neomycin, streptomycin, gentamicin, kanamycin, paromomycin, viomycin, polymyxin A and B, colistin, tetracycline, lincomycin, and clindamycin

ANTICHOLINESTERASE DRUGS

I. Reversal of neuromuscular block

    A. Anticholinesterase drugs such as edrophonium, physostigmine, pyridostigmine, and neostigmine can be used with or without anticholinergic drugs

        1. Atropine is used to block the undesirable muscarinic effects of anticholinesterase drugs; muscarinic effects include bradycardia and increased bronchial and salivary secretions, increased intestinal motility, and bradycardia

        2. This regimen is ineffective against depolarization block; in fact, it exacerbates the block because of additional depolarization by excess ACh

        3. This regimen may be effective when a depolarizing, blocking drug is producing a phase II block

    B. Reverse with 0.02 mg/lb neostigmine combined with 0.01 mg/lb atropine (average dose); do not repeat the neostigmine dose more than three times

    C. Edrophonium dose is 0.25 mg/lb IV; it may be repeated up to five times

    D. Complete reversal takes 5 to 45 minutes

CENTRALLY ACTING SKELETAL MUSCLE RELAXANTS

I. Guaifenesin (see Chapter 9)

    A. The mechanism of action is poorly understood but probably relates to depression of transmission through spinal polysynaptic pathways, which normally maintain SM tone

    B. No effect on cerebral arousal

        1. Mild sedation

        2. Variable, mild analgesia

    C. Clinical use: significantly reduces the dose of induction drug required to produce recumbency

    D. Dosage and route of administration

1. 25 mg/lb or to ataxic effect by IV infusion; 50 mg/lb for recumbency by IV infusion
2. Typically administered as a 5% solution

II. Benzodiazepines (see Chapter 3)

A. Mechanism of skeletal muscle relaxant activity is probably related to the ability to activate benzodiazepine receptors, activate chloride channels, and potentiate gamma-aminobutyric acid, a CNS inhibitory neurotransmitter

CHAPTER THIRTEEN

Anesthetic Toxicity, Oxygen Toxicity, and Drug Interactions

"Can we ever have too much of a good thing?"

DON QUIXOTE DE LA MANCHA

OVERVIEW

All drugs that produce chemical restraint and anesthesia have the potential to produce cytotoxic effects. These toxic effects, if allowed to continue or if sufficiently severe, can jeopardize the patient's life. Toxicity occurs when drugs are administered by individuals who are either unfamiliar with the pharmacologic properties of a drug or who have insufficient knowledge about how to counteract the toxic effects of the drug. Inhalation anesthetic drug toxicity is a major concern for operating room personnel. All inhalation anesthetics are central nervous system (CNS) depressants. When these agents are used, waste anesthetic vapors should be scavenged to minimize personnel exposure. Oxygen can be both beneficial and detrimental, depending on the tension of the oxygen and the duration of exposure. Drug interactions underscore the importance of obtaining a comprehensive history and preliminary physical examination.

GENERAL CONSIDERATIONS

I. All drugs used to produce chemical restraint and anesthesia are potentially toxic; toxicity is caused by the following:
   A. Inhibition of nervous system activity
   B. Alteration of normal physiology and depression of cardiopulmonary function

    C. Inhibition of enzyme systems

    D. Direct cytotoxic effects

    E. Differences in species' sensitivity to drugs

    F. Idiosyncratic reactions

II. The toxic manifestations of drugs used to produce chemical restraint and anesthesia are generally reversible

III. Many drugs used to produce chemical restraint and anesthesia can be antagonized

    A. Opioids by narcotic antagonists such as naloxone

    B. Xylazine by α_2-antagonists such as yohimbine, tolazoline, and atipamazole

    C. Nondepolarizing muscle relaxants by acetylcholinesterase inhibitors such as neostigmine and edrophonium

    D. Benzodiazepines by the antagonist flumazenil

    E. General anesthetic-induced depression can be partially antagonized by analeptics such as doxapram, yohimbine, tolazoline, and atipamazole

IV. Waste gas scavenging minimizes the potential danger of drug-induced toxicity

V. Drug interactions may significantly potentiate or inhibit the actions of drugs used for chemical restraint and anesthesia

VOLATILE ANESTHETICS

I. The anesthetic molecule is nontoxic; however, volatile anesthetics are not completely inert and are metabolized to varying degrees (except for nitrous oxide)

    A. Metabolites are believed to be responsible for drug toxicity

    B. Chloride, bromide, and fluoride metabolites have been reported

    C. Sevoflurane interacts with CO_2 absorbants (soda lime, bora lime) to produce Compound A

II. Metabolism of inhalation anesthetics occurs primarily in the liver; metabolites are excreted predominantly by the kidneys

III. Volatile anesthetics are amazingly uniform in distribution, except in areas high in fat, in the thymus, and in the adrenal gland

IV. Three general mechanisms of tissue injury are associated with inhaled anesthetics
   A. Toxic intracellular accumulation of metabolites
   B. Initiation of immune responses caused by hapten formation
   C. Destructive free-radical chain reactions initiated by reactive intermediate products of metabolism
V. Normal metabolic functions are affected as long as anesthetic is present; at normal metabolic rates, no toxic side effects may occur; however, some individual animals may have metabolic rates far below normal, which may augment toxic effects
   A. Animals in shock
   B. Hypothermic animals
VI. Metabolism of all inhalant anesthetics may be increased following the administration of enzyme-inducing agents (i.e., phenobarbital)
VII. Several inhalant anesthetic agents have demonstrated teratogenicity in mice when administered chronically or at high concentrations; further investigations are needed to clarify the importance of these findings and their relationship to other animals and humans
VIII. Materials that are properly prepared, stored, and used have not led to any known catastrophes attributable to contaminants; toxic impurities can be and have been caused by human error
   A. Cylinders of nitrous oxide (N_2O) have been mislabeled as nitrogen dioxide (NO_2)
   B. Improper storage can lead to decomposition of initially pure anesthetics
   C. Halogenated compounds are unstable in light

TOXICOLOGY OF ANESTHETIC DRUGS

I. Halothane toxicity
   A. Halothane sensitizes the myocardium to catecholamine-induced dysrhythmias
   B. Halothane predisposes some animals to hyperpyrexia and malignant hyperthermia

C. Halothane is extensively metabolized
   1. Major metabolites
      a. Trifluoracetic acid
      b. Fluoride ion
      c. Chloride ion
      d. Bromide ion
   2. Prolonged exposure to subanesthetic concentrations increases metabolism
D. Hepatotoxicity
   1. Many halogenated hydrocarbons are hepatotoxic
   2. Degree of halogenation increases the incidence of toxicity
   3. Hepatic necrosis is believed to be caused by toxic effects of the fluoride or bromide molecules released after halothane metabolism by the liver
   4. Toxic effects are potentiated by halothane-induced decreases in liver perfusion
   5. The National Study of Hepatic Necrosis was unable to identify any unique or consistent lesion resulting from halothane administration
E. Toxicity to halothane
   1. Dose related
   2. Increases with multiple uses
   3. Thymol preservative in commercially prepared halothane is potentially toxic to both the liver and the kidney; however, it is present in minute quantities

II. Methoxyflurane toxicity
   A. The primary metabolites of methoxyflurane metabolism
      1. Fluoride ions; all patients recovering from methoxyflurane anesthesia have elevated inorganic fluoride levels
      2. Dichloroacetic acid
      3. Methoxyfluroacetic acid (fluoride and oxalic acid)
      4. Carbon dioxide
   B. Renal and liver failure may occur following methoxyflurane anesthesia in dogs, particularly if the animal is receiving other potentially nephrotoxic drugs (tetracyclines, aminoglycosides)
   C. Nephrotoxicity
      1. Fluoride ions are excreted by the kidney and are known nephrotoxins that can cause tubular injury

      2. The degree of renal injury is dose related

      3. Adequate fluid replacement should be provided to ensure maximum excretion of fluoride ions

      4. Tetracyclines may impair renal function, leading to renal failure

      5. Both high- and low-output forms of renal failure may occur

      6. Clinical studies in normal dogs have not demonstrated renal dysfunction after clinical dosages of methoxyflurane

   D. Recommendations

      1. Methoxyflurane should be avoided in elderly and obese patients, especially those with impaired renal function

      2. Tetracycline or aminoglycoside antibiotics should not be administered concurrently with methoxyflurane

III. Isoflurane, enflurane, sevoflurane, and desflurane toxicity

   A. Metabolism

      1. Defluoridation of isoflurane and desflurane does not result in clinically significant concentrations of serum fluoride ions

      2. Metabolism of enflurane and sevoflurane results in higher fluoride concentrations, but they seldom reach the threshold for nephrotoxicity

      3. Sevoflurane interacts with CO_2 absorbants (e.g., soda lime), producing an olefin referred to as *Compound A*

         a. Toxic concentrations of Compound A have not been observed during small animal anesthesia

   B. Desflurane resists degradation by the liver

   C. All agents predispose some animals to malignant hyperthermia

   D. Future clinical and laboratory evaluation of these agents may reveal additional concerns

IV. Nitrous oxide toxicity

   A. Nitrous oxide is not metabolized in vivo

   B. It undergoes a physiochemical reaction with vitamin B_{12}

      1. This reaction results in megaloblastic bone marrow changes and neurologic disease

      2. Indirectly inhibits deoxyribonucleic acid synthesis, resulting in reproductive disorders

    C. Toxic effects appear after relatively long-term exposure (more than 10 hours)

    D. Clinical use is not associated with any direct toxic effects

       1. Diffusion hypoxia and diffusion into closed cavity spaces are discussed in Chapter 11

V. Barbiturate toxicity

    A. In general, clinical use of barbiturates does not manifest any direct cellular toxicities

       1. Barbiturates stimulate liver microsomal enzymes and may alter the metabolism of other drugs

       2. Some seemingly normal animals appear to be sensitive to the cardiorespiratory depressant effects of barbiturate anesthetics; this clinical observation is probably a result of inadvertent overdosage, but it may result from idiosyncracy (although unlikely)

       3. Thiobarbiturates increase the susceptibility to the development of ventricular arrhythmias

       4. Thiobarbiturates are metabolized slowly in sight hounds or animals with poor liver function, resulting in prolonged recovery from anesthesia

VI. Propofol toxicity

    A. Intravenous (IV) infusions administered for greater than 3 consecutive days result in significant Heinz body production, lethargy, anorexia, and diarrhea in normal cats

    B. Prolonged administration (more than 3 hours) will lead to drug accumulation and longer recovery from anesthesia

VII. Local anesthetic toxicity

    A. In general, the proper administration of local anesthetics has little or no deleterious effects on tissues

    B. Toxic reactions primarily affect the CNS and the cardiovascular system

       1. Acidosis and hypoxia potentiate toxicity

       2. Sensitivity is increased by rapidity of injection

    C. CNS toxicity

       1. Dose necessary to produce CNS toxicity is usually less than the dose that causes cardiovascular collapse

       2. Excessive levels of agents such as lidocaine can cause hypotension, anxiety, tremors, convulsions, or coma

    D. Cardiotoxicity

       1. Rapid IV injection of more potent local anesthetics (e.g., bupivacaine) may cause cardiovascular collapse

      2. Ventricular dysrhythmias and fatal ventricular fibrillation result

      3. Resuscitation is more difficult following bupivacaine

      4. Pregnant animals may be more sensitive

VIII. Narcotic, ataractic, and cyclohexamine toxicity

  A. These drugs have little or no toxic effect on the different organ tissues when administered in anesthetic dosages

  B. Deleterious side effects

    1. Narcotics

      a. The most common are hyperexcitability, respiratory depression, and bradycardia

      b. Anaphylactic reactions

      c. Blood dyscrasias, thrombocytopenia

    2. Ataractics

      a. Phenothiazine tranquilizers

        (1) Noted for their sympatholytic and hypotensive effects

        (2) Rarely cause extrapyramidal behavioral changes and bradycardia

      b. Butyrophenone tranquilizers can cause aggressive behavior and, rarely, excitement

      c. Benzodiazepines; propylene glycol, a preservative and diluent for diazepam, may cause bradycardia and cardiac arrest

      d. α_2-agonists cause significant respiratory depression and bradycardia

    3. Cyclohexamines

      a. Produce an apneustic pattern of ventilation and increased arterial PCO_2, resulting in respiratory acidosis

      b. Prolonged recovery from anesthesia may occur following the administration of Telazol to cats and pigs

WASTE ANESTHETIC GAS POLLUTION

  I. Waste anesthetic gases are the portion of fresh gases delivered through the anesthetic system that are not inhaled or absorbed by the patient

  II. Pollution and staff exposure occur when anesthetic waste gases leak into the environment

III. Health concerns
   A. Adverse effects associated with chronic exposure to trace levels of waste gases include increased incidence of spontaneous abortion, birth defects, neoplasia, hepatic and renal disease, neurologic disturbances, hematopoietic changes, infertility, and pruritus
      1. Individuals at highest risk
         a. Persons with preexisting hepatic or renal disease
         b. Persons with immune system compromise
         c. Women in the first trimester of pregnancy
   B. Anesthetics incriminated
      1. Nitrous oxide
      2. Halothane
      3. Methoxyflurane
      4. Enflurane
      5. Isoflurane
   C. Epidemiologic studies, animal studies, and human volunteer studies reveal conflicting evidence
      1. To date, there is no definitive cause-and-effect relationship between exposure to waste gases and disease
      2. Overall evidence implies a potential hazard
IV. Regulations regarding waste anesthetic gas levels
   A. Standards for maximum allowable concentrations have been established by the National Institute for Occupational Safety and Health
   B. Recommended acceptable levels
      1. Volatile agents used alone: less than 2 ppm
      2. Volatile agents combined with nitrous oxide: less than 0.5 ppm
      3. Nitrous oxide: less than 25 ppm
      4. Levels are time-weighted averages over the span of surgical procedure(s)
   C. These standards are used by the Occupational Safety and Health Administration (OSHA) when inspecting veterinary hospitals
V. Monitoring for waste gas levels
   A. Continuous sampling
      1. Instantaneous point sampling in many areas
      2. Immediate results
      3. Expensive equipment

B. Instantaneous (grab) sampling
   1. Room air aspirated into a container and sent to a laboratory for evaluation
   2. Delayed results
   3. Results may not reflect overall exposure
   4. Inexpensive and easy to perform
C. Time-weighted average sampling
   1. Samples absorbed by a collection device over a period of time
   2. Delayed results
   3. Best indication of overall exposure
   4. Inexpensive and easy to collect
VI. Collection and removal of waste gases
   A. Scavenging is the collection and removal of waste gases from the anesthetic system and the workplace (Fig. 13-1)
   B. Scavenging systems are made up of the following major components:
      1. Pressure relief valve (pop-off)
         a. Collects excess gases for conduction to removal system

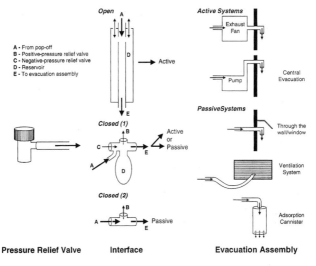

Fig. 13-1
Different methods of scavenging waste anesthetic gases.

b. May need to be modified or replaced for leak-free connection to transfer tubing
c. In nonrebreathing circuits, waste gases are collected from the reservoir bag
2. Interface
   a. Protects breathing circuit and patient from excessive positive or negative pressures
   b. Located between the pop-off valve and the disposal system
   c. Open interfaces contain no valves and are open to the atmosphere
      (1) Best suited for use with high-flow active evacuation systems
      (2) Must have reservoir to buffer pressure differences
      (3) Safety depends on the number of vents
      (4) Economical and easily made
   d. Closed interfaces contain mechanical pressure relief valves
      (1) Best suited for use with low-flow active or passive evacuation systems
      (2) Positive-pressure relief valve protects system from pressure buildup if the line is occluded
      (3) Negative-pressure relief valve required for use with active evacuation system
      (4) Does not require a reservoir, except when active evacuation is used
      (5) More costly, but safer and more versatile
3. Evacuation systems
   a. The evacuation system moves the collected waste gases to a remote area for release
   b. Passive evacuation systems
      (1) The flow of gases is controlled by ventilation
      (2) Gases are exhausted into a non-recirculating ventilation system, directly out into the atmosphere
      (3) Inexpensive and easy to install
      (4) Inefficient and a potential hazard to the patient because of potential resistance to exhalation

      c. Active evacuation systems
        (1) Mechanical flow-inducing devices
        (2) Consist of a central vacuum system or a dedicated fan or pump
        (3) Negative pressure produced requires an interface with a negative pressure relief valve
        (4) More costly and complex than passive systems
        (5) More effective than passive systems
      d. Activated charcoal absorption cannisters
        (1) Remove hydrocarbons
        (2) Do not remove nitrous oxide
        (3) Require frequent replacement
    4. Transfer tubing
      a. Connects the different components of the system
      b. Tubing should be resistant to kinking, easily differentiated from the breathing circuit, and able to transfer high flows
      c. Tubing for passive systems should be as short and wide as practical

VII. Additional control methods
  A. Pressure check all breathing circuits and machines for leaks (see Chapter 15)
  B. Use agent-specific bottle cap adaptors when filling vaporizers to avoid spillage, and fill at the end of the work day when fewer people are present
  C. Use low flow or closed-system techniques whenever possible
  D. Check endotracheal tube cuff before use and be sure it is adequately inflated during use
  E. Avoid chamber and mask inductions; when they cannot be avoided, use tight-fitting mask and attach scavenger tubing to chamber
  F. Ventilate areas where inhalation anesthesia is commonly used and areas where animals are recovering; remain at least 3 feet from the recovering patient's head
  G. Do not turn on vaporizer until patient is connected to the circuit
  H. When disconnecting the patient from the breathing circuit, turn off flowmeter and vaporizer, occlude Y piece, and evacuate remaining gas in the system into the scavenger

I. Wear a half-mask respirator if waste gases cannot be avoided

J. Inform all employees of potential risks associated with waste gas exposure and emphasize measures to reduce exposure

OXYGEN TOXICITY (HYPEROXIA)

I. Tolerance to oxygen

A. Exposure of animals to increased oxygen tensions (more than 40%) at atmospheric pressures for prolonged periods (more than 24 hours) causes metabolic derangements resulting in pulmonary dysfunction; changes include decreases in vital capacity, lung compliance, minute ventilation, respiratory rate, pH, arterial oxygen partial pressure, total lung volume, and carbon dioxide-diffusing capacity

B. Animals show considerable variation in the susceptibility to oxygen toxicity

C. The rate of onset of the disease process is proportional to the inspired tension of oxygen and the duration of exposure

D. Reductions in vital capacity and pulmonary compliance are the best criteria for identifying the onset of toxicity

II. Mechanisms of pulmonary oxygen toxicity

A. Although oxygen is necessary for the production of energy and survival of all aerobic cells, it is also a cellular poison

1. Cellular injury results from the metabolic processing of oxygen itself

2. The majority of oxygen entering the body is metabolized to create adenosine triphosphate and enzymatically reduced to form water

3. Free radicals are active products of this process: superoxide anion (O_2^-), the hydroxyl radical (OH^-), and hydrogen peroxide (H_2O_2)

4. Elevated levels of these products released when increased tensions of oxygen are administered and thought to be the cause of biologic membrane damage related to oxygen toxicity

5. Interaction of free radicals with side chains of membrane lipids results in the formation of lipid peroxides, which

inhibit many enzyme activities and further by-products that can create holes in cell membranes

6. Damaged membranes leak fluids into extracellular spaces

7. Inflammation and phagocytosis occur, producing additional free radicals

III. Lesions

  A. Pulmonary responses to increased oxygen tension

    1. Low doses of oxygen (25% to 60%) are associated with proliferative changes in endothelium and epithelium and permanent widening of the interstitium caused by increased collagen and elastin fiber deposition

    2. Exposure to high concentrations (more than 60%) of oxygen for more than 12 hours results in the following:

      a. Pulmonary capillary endothelial congestion and hyaline accumulation, type 1 epithelial cell death

      b. Enhanced alveolar epithelial permeability

      c. Interstitial and alveolar edema

      d. Atelectasis; increased shunting

      e. Intraalveolar hemorrhage

    3. Bronchiolar epithelium is also damaged to a lesser degree

  B. Hemolysis

  C. Multi-organ damage (retinal, hepatic, renal, and myocardial)

IV. Signs of toxicity

  A. Early signs

    1. Restlessness

    2. Coughing

    3. Anorexia and lethargy

    4. Dyspnea

  B. Late signs

    1. Respiratory insufficiency

    2. Cyanosis

    3. Frothy or bloody fluid from mouth

    4. Asphyxia

V. Conditions contributing to toxicity

  A. General rate of metabolism affects the response to oxygen toxicity

  B. Hyperthyroidism and elevations of adrenocortical hormones hasten toxicity

    C. The depression of cellular activity by anesthesia decreases susceptibility to oxygen toxicity

    D. Preexisting pulmonary disease and hypoxia may help protect against rapid onset

    E. Increased susceptibility may result from extremes in humidity, hypercapnia, acidosis, hyperthermia, and pulmonary edema

VI. Recommendations

    A. Do not overreact to the use of oxygen

        1. Hypoxia is commonly associated with anesthesia and hypoventilation, and the damage it causes occurs rapidly

        2. Pulmonary injury from oxygen is uncommon, and onset is slow

        3. Early symptoms are fully reversible on termination of oxygen administration

    B. There are no known contraindications to the use of pure oxygen for brief periods or in emergencies; in the normal lung, no significant toxicity develops if pure oxygen is given for 12 hours or less

ANESTHETIC DRUG INTERACTIONS

I. Pharmacologic drug interactions: combinations of two or more drugs may be additive, supra-additive (synergistic), or antagonistic, thereby enhancing or negating expected effects and side effects; experience with tested drug combinations is the best way to avoid problems; for example, the combination of opioids (morphine) and α_2-agonists (medetomidine) can produce bradycardia and apnea

    A. Blood or blood products with calcium-containing solutions other than saline

    B. Acidic drug with basic drug

        1. Thiobarbiturate plus lidocaine

        2. Sodium bicarbonate with calcium-containing solutions

        3. Diazepam with oxymorphone or butorphanol

II. Pharmacokinetic interactions: interactions affecting absorption, distribution, or elimination of a drug

    A. Protein-binding effects

        1. Phenylbutazone displaces thiobarbiturates from binding sites, resulting in relative barbiturate overdose

        2. Decreased protein binding is caused by hemodilution of intravenous fluid administration

   B. Alterations in biotransformation

        1. Barbiturates enhance liver microsomal enzyme activity

        2. Organophosphates inhibit plasma cholinesterase, prolonging the duration of action of ester-linked local anesthetics and depolarizing muscle relaxants

        3. Cimetidine and chloramphenicol reduce hepatic microsomal enzyme activity, thus prolonging the duration of action of some drugs

        4. Epinephrine prolongs local anesthetic duration of action, and hyaluronidase increases the area of local anesthetic spread

III. Chemical interactions: combining two or more drugs in solution may result in a chemical incompatibility; unless you are certain there is not incompatibility, do not combine drugs

IV. Pharmacodynamic interactions: the actions of a drug on a particular organ system or on the body as a whole can be altered by concurrently administered drugs

   A. Agonist-antagonist interactions

        1. Narcotic agonists-antagonists

        2. α_2-agonists: yohimbine/tolazoline/atipamazole

        3. Nondepolarizing muscle relaxants-cholinesterase inhibitors

        4. Benzodiazepines: flumazenil

        5. Autonomic receptor agonists-antagonists

   B. Other alterations in pharmacodynamics

        1. Arrhythmogenicity of halothane in presence of catecholamines

        2. Enhancement of halothane-catecholamine arrhythmias by certain drugs, such as barbiturates, xylazine, or ketamine

        3. Decrease in digitalis-induced arrhythmias by halothane

        4. Epinephrine induces hypotension after acepromazine administration

        5. Aminoglycoside antibiotics prolong effects of muscle relaxants

        6. Tetracyclines enhance nephrotoxicity of methoxyflurane

        7. The development of acute (thiobarbiturates) and delayed tolerance (opioids) to drugs

CHAPTER FOURTEEN

Anesthetic Machines and Breathing Systems

"Give the tools to him that can handle them."
NAPOLEON BONAPARTE

OVERVIEW

A variety of equipment is used to deliver inhalation anesthetic drugs. Volatilizing the anesthetic and safely delivering it to the patient, while minimizing environmental pollution, requires relatively sophisticated, expensive, and, at times, cumbersome devices. Regardless of their apparent complexity, most inhalation anesthetic delivery systems use similar, simple designs for the delivery of oxygen, safe anesthetic concentrations, and the removal of carbon dioxide. This chapter describes the anesthetic machine, breathing circuits, and ancillary equipment for delivering inhalation anesthetics to animals.

GENERAL CONSIDERATIONS

Most anesthetic delivery systems contain the same components. They reduce the pressure of stored oxygen and nitrous oxide and precisely mix these gases with potent inhalation anesthetics for delivery through a breathing system.

ANESTHETIC EQUIPMENT

I. Compressed gases: oxygen, nitrous oxide, and other select gases come in color-coded cylinders of varying size (Table 14-1). They are used as carrier gases for delivering inhaled anesthetics

TABLE **14-1**
COMPRESSED GASES

CYLINDER SPECIFICATION (LITERS, STP)

AGENT	COLOR	E (4 IN × 30 IN)	G (8 IN × 55 IN)	H (9 IN × 55 IN)	FILLING PRESSURE (PSI)
Oxygen	Green	655	5290	6910	2200
Nitrous oxide	Blue	1590	12,110	14,520	750
Carbon dioxide	Gray	1590	4160		800
Helium	Brown	500	4350	5930	1650

STP, Standard temperature and pressure; *psi,* pounds per square inch.

A. Cylinders should be handled carefully
   1. Never leave a cylinder sitting upright
      a. Store E cylinders in a rack
      b. Secure H cylinders to the wall or a transport cart with a chain
   2. If it is dropped, a cylinder may explode because it is under high pressure
   3. Open cylinder valves slowly and completely
   4. Crack the cylinder valve (open and shut quickly) before attaching it to the machine to remove dust from the connecting port
   5. Install a new gasket supplied with each full cylinder to the connecting port
B. Most machines have a hanger yoke for attaching one or more E cylinders; hanger yokes and E cylinders are keyed (coded) with a pin index safety system that prevents inadvertent connection of the wrong cylinder to the wrong gas yoke on the machine (Fig. 14-1)
C. Centralized oxygen sources usually use G or H cylinders
   1. H cylinders require an individualized pressure regulator (thread size and connection are coded for different types of gas)
   2. These cylinders are attached to the machine by a length of high-pressure hose connected to the Diameter Index and Safety System (DISS) fitting of the machine

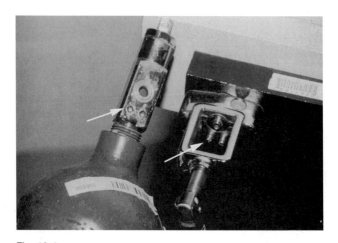

Fig. 14-1
The pin index system ensures that the appropriate tank is properly secured to the anesthetic machine.

       3. In other systems, the high pressure hose is connected to a special yoke-block connector that attaches to the pin index system in the hanger yoke

    D. Oxygen and nitrous oxide

       1. Oxygen is present within the cylinder only as a gas, and its pressure is proportional to gas volume

       2. Nitrous oxide is present within the cylinder as a liquid and a gas; pressure within the tank remains constant at 750 psi until all the liquid is gone and then falls

    E. Oxygen generators can be installed for central gas supply; they extract oxygen from room air to 90% to 95% O_2

  II. Hanger yoke site of E-cylinder attachment

    A. Pin index system configuration avoids improper cylinder connection

    B. A brass filter prevents particulate contamination of the anesthetic machine's gas lines

    C. Pressure gauges located at the back of the anesthetic machine measure cylinder pressure

    D. One-way valves prevent transfilling of cylinders or cylinder into pipeline supply

III. Pressure-reducing valves (pressure regulators) are built into most anesthetic machines
    A. Reduces the pressure of the gas within the cylinder to a constant pressure of approximately 50 psi
    B. Provides constant pressure to the flowmeter
    C. Allows a wide range of flowmeter settings
    D. Ensures that the flowmeter does not have to operate at high pressures
    E. Hospital supply cylinders (G & H) require individualized regulators (see I,C,1 p. 211)

IV. Oxygen "fail-safe" system
    A. If the oxygen supply is interrupted, nitrous oxide and any other gas flow is automatically interrupted
    B. An audible oxygen supply failure alarm is also activated on some machines

V. Flowmeters
    A. A flowmeter (ml/min; L/min) controls the rate at which a specific gas is delivered; the most common gas flowmeter is the rotameter; it contains a ball or bobbin that rises within a glass tube to a height proportional to the flow of gas through the tube; the gas flow rate is read at the widest diameter of the ball or bobbin
    B. Ideally, the oxygen flowmeter should be the last in a series of flowmeters (a hypoxic gas mixture is less likely to develop if a flowmeter tube is cracked)
    C. Avoid excessive torque when closing flowmeters, because the knobs can be twisted off
    D. Flowmeter tubes are gas specific; an N_2O flow tube cannot be substituted for an O_2 tube
    E. Individual gas flows are combined downstream from the flowmeters; from here, gases move to an out-of-circuit vaporizer or directly to the anesthetic circuit or circle
    F. Some machines are equipped with two oxygen flowmeters
        1. They are typically connected in series; the flow from both is additive
            a. One flowmeter is used for low flows (up to 1 L/min)
            b. The other is used for flows greater than 1 L/min

VI. Oxygen flush valve
- A. Bypasses the vaporizer and delivers oxygen directly to the common gas outlet or anesthetic circle
- B. Delivers oxygen to the circle at 35 to 75 L/min
- C. Dilutes the anesthetic gases in the system

VII. Common gas outlet: the point-of-gas-exit from the machine for oxygen, nitrous oxide, and vaporized (out-of-circuit) gas anesthetic; has a 15-mm connector

VIII. Anesthetic vaporizers
- A. Vaporizers are designed to volatilize liquid and inhaled anesthetics and to deliver clinically useful concentrations of anesthetic vapor
- B. Vaporizers are located near the flowmeters out of the anesthetic circle (vaporizer out of circle, VOC) or within the anesthetic circle (vaporizer in the circle, VIC)
- C. Vaporizers out of the circle (VOCs)
  1. Variable bypass vaporizers (i.e., gas flow within the vaporizer is split between the bypass and vaporization chamber); the splitting ratio is determined by the desired output (%) of anesthetic vapor and the specific anesthetic
  2. Precision-type vaporizers
     a. Deliver precise anesthetic concentrations (%) of anesthetic vapor that are relatively independent of temperature and flow rate; the manufacturer specifies limits of temperature and flow
     b. Can change anesthetic concentration relatively rapidly
  3. VOCs are agent specific
     a. Isoflurane vaporizers
        (1) Ohio Calibrated Vaporizer for Isoflurane (Ohmeda)
        (2) Vapor 19.1 (Dräger)
        (3) Fortec and Fortec 4 and Isotec 5 also sold as Isotec (Cyprane, serviced by Ohmeda)
        (4) Isoflurane can be used in halothane vaporizers if the vaporizer is completely drained and the wick is thoroughly dried
        (5) Halothane vaporizers that have been recalibrated for isoflurane use are available from several suppliers

b. Halothane vaporizers
  (1) Fluotec Mark II, III, IV, V (Cyprane, Matrix)
  (2) Vapomatic (old Foregger Fluomatic; A.M. Bickford)
  (3) Vapor and Vapor 19.1 Halothane (Dräger)
  (4) Ohio Calibrated Vaporizer for Halothane (Ohmeda)
c. Sevoflurane vaporizers
  (1) Tec III (converted enflurane vaporizers); Sevoflurotec (Tec 5)
  (2) Sevomatic (A.M. Bickford)
d. Desflurane vaporizer
  (1) Tec 6 vaporizer (Ohmeda): electronically heated vaporizer; unique construction because of the physical-chemical properties of desflurane
e. Methoxyflurane vaporizers
  (1) Pentec Mark II (Cyprane, serviced by Fraser Harlake)
  (2) Pentomatic (Foregger)
  (3) Vapor-Methoxyflurane (Dräger)
f. Enflurane vaporizers
  (1) Enfluratec (Cyprane, serviced by Ohmeda)
  (2) Enflurane Vapor 19.1 (Dräger)
  (3) Ohio Vaporizer for Enflurane (Ohmeda)
g. Vaporizers used for various inhalation agents (measured flow, nonagent specific) except desflurane
  (1) Vernitrol (Ohio Medical)
  (2) Copper Kettle (Foregger)
  (3) A separate flowmeter controls carrier gas flow through vaporizer
  (4) Slide rule or calculator needed to determine vaporizer flowmeter setting
    (a) Vapor pressure (depends on inhalant anesthetic chosen and temperature)
    (b) Desired total gas flow
    (c) Desired anesthetic percent
  (5) A slide rule is provided by most manufacturers for calculating flow rate through the vaporizer; an exception is the old Metomatic 980; it is a Vernitrol with specific calibration marks for

methoxyflurane that should not be used for other inhaled anesthetics

h. Maintenance

(1) Vaporizers should be sent to the manufacturer yearly for cleaning and recalibration

(2) They should also be serviced whenever the control dial becomes "sticky" or whenever the dial setting (%) does not match clinical perception

D. Vaporizers in the circle (VICs) (also called draw-over vaporizers); the animal's breathing moves the gas through the vaporizer and volatizes the anesthetic

1. Draw-over vaporizers are not agent specific

2. Output depends on the following:

a. The inhalant anesthetic's volatility

(1) Less volatile agents (e.g., methoxyflurane) require a wick; more volatile inhalants (halothane, isoflurane, sevoflurane) need no wick

b. Temperature

(1) Vapor pressure and therefore vaporizer output increases or decreases with ambient temperature

(2) Overdose can occur at high ambient temperatures

(3) Animals may be difficult to keep anesthetized at low ambient temperatures

c. Flow-through vaporizer

(1) Controlled by animal's minute ventilation; increases in depth and rate of ventilation (spontaneous or assisted) increase the vaporizer output

d. Vaporizer construction

(1) Wick versus no wick; adjustable sleeves; distance between the surface of the liquid and the gas flow

e. Location of vaporizer in the breathing circuit

(1) The vaporizer should be mounted on the inspiratory side to reduce the condensation of water in the vaporizer

3. Calibration marks on top of the vaporizer are not synonymous with the percentage output of VIC vaporizers

4. Types
   a. Ohio No. 8 Vaporizer (Pitman-Moore); wick must be removed when using with halothane, isoflurane, or sevoflurane
   b. Stephens Universal (Henry Schein); wick must be removed when using with halothane, isoflurane, or sevoflurane
   c. Komasarof
   d. Others: Goldman, EMO, McKesson, Rowbotham

5. Maintenance: wick should be allowed to dry weekly to rid system of excess water vapor

E. General comments
   1. Vaporizers should ideally be filled with anesthetic at the beginning or end of the day to minimize exposure of personnel to vapor
   2. Vaporizers must be in the off position when filling or draining
   3. Special filling devices are available to minimize spills and escape of vapors into the environment
   4. Vaporizers should not be tilted or laid on their sides unless completely drained; dangerously high concentrations can result during subsequent use

ANESTHETIC BREATHING SYSTEMS

I. Purpose
   A. The safe delivery of inhaled anesthetics and oxygen
   B. Removal of carbon dioxide and excess anesthetic gases by one of three methods
      1. Dilution (e.g., T-piece systems)
      2. Nonrebreathing one-way valve systems are rarely used because disadvantages outweigh advantages (currently used in manual resuscitators)
      3. Carbon dioxide absorbants (baralyme, sodasorb)

II. Types of systems

    A. Open drop or cone system (Fig. 14-2)

        1. Features

            a. No reservoir

            b. Minimal or no rebreathing of expired gases

            c. Carbon dioxide removal by dilution

        2. Advantages

            a. Low cost of equipment

            b. Minimal or no rebreathing of expired gases

            c. Minimal resistance to breathing (especially open drop)

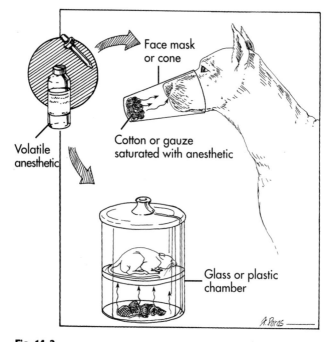

Fig. 14-2

Open system. Gauze or cotton is saturated with anesthetic and placed in a cone or chamber from which the animal breathes.

3. Disadvantages
   a. Wasteful because so much anesthetic is vaporized
   b. Difficult to control anesthetic concentration delivery
   c. No ventilation method
   d. Difficult or impossible to scavenge waste gas
   e. Vaporization of anesthetic depends on room temperature (open drop and cone)

B. Non-rebreathing systems (Mapleson) rely on a relatively high, fresh gas flow rate (Table 14-2) to remove carbon dioxide; the following classifications are based on the location of fresh gas inlet and opening (or valve) for exit of exhaled gas

1. Types
   a. Rees modification of Ayre's T piece (Fig. 14-3) (Mapleson F: fresh gas enters near the patient and exits from the reservoir bag)
   b. Bain circuit (modified Mapleson D): fresh gas enters circuit near the bag, but in the coaxial (tube in a tube) design, it delivers anesthetic near the patient; exhaled gas passes around the fresh gas line to exit near the bag (Fig. 14-4 and Fig. 14-5)
   c. Lack system (modified Mapleson A): fresh gas is delivered via a large bore corrugated tube surrounding a

---

TABLE **14-2**

RECOMMENDED OXYGEN FLOW RATES FOR ANESTHETIC SYSTEMS

Non-rebreathing systems	
Mapleson systems	
Magill system	100 ml/lb/min
Lack system	75 ml/lb/min
Ayre's T piece	0.5-2 L/min*
Bain circuit	100-150 ml/lb/min
Insufflation	100-150 ml/lb/min
Rebreathing or circle systems	
Closed	2-5 ml/lb/min†
Semi-closed low flow	5-10 ml/lb/min‡
Semi-closed high flow	10-50 ml/lb/min‡

*Indicates total flow rate for non-rebreathing (O_2 plus N_2O).
†Cannot use nitrous oxide in a closed circle.
‡If using nitrous oxide, add to the O_2 flow.

Ayres Y or T piece system

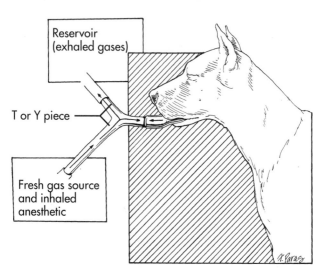

Reservoir
(exhaled gases)

T or Y piece

Fresh gas source
and inhaled
anesthetic

Fig. 14-3
Mapleson F (Ayres T piece). Low resistance method of delivering anesthetic and oxygen. High, fresh gas flow rates are used to minimize or eliminate the rebreathing of exhaled gas. Exhaled gas flows through corrugated tubing into a rebreathing bag. Excess gas is vented through an opening in the bag.

smaller inner tube that carries exhaled gas to a pop-off valve at the distal end of the circuit (opposite of the Bain; Fig 14-4)

d. Magill system (Fig. 14-6) (modified Mapleson A): fresh gas enters near bag and exhaled gas exits through a pop-off valve located near the patient
    (1) Efficient during spontaneous ventilation
    (2) Very inefficient during controlled ventilation
    (3) Advantages: low equipment dead space, low resistance to breathing
    (4) Disadvantages: wasteful; rapidly decreases patient's temperature; difficult to scavenge

Bain (modified Mapleson D)

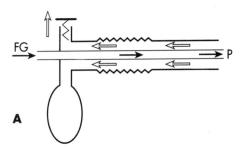

A

Lack (modified Mapleson A)

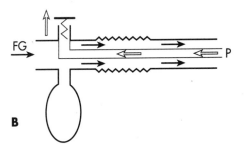

B

Fig. 14-4
Examples of non-rebreathing systems. *FG,* Fresh gas; *P,* patient.

C. Rebreathing systems allow rebreathing of exhaled gases minus carbon dioxide; amount of rebreathing depends on the fresh gas flow rate
   1. Circle system (Figs. 14-7 and 14-8)
      a. Components
         (1) Pop-off (pressure relief) valve
            (a) Allows the release of excess pressure from the system; the volume of gas in excess of the animal's minute oxygen consumption is vented from the system
            (b) Fitted with spring-loaded or variable orifice valves; modern valves usually "pop off" or

Bain circuit

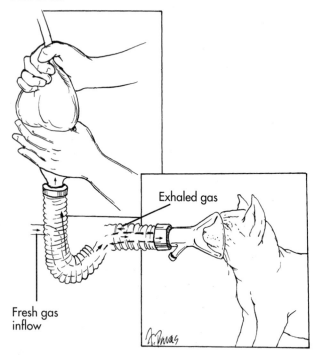

Exhaled gas

Fresh gas
inflow

Fig. 14-5

Modified Mapleson D Bain circuit. Functions similarly to Ayres T-piece system. It is designed to minimize equipment dead space and facilitate warming of the inspired gases.

open when pressure exceeds 0.5 to 1 cm H_2O; as valve is tightened down, more pressure is required to open valve

(c) Fitted with orifice for scavenging waste gas
2. Carbon dioxide absorbant canister
   a. Removes carbon dioxide from the expired gases
   b. Capacity should be one to two times tidal volume (5 ml/lb)

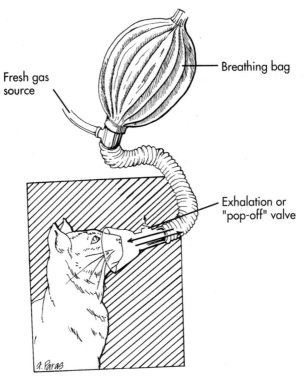

Fig. 14-6
Mapleson A Magill system. Low, fresh gas flow rates can be used during spontaneous ventilation because of the presence of a pop-off valve near the patient that preferentially exhausts alveolar gas.

  c. Absorbant used is either soda-lime or barium hydroxide-lime; Na^+, K^+, Ca^{++}, and Ba^{++} hydroxide reacts with exhaled CO_2 and water to form carbonate; heat is liberated, pH decreases

  d. Uses 4- to 8-mesh, granule-size soda-lime

  e. Absorbant has a pH color-change indicator (ethyl violet) that turns blue on consumption; the indicator may revert to its original color when allowed to rest; it should be changed after 6 to 8 hours of use, depending on fresh gas flow rates and size of the animal

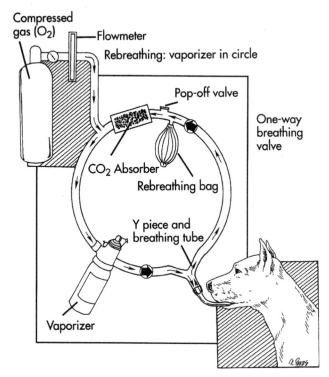

Compressed
gas (O$_2$) — Flowmeter
Rebreathing: vaporizer in circle
Pop-off valve
One-way
breathing
valve
CO$_2$ Absorber
Rebreathing bag
Y piece and
breathing tube
Vaporizer

Fig. 14-7
Anesthetic circle system with the vaporizer in circle

   f. Absorbant becomes brittle, dusty, and clumps together
       when no longer useful
3. Two unidirectional flow valves prevent exhaled gas from
   being rebreathed before it passes through the absorbant
   canister
4. Vaporizer (in or out of the circle; see Figs. 14-7, 14-8)
5. Rebreathing bag (reservoir bag) is available in the following sizes:
   1L: for animals less than 15 lb
   2L: for animals more than 15 lbs but less than 40 lbs
   3L: for animals more than 40 lbs but less than 120 lbs

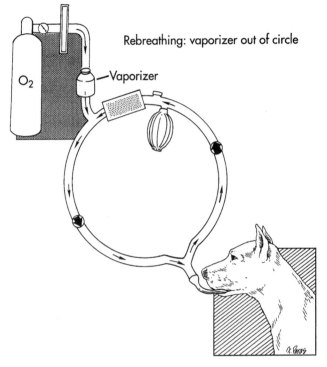

Fig. 14-8
Anesthetic circle system with the vaporizer out of circle.

        5L: for animals more than 120 lbs but less than 300 lbs
        35L (large-animal system): for animals more than 300 lbs
  6. Pressure manometer
     a. Monitors pressure within breathing system
     b. Typically calibrated from -30 to $+50$ cm H_2O
     c. Pressure within circle increases when bag is squeezed,
       particularly when the "pop-off" valve is closed
  7. Corrugated breathing tubes and Y piece
     a. Generally 1 m long and 22 mm in diameter
     b. Longer tubes are used when machines cannot be lo-
       cated near the patient's head

    c. Shorter tubes with small diameter (13 mm) are used for animals less than 10 lbs

    d. Large animal tubes are 50 mm in diameter

    e. Advantages:

       (1) Relatively low gas flow rates can be used (economical and minimize pollution)

       (2) Carbon dioxide-absorbent canister is located away from patient, as opposed to to-and-fro system

       (3) Ventilation is readily observed and controlled by reservoir bag

       (4) Minimal heat loss and airway drying

       (5) Absence of abrupt fluctuations in anesthetic depth

    f. Disadvantages:

       (1) System is bulky

       (2) Parts may be rearranged or may malfunction

       (3) Resistance to gas flow is greater than with Mapleson systems; conventional circle systems should not be used in animals less than 5 lb

       (4) Some components are difficult to clean

       (5) Cross-infection of patients is possible; bag and hoses should be disinfected after each use

       (6) Concentration within system typically is less than the vaporizer setting

       (7) System concentration slowly changes with changes in vaporizer setting

8. To-and-fro systems (Fig. 14-9); exhaled gas passes through the absorbant into the reservoir bag and during inhalation returns through the absorbant to the animal

    a. Same components as circle system minus the unidirectional valves

    b. Heat accumulates in the system because the carbon dioxide canister is attached near the endotracheal tube; alkaline dust from carbon dioxide absorbant may be inhaled

    c. Canister dead space increases with time because of the exhaustion of absorbant near the patient

    d. Advantages:

       (1) Low resistance and efficient carbon dioxide absorption

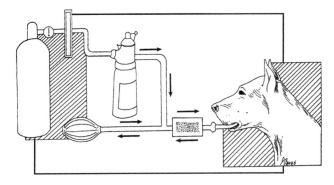

Fig. 14-9
The to-and-fro anesthetic system maximizes carbon dioxide removal and helps maintain body temperature

      (2) Maintains higher patient temperatures
      (3) Portable
      (4) Easily cleaned and disinfected
    e. Disadvantages:
      (1) Cumbersome because apparatus is near the animal's head
      (2) Different-sized canisters needed for different-sized animals
      (3) Possible inhalation of alkaline dust
  9. Fresh gas flow rates for rebreathing systems (see Table 14-2)
    a. Minimum flow rate equals minute oxygen consumption
      (1) Approximately 2 to 3 ml/lb/min
      (2) Because the volume of fresh gas delivered equals patient uptake, the volume of the system will not change; the pop-off valve can remain closed
      (3) Advantages of closed system
        (a) Minimal pollution
        (b) Economical
        (c) Breathing system warmth and humidity maximized

(4) Disadvantages

(a) Difficult to rapidly change concentration with VOC; VOC cannot be used with closed-system flow rate for the first 10 to 20 minutes because anesthetic uptake is too great; VOC can be used with closed-system flow rates from the beginning of anesthesia

(b) System volume must be more closely monitored

(c) Increased CO_2 absorbant use

(d) N_2O cannot be used without an oxygen monitor in the system

b. Flow rates in excess of 2 to 3 ml/lb/min require an open pop-off valve (semi-closed)

VETERINARY ANESTHETIC MACHINES

I. Machines are currently manufactured for veterinary use by the following companies:

A. Anesco: a variety of machines and ventilators for small and large animals

B. A.M. Bickford: several small-animal models

C. Bowring Engineering (United Kingdom): to-and-fro, circle systems for large and small animals

D. DRE: small-animal machine

E. Engler: small animal combination ventilator/anesthetic machine

F. J. D. Medical: several large-animal machines with ventilators

G. Mallard Medical: large-animal machines and ventilators

H. Matrix: several small-animal machines and ventilators and one large-animal machine

I. Minerve (France): small- and large-animal machines

J. Stephens anesthetic machine: in-circle vaporizer for small animals

K. Summit Hill: a variety of small-animal machines

II. Veterinary machines no longer manufactured
   A. Dupaco compact 78: small-animal machines
   B. North American Dräger Narkovet: small- and large-animal machines
   C. Pitman-Moore: 970, 980, and Vetaflex-5
III. Used human anesthesia machines are available through most anesthesia equipment dealers

CLEANING AND DISINFECTION

I. Breathing hoses and reservoir bags should be cleaned and disinfected after each use
   A. Wash with hot, soapy water and rinse
   B. Soak in a cold disinfectant solution such as Nolvasan or Cidex and thoroughly rinse
   C. Clean the external surfaces of the anesthetic machine daily with a spray cleaner
   D. Occasionally disassemble the dome valves and absorbant canister and wipe dry
II. Gas or steam autoclaving is not necessary unless gross contamination is present
III. Anesthetic machine check (Table 14-3)
   A. Verify proper machine function before each use; some checks should be performed daily, others before each use
   B. Consult the owners' manual for manufacturer's recommendations

TROUBLESHOOTING ANESTHETIC EQUIPMENT PROBLEMS

I. Rebreathing bag empty
   A. Flow rate is too low or the flowmeter control knob is turned off
   B. System leak
      1. Gasket on carbon dioxide canister improperly installed
      2. Hole in rebreathing bag or tubing
      3. Leak in endotracheal tube cuff
      4. Waste-gas scavenging system using active suction improperly regulated

TABLE 14-3
GENERIC ANESTHESIA MACHINE AND BREATHING CIRCUIT CHECK

I. Inspect machine
   A. Fill vaporizers, tighten filler caps, turn off vaporizers
   B. Fill CO_2 canister, and confirm that absorbant is functional
   C. Confirm proper function of unidirectional valves in circle-with surgical mask inhale and exhale through Y piece*

II. Confirm oxygen supply and failsafe
   A. Check cylinder pressure
   B. Turn on N_2O cylinder and flowmeter; turn O_2 cylinder off; N_2O float should drop to zero; reopen O_2 cylinder*

III. Verify proper flowmeter functions-bobbin or float should move freely throughout length of tube*

IV. Check breathing circuit
   A. Proper, tight connections
   B. Occlude Y piece, close pop-off valve, pressurize circuit to 30 cm H_2O; check for leaks; open pop-off valve and confirm release of pressure

V. Check waste gas scavenging system (if attached)*
   A. Confirm that scavenging system is connected to pop-off valve
   B. Turn on vacuum pump or verify patency of passive system

VI. Check ventilator function*
   A. Verify connection to breathing circuit
   B. Check for leaks according to manufacturer

*Need only be performed daily.

     5. Water drain near carbon dioxide absorbant canister is open

II. Rebreathing bag overly distended (positive pressure in circuit)
   A. Pop-off valve inadvertently left closed
   B. Flow rate too high in closed system
   C. Waste-gas scavenging system improperly regulated

III. Patient seems "light"
   A. Vaporizer empty, not working properly, or on an inadequate setting
   B. Excessive carbon dioxide buildup
      1. Exhausted carbon dioxide absorbant
      2. Sticky unidirectional valve
   C. Vaporizer needs service
      1. Water buildup on wick
      2. Recalibration necessary

    D. Patient receiving hypoxic gas mixture
      1. Nitrous oxide flowmeter set too high relative to oxygen flow
IV. Patient seems "deep"
    A. Vaporizer set too high or not working properly
    B. Patient severely hypercarbic or hypoxic
    C. Patient is hypotensive

CHAPTER FIFTEEN

Ventilation and Mechanical Assist Devices

"You don't need a weatherman to know which way the wind blows."

BOB DYLAN

OVERVIEW

One of the most crucial aspects of providing safe general anesthesia is the maintenance of normal ventilation. Normal ventilation is defined as the maintenance of arterial carbon dioxide levels within normal limits (35 to 40 mm Hg). Generally, respiratory effort can be verified by observing the movements of the patient's chest and abdominal wall. Although these movements may be regular and give the appearance of satisfactory gas exchange, they do not ensure adequate movement of air in and out of the lungs. Adequate gas exchange can be provided by inflating the lungs to a predetermined pressure or predetermined volume by manually squeezing a rebreathing bag on an anesthetic machine or using a mechanical ventilatory-assist device. Controlled ventilation helps to maintain a more stable plane of anesthesia since the lungs serve as the exchange site for inhalant anesthetic uptake and elimination. High-frequency ventilation of patients is a unique procedure based on the principle that diffusion is the primary means by which fresh gases are delivered to peripheral airways and gas exchange sites.

GENERAL CONSIDERATIONS

I. Artificial ventilation can do more harm than good if improperly used

II. Anyone attempting artificial ventilation should be thoroughly familiar with the equipment, procedure, and normal cardiopulmonary physiology and blood gas interpretation

III. Generally, mechanical ventilatory-assist devices do no more than compress a rebreathing bag to inflate the lungs; they are an extra pair of hands

IV. The use of artificial ventilation should be considered in patients who are not breathing adequately or are difficult to keep anesthetized

V. Blood gas determinations are the best test of ventilatory adequacy

REASONS FOR RESPIRATORY INADEQUACY

I. Depression of respiratory centers
   A. Drug induced
      1. Anesthetic
      2. Drug toxicities
   B. Metabolic
      1. Acidosis
      2. Coma
      3. Toxic metabolites (endotoxins)
   C. Physical
      1. Head trauma (increased intracranial pressure)

II. Inability to adequately expand the thorax
   A. Pain (splinting of chest)
   B. Chest trauma
   C. Thoracic surgery
   D. Abdominal distention
   E. Muscle weakness
   F. Obesity
   G. Bony deformities of the chest wall
   H. Positioning
      1. Weight of viscera may impede expansion
      2. Abdominal compression may impede expansion
   I. Neuromuscular blocking drugs (NMBDs)
   J. Severance of nerves
   K. Nerve trauma (edema)

III. Inability to adequately expand the lungs
   A. Pneumothorax (especially tension pneumothorax)
   B. Pleural fluid

    C. Diaphragmatic hernia
    D. Lung disease
    E. Neoplasia
    F. Pneumonia
    G. Atelectasis
    H. Positioning
    I. Airway obstruction
IV. Acute cardiopulmonary arrest
 V. Pulmonary edema or insufficiency

MANAGEMENT OF VENTILATION IN ANESTHESIA

  I. Anesthetics are respiratory depressants; therefore, ventilation may need to be assisted if hypoventilation occurs
 II. Special indications for artificial ventilation in anesthesia
    A. Thoracic surgery
       1. Controlled respiration minimizes extraneous chest wall movements, which aids the surgeon
       2. With the chest open, the patient cannot adequately expand the lungs (pneumothorax)
    B. Neuromuscular blockers (see Chapter 12): clinical doses of NMBDs, which produce muscular relaxation, also paralyze the diaphragm and intercostal muscles
    C. Prolonged anesthesia (more than 90 minutes), especially in the horse
    D. Trauma
       1. Flail chest
       2. Diaphragmatic hernia
    E. Maintain a more stable plane of anesthesia
    F. Drug overdose
    G. Convenience: eliminate concerns about hypoventilation and poor gas exchange (low O_2; high CO_2)

PHYSIOLOGIC CONSIDERATIONS

  I. Pulmonary system
    A. Normal lungs are well ventilated during spontaneous breathing due to the generation of different pressures, volumes, and flow rates (Fig. 15-1)

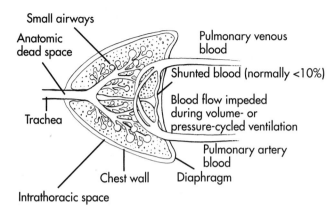

Small airways

Anatomic dead space

Pulmonary venous blood

Shunted blood (normally <10%)

Blood flow impeded during volume- or pressure-cycled ventilation

Trachea

Pulmonary artery blood

Chest wall   Diaphragm

Intrathoracic space

Fig. 15-1

Lung volume and airway pressure can augment or impede blood flow through the lung.

  B. During spontaneous ventilation, the portions of the lung in closest contact with moving surfaces (i.e., the peripheral lung field) undergo the greatest volume changes

  C. During artificial ventilation, pressure is introduced into the trachea, which inflates the peribronchial and mediastinal areas of the lung; the peripheral segments remain relatively hypoventilated compared to normal spontaneous breathing; pressure or volume ventilation increases airway diameter and thus anatomic dead space, further reducing alveolar ventilation

  D. Positive-pressure ventilation results in a significant reduction in lung compliance; the lung becomes stiffer, which can lead to atelectasis and hypoxemia

   1. Small airway closure can occur

   2. The distribution of ventilation is altered

   3. Volume-cycled ventilators compensate for worsening lung mechanics to a greater degree than do pressure-cycled ventilators (by ensuring delivery of a constant volume); pressure-cycled ventilators must be reset to compensate for "stiffened" lungs (periodic "sighs" are important)

TABLE 15-1
CARDIOVASCULAR SYSTEM: EFFECTS OF BREATHING AND INTERMITTENT POSITIVE-PRESSURE VENTILATION

PHASE OF CYCLE	INTRATHORACIC PRESSURE	TOTAL THORACIC BLOOD VOLUME	LEFT VENTRICLE CARDIAC OUTPUT
Normal breathing			
Inspiration active	$(-5$ cm of $H_2O)$	↑	↓
Expiration passive	↑ $(-2$ cm $H_2O)$	↓	↑
IPPV			
Inspiration passive	↑ (10-20 cm H_2O)	↓	↑ (↓ if IPP prolonged)
Expiration generally passive	↓ To atmospheric pressure	↑	↓

IPPV, Intermittent positive-pressure ventilation; *IPP,* intermittent positive pressure.

II. Cardiovascular system (Table 15-1)
   A. During spontaneous ventilation, the subatmospheric pressure within the thorax augments venous return; this subatmospheric pressure is reduced (made more negative) during inspiration by downward movement of the diaphragm
   B. During artificial ventilation, the pressure in the trachea and lung is transmitted to the thoracic cavity, thus impeding venous return and potentially decreasing cardiac output (Fig. 15-2; also see Fig. 15-1)
   C. Artificial ventilation decreases arterial blood pressure and cardiac output in any of the following instances:
      1. Average airway pressure consistently more than 10 mm Hg
      2. Low circulating blood volume caused by dehydration, anemia, and blood loss
      3. Impaired sympathetic nervous system activity caused by anesthesia, local anesthetics, and shock
   D. Artificial ventilation decreases pulmonary blood flow, and therefore, may lead to ventilation-perfusion abnormalities
   E. Circulatory changes during artificial ventilation are caused by prolonged increases in mean airway pressure and decreased CO_2

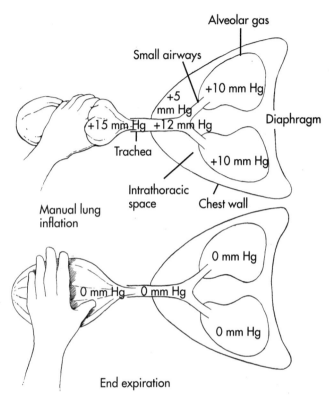

Fig. 15-2
Manual lung inflation produces a positive pressure in the lung and thoracic cavity, which impedes lung blood flow and lowers cardiac output.

III. Important normal values to remember
   A. Tidal volume (V_T): the amount of gas exchanged in one respiratory cycle
      1. 15 ml/kg in animals weighing less than 400 pounds
      2. 10 ml/kg in animals weighing more than 400 pounds
      3. Ventilator bellows volume is usually increased by 2 to 4 ml/kg over V_T during intermittent positive-pressure breathing (IPPV) to compensate for the increased positive pressure-induced volume of the breathing hoses and conducting airways (wasted ventilation)

B. Minute volume (V^m): the volume of gas exchanged in 1 minute
   1. Dependent on V_T and breaths per minute (BPM): $V_T \times$ BPM = V^m
C. Adequate inflation of the lungs of a normal animal requires approximately 15 to 20 cm H_2O pressure; lung compliance (volume/pressure/kg) is important in determining the pressure required to inflate the lung
D. The spontaneous ventilatory cycle
   1. Inspiration (I) is active
      a. 1 second in small animals
      b. 1.5 to 2 seconds in large animals
E. Guides to adequate mechanical artificial ventilation in the normal patient
   1. V_T (under normal conditions)
      a. Up to 10 to 15 ml/kg in small animals
      b. Up to 14 to 16 ml/kg in large animals
   2. Pressures
      a. 15 to 20 cm H_2O in small animal species with normal lungs; 20 to 30 cm H_2O in large animal species with normal lungs
      b. During open-chest procedures or in the presence of "stiff" or mechanically inhibited lungs, pressure must be increased
   3. I/E (inspiration/expiration) ratios
      a. 1:2 to 1:4.5 in small animals
      b. 1:1 to 1:4.5 in large animals
   4. Inspiratory times during artificial ventilation
      a. Less than 1.5 seconds in small animals
      b. Less than 2 to 3 seconds in large animals (e.g., 2 seconds in a 450-kg horse)
      c. Observation of chest wall movements is a reliable indicator for lung inflation

CLASSIFICATION OF VENTILATORS

I. Volume preset (Fig. 15-3)
   A. A gas or gas mixture is delivered to a preset volume by the ventilatory-assist device

Volume-cycled Ventilation

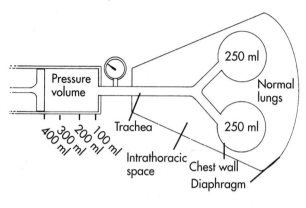

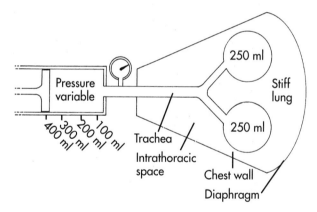

Fig. 15-3
Volume-preset ventilators deliver a predetermined volume regardless of the pressure developed.

B. Advantages
1. Delivers a known V_T regardless of the pressure imposed
    a. Most volume-cycled ventilators are equipped with a blow-off safety valve to prevent the development of extremely high pressure (more than 60 cm H_2O)

        b. Delivers a constant volume despite changes in compliance and resistance of the lungs during anesthesia

    2. Relatively simple machine

C. Disadvantages

    1. High airway pressures may develop

    2. Volume ventilators do not compensate for small leaks in the system; eliminating them requires an airtight system; a major leak prevents the patient from receiving an adequate V_T

D. Piston or bellows-type ventilator delivers a predetermined volume

E. Some are equipped with the ability to select a maximum pressure

II. Pressure preset (Fig. 15-4)

A. A gas or gas mixture is delivered by a ventilatory-assist device during the inspiratory phase until the system reaches a preset pressure

B. Advantages

    1. High safety factor; high pressure will not develop unless preset by the operator

    2. Compensates for small leaks; large leaks prolong inspiratory time

C. Disadvantages

    1. Volume delivered is variable and depends on the following:

        a. Lung compliance

        b. Airway resistance

        c. Number of functional alveoli

        d. Pressure within the thorax

    2. Measurement of tidal volume may be difficult if the ventilator is not equipped with bellows or a respirometer

    3. Pressure may need to be increased during a procedure to maintain adequate V_T

III. Time cycled: most volume-preset ventilators can be adjusted to limit the volume delivered through a combination of adjustments to the I : E ratio, frequency or respiratory rate (f), and inspiratory flow rate (most modern anesthesia ventilators are this type)

Pressure-cycled Ventilator

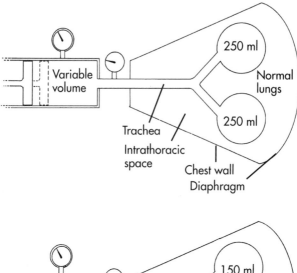

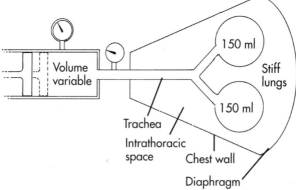

Fig. 15-4
Pressure-preset ventilators deliver a predetermined pressure regardless of the volume delivered.

IV. Volume-preset ventilators classified by bellows movement during expiration
   A. Ascending: preferred design since leaks are easily identified; bellows rise during expiratory phase
   B. Descending: bellows fall during expiratory phase

MODES OF OPERATION OF VENTILATORY-ASSIST DEVICES

I. Assist mode: patient triggers the ventilatory device by initiating an inspiratory effort

II. Controlled mode
  A. Operator sets the desired respiratory rate
  B. Ventilator is insensitive to the patient's inspiratory efforts
  C. If the patient resists controlled ventilation ("bucks" the ventilator), severe cardiopulmonary embarrassment may occur

III. Assist-controlled mode: a minimal respiratory rate is set by the operator, which the patient may override by initiating spontaneous ventilatory efforts at a faster rate

IV. Intermittent mandatory ventilation (IMV): used in intensive care unit ventilation; a predetermined number of positive breaths is set by the operator; the patient also breathes spontaneously through a parallel breathing circuit

TERMS USED FOR VARIABLE MODES OF OPERATION DURING MECHANICAL VENTILATION

I. **IPPV** (intermittent positive pressure ventilation): positive pressure maintained only during inspiration

II. **CPPV** (continuous positive pressure ventilation): mechanical ventilation with positive pressure maintained during inspiration and at lower pressure on expiration

III. **PNPV** (positive/negative pressure ventilation): positive pressure during inspiration and negative pressure during expiration

IV. **PEEP** (positive end-expiratory pressure): used to open small airways following lung trauma or pulmonary edema

V. **ZEEP** (zero end-expiratory pressure): normal passive expiration

VI. **NEEP** (negative end-expiratory pressure): used to hasten expiration

VII. **CPAP** (continuous positive airway pressure): spontaneous breathing with positive pressure during both inspiratory and expiratory cycles

VIII. **IMV** (intermittent mandatory ventilation): breaths supplied by ventilator, in addition to normal negative pressure breaths supplied by the patient

VENTILATORS COMMONLY USED IN VETERINARY MEDICINE

Most ventilators used during general anesthesia connect to the anesthesia breathing system where the rebreathing bag attaches; other free-standing ventilators are used without a breathing circuit

    I. Mallard medical microprocessor-controlled large animal anesthesia ventilator (Fig. 15-5)

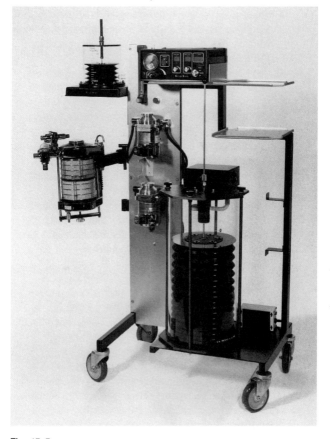

Fig. 15-5
Mallard anesthesia ventilator system shown with small and large animal ascending (standing) bellows and small animal circle attachment.

A. Classification: ascending bellows; time cycled, microprocessor controlled
B. Controls
   1. Inspiratory flow rate is adjustable between 10 and 600 L/min
   2. Respiratory rate
   3. Inspiratory time
C. Volume and pressure delivered are a function of adjustments in inspiratory flow rate, frequency, and inspiratory time
D. Ventilator bellows connect to rebreathing bag port of large animal circle system
E. PEEP capability

II. Anesco Large Animal Ventilator
   A. Classification: volume preset; descending bellows; time cycled
   B. Volume delivered depends on frequency, inspiratory flow rate, and inspiratory time

III. Hallowell EMC 2000-Volume Preset Small Animal Ventilator (also sold by Matrix, Inc. as model 3000)
   A. Ascending (standing) bellows
   B. V_T adjustable from 0 to 3000 ml
   C. Volume and pressure delivered are a function of adjustments in frequency and inspiratory time
   D. Interchangeable bellows for animals weighing 1 kg to 200 kg

IV. Anesco Small Animal Anesthesia Ventilator
   A. Ascending (standing) bellows
   B. Similar to Hallowell ventilator

V. Engler ADS 1000
   A. Microprocessor controlled
   B. Can be used with a vaporizer for anesthesia or without a vaporizer
   C. Nonrebreathing circuit principle of operation
      1. No CO_2 absorbant necessary
      2. No conventional anesthesia breathing circuit necessary
   D. Machine automatically selects ventilation parameters based on patient weight
   E. PEEP capability

VI. North American Dräger Large and Small Animal Anesthetic Ventilator
   A. Classification: volume-preset ventilator; time cycled; descending bellows
      1. Volume is adjusted by raising and lowering bellows support to appropriate level
      2. Pressure manometer indicates the pressure within the system
   B. Controls
      1. On/off switch
      2. Frequency is adjusted to breaths/minute
      3. Flow is adjustable; inspiratory flow rate determines inspiratory time
      4. I:E ratio is adjustable from 1:1 to 1:4.5
      5. Adjustment of flow rate, I:E ratio, and inspiratory time determine delivered volume
      6. Operates only in the control mode
   C. Pop-off valve
      1. Manual pop-off valve of breathing system must be closed during ventilator use
      2. Automatic pop-off closes with the inspiratory cycle
VII. Bag-in-a-barrel type ventilator, generally powered by a Bird pressure-cycled ventilator (J. D. Medical anesthetic machine)
   A. Classification: pressure-preset ventilator; descending bellows
   B. Large-animal ventilator
      1. Bag or bellows in a cylinder is compressed by the flow generated by a modified Bird Mark 7 ventilator
      2. Volume is indicated on the chamber encasing the bellows
      3. The pressure and f can be adjusted for the desired volume
   C. Mode
      1. Assisted: the sensitivity can be adjusted so that the patient can trigger the machine
      2. Controlled: the value of sensitivity can be decreased so that the patient cannot trigger the machine
      3. Assist-controlled: the operator can control the minimum number of breaths delivered; the patient can also trigger ventilator operation

D. Controls
  1. Inspiratory pressure
    a. Usually set at 20 to 30 cm water
    b. Adjusted for the desired tidal volume
  2. Expiratory time
    a. Controls respiratory rate by controlling time between breaths
    b. Rate usually set at 6 to 10 breaths/minute for horses
  3. Flow rate (adjust to an inspiratory time of 1.5 to 2 seconds for horses)
  4. Air mix: pull air mix knob to "out" position
    a. Set at 50% to conserve oxygen
    b. Does not affect oxygen supply to the animal
  5. Sensitivity
    a. Governs the animal's ability to trigger the ventilator
    b. Numbers are merely a rough guide to indicator of position

VIII. Bird Mark 7 and Bird Mark 9 ventilators
  A. Classification: pressure preset ventilator; volume delivered is controlled by the pressure developed unless the machine is equipped with a bellows
  B. Must be equipped with a bag-in-a-barrel or a bellows to be used as an anesthetic system; otherwise, it can stand alone as an intensive care ventilator
  C. Controls
    1. Inspiratory pressure
      a. Controls peak pressure
      b. Normally set at 15 to 30 cm water
    2. Sensitivity
      a. Controls animal's ability to trigger the machine
      b. Low numbers; easily triggered
      c. High numbers; difficult to trigger
    3. Inspiratory flow rate
      a. Controls inspiratory time
      b. Set equal to or less than expiratory time
    4. Expiratory time
      a. Controls respiratory rate by controlling expiratory time
      b. Respiratory rate is normally 6 to 12 breaths/minute

5. Air mix
    a. Varies percentage of inspired oxygen from 50% (knob out) to 100% (knob in)
    b. Negative pressure: (Bird Mark 9 only) allows the operator to produce NEEP

IX. Metomatic (Ohio) veterinary ventilator (small animals only)
    A. Classification: volume-preset ventilator; descending bellows; pressure limited
    B. Controls
        1. Tidal volume
            a. Controlled by adjustable knob
            b. Indicated on the front of the bellows
        2. Inspiratory flow rate
            a. Controls inspiratory time
            b. Adjusted to be equal to or less than expiratory time
        3. Expiratory time
            a. Controls rate by controlling length of expiratory phase
            b. Usually 6 to 12 breaths/minute
        4. Inspiratory hold
            a. Holds ventilator at peak pressure; used to eliminate atelectasis
            b. Can cause cardiovascular embarrassment if the chest is closed
        5. Inspiratory pressure
            a. Can limit maximal pressure
            b. Reduces the possibility of extreme pressure being placed on the chest
        6. Inspiratory trigger effort
            a. Governs an animal's ability to initiate inspiration
            b. Minimal trigger effort setting allows the ventilator to be used in assist or assist-control mode
        7. Expiratory flow rate
            a. Governs rate of fall of the bag (and therefore expiration)
            b. Adjusted to regulate impedance to expiration

HIGH-FREQUENCY VENTILATION (HFV)

I. HFV is a form of mechanical ventilation in which f is greater than 1 Hz (hertz), and V_T is less than anatomic dead space; generally one of three modes is used
   A. High-frequency, positive-pressure ventilation: f = 1 to 2 Hz; positive pressure maintained throughout the respiratory cycle
   B. High-frequency jet ventilation: f = 2 to 7 Hz; a small cannula is used to deliver jets of gas into the airway
   C. High-frequency oscillating ventilation: f = 6 to 40 Hz; bias flow of fresh gas entrained by oscillating the column of gas
II. Potential uses include acute respiratory distress syndrome, hyaline membrane disease, bronchopleural fistula, and pulmonary contusion

WEANING THE PATIENT OFF THE VENTILATOR

The initiation of spontaneous respirations following controlled ventilation can be hastened by the following methods:
   I. Decreasing the rate of controlled respiratory frequency
  II. Decreasing anesthetic depth
 III. Reversing neuromuscular blockade
  IV. Antagonism of opioid-induced respiratory depression
   V. Long-term ventilation patients require a more sophisticated approach to weaning from a ventilator (e.g., use of IMV)
  VI. Physical manipulation: rolling the patient, twisting an ear, pinching a toe
 VII. Respiratory stimulants: doxapram administration, 0.2 to 0.5 mg/kg intravenously

HAZARD PREVENTION

 I. Always be prepared to convert the anesthesia system back to the nonventilator mode in case of unforeseen ventilator problems; keep the rebreathing bag near the ventilator
II. Verify proper ventilator function before use; follow manufacturer's recommendations
   A. Verify that all controls are operational
   B. Perform a leak test

1. Ascending bellows: fill bellows using O_2; flush valve on anesthesia machine; occlude ventilator delivery hose; bellows will remain in fully ascended position if no leaks are present
2. Descending bellows: fully contract bellows; occlude ventilator delivery hose; bellows will remain fully contracted if no leaks are present

RESPIRATORY ASSIST DEVICES

I. Manual resuscitators
   A. Several models available
   B. Self-inflating bags and one non-rebreathing valve
   C. Useful for rapid emergency ventilation
II. Demand valves
   A. An apparatus that can be inserted into the proximal end of an endotracheal tube and is capable of delivering oxygen on demand from a patient-initiated breath or from operator assistance
   B. Inspiration is passive or assisted
   C. Expiration is passive
   D. Adapters are available for large and small animal use

CHAPTER SIXTEEN

Patient Monitoring During Anesthesia

"You see only what you look for, you recognize only what you know."

MERRIL C. SOSMAN

"Diligence is the mother of good fortune."

MIGUEL DE CERVANTES

OVERVIEW

A variety of simple and complex equipment is available for monitoring patients during anesthesia. Machines can record the electroencephalogram, the electrocardiogram (ECG), and the electromyogram (EMG) and facilitate their interpretation. Other machines monitor blood pressure (arterial or central venous pressure [CVP]); record and audibly transmit heart sounds; record peripheral blood flow; and measure arterial and venous pH, oxygen and carbon dioxide tensions, and arterial or capillary blood oxygen saturation (pulse oximetry). End-expired samples of respiratory gases can be monitored for oxygen/carbon dioxide content as well as inhalation anesthetic concentration. "Point of care" concepts and devices are available that permit patient side evaluation of the hemogram, pH and acid-base values, blood chemistries, and serum enzyme values within minutes of collecting a peripheral blood sample. All the monitoring equipment in the world, however, cannot replace an educated, attentive anesthetist.

GENERAL CONSIDERATIONS

  I. A patient's physiology and compensation mechanisms are altered by anesthetic drugs and by the pathophysiologic processes of disease
 II. Intraoperative patient monitoring optimizes anesthetic procedures in the following ways:
    A. Facilitates informed, flexible, and timely responses to changes in patient status by tracking physiologic variables
    B. Provides a data base for comparison to subsequent anesthetic procedures
III. Prerequisites for intraoperative monitoring
    A. Knowledge of pharmacodynamics, pharmacokinetics, and toxicity of anesthetic drugs and adjuncts
    B. Applied understanding of normal physiology and pathophysiology
    C. Thorough, accurate knowledge of the patient's physiologic status
    D. Availability of a convenient system for recording observations (anesthetic record)
    E. A thorough knowledge of the monitoring devices, their operation and limitations, and the inherent assumptions associated with their use

BASIC PRINCIPLES

  I. Monitor body functions (see Chapter 1 for normal values)
    A. Formulate a monitoring plan based upon the following:
      1. Patient's health status and disease(s)
      2. Specific procedure and duration
      3. Available monitoring equipment
      4. Anticipated duration of anesthesia
    B. Intraoperative decisions are based on comparisons to normal values (i.e., Are observed responses qualitatively and/or quantitatively appropriate? Are measured variables within normal limits?)
 II. Monitor more than one body system and more than one variable per body system, if possible
    A. Evaluating several values (e.g., heart rate, respiratory rate) rather than fragments of information increases the likelihood of correct assessment

B. Determining trends in the individual variables facilitates an early response

III. Use monitoring techniques that are specific, accurate, and complementary

A. Use simple, reliable techniques (e.g., visual inspection, palpation, auscultation)

B. Check instrument calibrations frequently; instruments may provide specific data, but inaccurate information may be confusing, misleading, and dangerous

C. Never totally depend on one piece of monitoring equipment

NONINVASIVE (INDIRECT) MONITORING TECHNIQUES

I. Information is gathered by observing readily apparent variables (e.g., counting respiratory rate) and/or noninvasive diagnostic testing (e.g., ECG, pulse oximeter, arterial blood pressure)

A. Advantages

1. Techniques are simple, reliable, and informative
2. Patient is not placed at risk for complications secondary to the monitoring technique

B. Disadvantages

1. Certain potentially useful physiologic variables cannot be accurately monitored noninvasively
2. Inaccurate information (highly variable) is sometimes gathered when a noninvasive technique (e.g., noninvasive arterial blood pressure) is substituted for a more invasive procedure (e.g., arterial catheterization) to determine the same information

INVASIVE (DIRECT) MONITORING TECHNIQUE

I. Information is gathered by placing instruments inside the body (e.g., intravascular pressure catheters)

A. Advantages

1. Physiologic data base is increased
2. Many techniques are accurate, reliable, and simple to perform
3. A direct measurement of a physiologic variable is often provided with fewer assumptions

B. Disadvantages
   1. Patient is at risk for secondary complications depending on technique; these complications include the following:
      a. Sepsis
      b. Direct tissue damage
      c. Inflammation with subsequent tissue damage
      d. Acute perturbation of tissue function (e.g., cardiac dysrhythmias)
   2. Some monitors require advanced technical knowledge and skills

PHYSIOLOGIC CONSIDERATIONS

I. Homeostasis
   A. Monitoring compensatory responses to anesthesia and surgical stimulation (Fig. 16-1; Tables 16-1 and 16-2)
      1. Responses observed
         a. Individual organ systems
         b. Integrated responses
      2. Invasive monitoring techniques may evoke additional responses

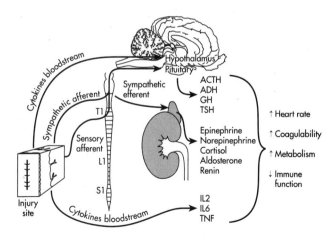

Fig. 16-1
Physiologic response to surgical stimulation; implications for patient monitoring.

TABLE 16-1
AMERICAN COLLEGE OF VETERINARY ANESTHESIOLOGISTS SUGGESTIONS FOR MONITORING

Circulation

Objective: to ensure that blood flow to tissues is adequate

Methods:
1. Palpation of peripheral pulse
2. Palpation of heart beat through chest wall
3. Auscultation of heart beat (stethoscope, esophageal stethoscope, or other audible heart monitor)
4. Electrocardiogram (continuous display)
5. Noninvasive blood flow or blood pressure monitor (e.g., Doppler ultrasonic flow detector, oscillometric flow detector)
6. Invasive blood pressure monitor (arterial catheter connected to transducer/oscilloscope or to anaeroid manometer)

Oxygenation

Objective: to ensure adequate oxygen concentration in the patient's arterial blood

Methods:
1. Observation of mucous membrane color
2. Pulse oximetry (noninvasive estimation of hemoglobin saturation)
3. Oxygen analyzer in the inspiratory limb of the breathing circuit
4. Blood gas analysis (PaO_2)
5. Hemoximetry (measurement of hemoglobin saturation in the blood)

Ventilation

Objective: to ensure that the patient's ventilation is adequately maintained
Methods:
1. Observation of chest wall movement
2. Observation of breathing bag movement
3. Auscultation of breath sounds
4. Audible respiratory monitor
5. Respirometry (measurement of tidal volume ± minute volume)
6. Capnography (measurement of CO_2 in end-expired gas)
7. Blood gas monitoring ($PaCO_2$)

Anesthetic record

Objective: to maintain a legal record of significant events and to enhance recognition of trends in monitored parameters
Methods:
1. Record all drugs administered to each patient, noting the dose, time, and route of administration
2. Record monitored parameters (minimum: heart rate, respiratory rate) on a regular basis (minimum: every 10 min) during anesthesia

Continued

TABLE 16-1

AMERICAN COLLEGE OF VETERINARY ANESTHESIOLOGISTS SUGGESTIONS FOR MONITORING—cont'd

Personnel

Objective: to ensure that a responsible individual is aware of the patient's status at all times during anesthesia and recovery, and is prepared either to intervene when indicated or to alert the veterinarian in charge about changes in the patient's condition

Methods:

1. If a veterinarian, technician, or other responsible person is unable to remain with the patient continuously, a responsible person should check the patient's status on a regular basis (at least every 5 minutes) during anesthesia and recovery

2. A responsible person may be present in the same room, although not necessarily solely occupied with the anesthetized patient (for instance, the surgeon may also be responsible for overseeing anesthesia)

3. In either of the above situations, audible heart and respiratory monitors are suggested

4. A responsible person, solely dedicated to managing and caring for the anesthetized patient during anesthesia, remains with the patient continuously until the end of the anesthetic period

TABLE 16-2
COMMONLY MONITORED PARAMETERS AND POTENTIAL CAUSES OF ABNORMAL RESPONSES

Heart rate

Tachycardia	Too "light," pain, hypotension, hypoxemia, hypercarbia, ischemia, acute anaphylactoid reactions, anemia, drug effects (e.g., thiobarbiturates, ketamine, catecholamines), fever, hypokalemia
Bradycardia	Too "deep," hypertension, elevated intracranial pressure, surgically induced vagal reflexes (e.g., visceral stretch responses), hypothermia, hyperkalemia, myocardial ischemia/anoxia, drug effects (e.g., xylazine, narcotics)

Respiratory rate and pattern

Tachypnea	Too "light," pain, hypoxemia, hypercarbia, hyperthermia, true or paradoxical CSF acidosis, drug effects (e.g., doxapram)
Apnea	Too "deep," hypothermia, recent hyperventilation (especially while breathing O_2-enriched gases), musculoskeletal paralysis (pathologic or pharmacologic), drug effects (e.g., ketamine, thiobarbiturates, propofol)

Arterial blood pressure

Hypotension	Too "deep," relative or absolute hypovolemia, sepsis, shock, drug effects (e.g., thiobarbiturate boluses, inhalation anesthetics)
Hypertension	Too "light," pain, hypercarbia, fever, drug effects (e.g., catecholamines, ketamine)

Corneal reflexes*

Hyperactive	Too "light," pain, hypotension, hypoxemia, hypercarbia, drug effects (ketamine)
Hypoactive	Too "deep," CNS depression (e.g., excessively deep anesthesia, acidosis, hypotension)

*Pertains to horses and ruminants only; not useful in pigs, dogs, and cats.
CSF, Cerebral spinal fluid; *CNS,* central nervous system.

II. Individual organ systems

    A. Central nervous system (CNS)

        1. Observe reflex activity to monitor degree of CNS depression

            a. Eye reflexes

                (1) Palpebral

                (2) Corneal

                (3) Nystagmus

                (4) Lacrimation

            b. Jaw tone

            c. Anal reflex

            d. Pedal reflex

        2. Monitor skeletal muscle relaxation

        3. Electroencephalography

            a. Records and averages brain activity

            b. Correlates to depth of anesthesia

        4. End-tidal concentration of anesthetic gases can be monitored and correlated to anesthetic depth (Fig. 16-2)

    B. Respiratory system (see Tables 16-1 and 16-2; Fig. 16-3 through 16-6)

        1. Noninvasive measurements

            a. Respiratory frequency

            b. Respiratory pattern

            c. Changes in tidal volume, noted by observing thorax and rebreathing bag

        2. Noninvasive equipment

            a. Esophageal or precordial stethoscope

            b. Breathing frequency monitors (see Fig. 16-4)

                (1) Activated by changes in airway temperature or gas flow

                (2) Some emit an audible tone

                (3) Some units contain alarms

            c. Pulse oximetry (see Fig. 16-5, *A*)

                (1) Measures pulse rate and functional oxygen saturation (SaO_2)

                (2) A spectrophotoelectric device applied directly to nonhaired skin over a pulsating vascular bed; light absorbance of oxygenated versus reduced hemoglobin detected and percentage of saturated hemoglobin are displayed numerically

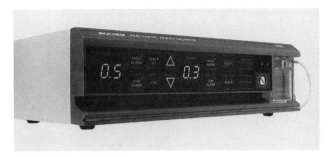

Fig. 16-2
Monitor that measures end-tidal concentration of inhalant anesthetics (halothane, isoflurane, sevoflurane) to ensure that proper anesthetic concentrations are being delivered to the patient.

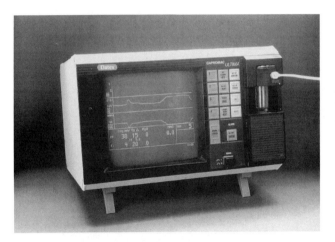

Fig. 16-3
This machine monitors end-tidal anesthesia concentration, CO_2, O_2, and pulmonary function.

(a) Inaccurate in the presence of carboxyhemoglobin or methemoglobin
(b) The pulsatile signal is reduced by hypotension, hypothermia, and altered vascular resistance, which limits SaO_2 determination

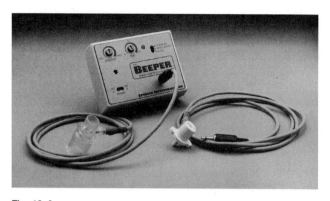

Fig. 16-4

Monitors that detect breathing frequency may be activated by changes in airway temperature (exhaled air is warmer).

        d. Analysis of inspired oxygen concentration

        e. Analysis of inspired or expired carbon dioxide concentration (capnography) (see Fig. 16-5, *B* and Figs. 16-6, *A, B*)

          (1) End tidal carbon dioxide ($ETCO_2$) measurements estimate alveolar concentrations

          (2) Useful when controlled ventilation is used

          (3) True alveolar concentrations are underestimated by 5 to 10 mm Hg

          (4) Measurements become more inaccurate during hypoventilation

        f. Spirometry (Fig. 16-7)

    3. Invasive measurements

        a. Hematocrit (packed cell volume percentage) and/or hemoglobin concentration

        b. Arterial and/or venous blood gas pH and lactate analysis (Fig. 16-8) (also see Chapter 17)

        c. Oximetry (oxygen saturation)

  C. Cardiovascular system (see Tables 16-1, 16-2)

    1. Heart rate

        a. Range of normal heartbeats, by species

          (1) Dog: 70 to 180

          (2) Cat: 145 to 200

Text continued on p. 265

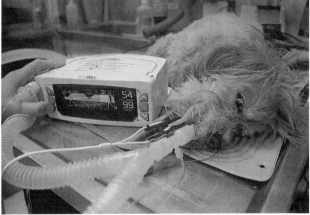

Fig. 16-5
A, Noninvasive, portable, battery-operated pulse oximeter for determining the oxygen saturation of hemoglobin (SpO_2). **B,** Capnograph for determining end-tidal carbon dioxide.

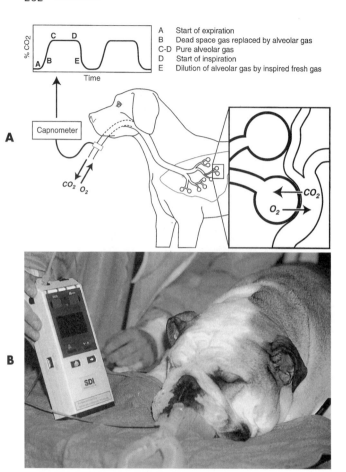

A Start of expiration
B Dead space gas replaced by alveolar gas
C-D Pure alveolar gas
D Start of inspiration
E Dilution of alveolar gas by inspired fresh gas

Fig. 16-6
ETCO$_2$ is an indirect method of assessing arterial CO$_2$.

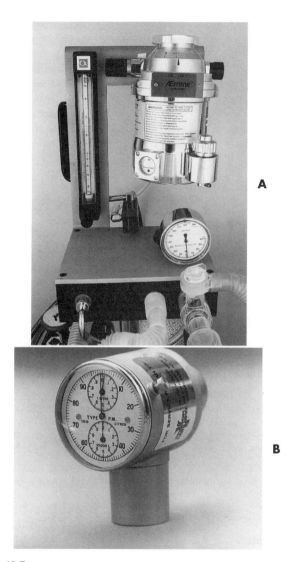

Fig. 16-7
Respiratory monitors used in anesthesia practice. **A,** P-N pressure gauge used
to monitor inspiratory pressure during ventilation. **B,** Ventilometer used to
measure tidal volume and minute volume.

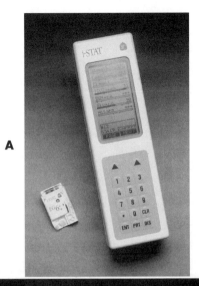

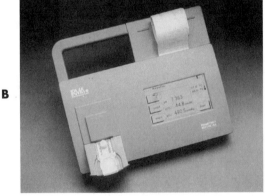

Fig. 16-8
Point of care blood chemical analyzers. **A,** i-STAT (Heska/Sensor Devices, Inc.). **B,** IRMA (Diametrics Medical, Inc.).

        (3) Horse: 30 to 45; up to 80 in foals

        (4) Cow: 60 to 80

        (5) Sheep, goat: 60 to 90

        (6) Pig: 60 to 90

        (7) Llama: 50 to 100

b. Limits of heart rate during anesthesia (values outside these limits indicate that cardiovascular function may be impaired)

        (1) Dog: $<50, >180$

        (2) Cat: $<100, >220$

        (3) Horse: $<28, >50$

        (4) Cow: $<48, >90$

        (5) Sheep, goat: $<60, >150$

        (6) Pig: $<50, >150$

        (7) Llama: $<50 >150$

c. Techniques for monitoring heart rate

        (1) Direct palpation of arteries or the heart

            (a) Dog: femoral, dorsal pedal, digital, and lingual arteries; precordium

            (b) Cat: femoral artery, precordium

            (c) Cow, sheep, and goat: auricular, digital, coccygeal, and dorsal metatarsal arteries

            (d) Horse: facial, transverse facial, dorsal metatarsal, and palatine arteries

            (e) Pig: femoral and auricular arteries

            (f) Llama: auricular, femoral artery

        (2) Indirect method uses esophageal stethoscope (Figs. 16-9 and 16-10)

            (a) Coupled to earpieces or to an electronic amplifier

            (b) Advantages: inexpensive; can detect abnormalities in rhythm as well as rate; can monitor breath sounds

            (c) Disadvantages: difficult to use for surgeries involving the mouth or throat

d. Peripheral pulse amplifiers

        (1) Applied over peripheral arteries; audible beep heard with each pulse

        (2) Advantages: can determine heart rate and rhythm

        (3) Disadvantages: prone to electrical interference; difficult to keep in place

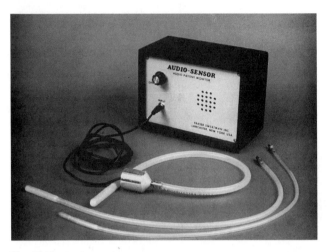

Fig. 16-9
Esophageal catheters are attached to a stethoscope or audio monitor to hear heart sounds and determine heart rate.

    e. Ultrasonic Doppler device
      (1) Doppler crystal applied over peripheral pulse; sound of blood flow amplified
      (2) Advantages: detects abnormalities in rhythm as well as rate; can also be used to estimate systolic BP
      (3) Disadvantages: accurate for systolic blood pressure only
    f. ECG, hand-held monitors are available; examples include Schiller Miniscope MS-3 (Heska/Sensor Devices, Inc.; Fig. 16-11, *A*); Biolog (Micromedical Industries, Inc.; Fig. 16-11, *B*)
      (1) Direct visualization of ECG, or sound amplifier that beeps with each R wave
      (2) Advantages: direct visualization of ECG allows interpretation of heart rate and rhythm
      (3) Disadvantages: ECG activity can continue to look and sound normal in the absence of a perfusing blood pressure (pulseless electrical activity)

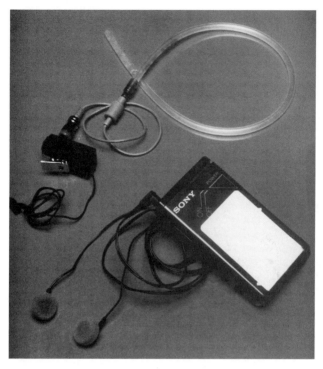

Fig. 16-10
Esophageal stethoscopes are attached to a transmitting device, which gives the anesthetist more freedom of movement.

      g. Pulse oximeters
        (1) Most units include heart rate
      h. Reasons for abnormal heart rates (see Table 16-2)
        (1) Bradycardia
          (a) Drugs: opioids, α_2-agonists (e.g., xylazine, medetomidine, detomidine, romifidine), anticholinesterases (e.g., neostigmine)
          (b) Excessive anesthetic depth
          (c) Hyperkalemia
          (d) Preexisting heart disease (second- or third-degree heart block)

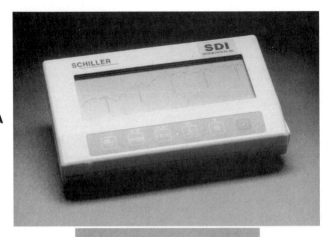

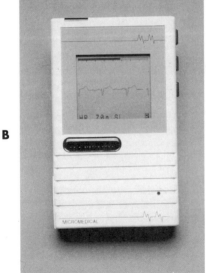

Fig. 16-11
Hand-held ECG monitors. **A,** Schiller Miniscope MS-3 (Heska/Sensor Devices, Inc.). **B,** Biolog (Micromedical Industries, Inc.).

      (e) Vagal reflex (intubation, oculocardiac reflex)

      (f) Terminal stages of hypoxemia

      (g) Hypothermia

   (2) Tachycardia

      (a) Drugs: ketamine, thiobarbiturates, anticholinergics, sympathomimetics, pancuronium

      (b) Hypokalemia

      (c) Hyperthermia

      (d) Inadequate anesthetic depth

      (e) Hypercarbia and hypoxemia

      (f) Anemia, hypovolemia

      (g) Hyperthyroidism, pheochromocytoma

      (h) Anaphylaxis

2. Peripheral perfusion
   a. A function of arterial BP and local vasomotor tone
   b. Assessment
      (1) Capillary refill time
         (a) Normal: less than 1 to 2 seconds
         (b) Assess on oral or vulvar mucous membranes
      (2) Urine production
         (a) Palpation of bladder
         (b) Urinary catheterization
         (c) Dog and cat: 1 to 2 ml/kg/hr
3. Central venous pressure (CVP) is obtained by measuring the mean right atrial pressure; awareness of the CVP value and monitoring its changes can be important in some clinical situations (Fig. 16-12)
   a. Physiologic significance
      (1) Right atrial pressure is a balance between the following:
         (a) Cardiac output: the forward flow of blood
         (b) Venous return: tendency for blood to flow from the peripheral veins back into the right atrium
   b. Range of normal values
      (1) 0 to 4 cm H_2O: standing, awake animals
      (2) 2 to 7 cm H_2O: anesthetized small animals
      (3) 15 to 25 cm H_2O: anesthetized large animals

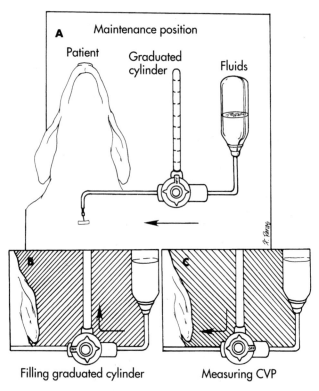

Fig. 16-12

A, CVP monitoring. **B,** A graduated cylinder at or below the level of the heart is filled with saline. **C,** The cylinder is then opened to the patient.

    c. Indications
        (1) Monitoring fluid therapy
        (2) Assessing cardiac output
            (a) Shock
            (b) Heart failure
            (c) Anesthesia
    d. Primary factors affecting CVP
        (1) Blood volume

      (a) Increase in circulating blood volume may cause an increase in CVP, as in overzealous intravenous fluid administration

      (b) Decrease in effective circulating blood volume may cause a decrease in CVP, as in dehydration and acute hemorrhage

  (2) Vascular tone

      (a) Venous dilation (e.g., acepromazine) may cause CVP to decrease because of peripheral pooling of blood and decreased venous return; venous constriction (e.g., alpha-2 agonists) produces the opposite effect

  (3) Cardiac contractility

      (a) Decreased by most anesthetic agents

      (b) Decreases may cause CVP to increase because of the decreased pumping of the heart

  (4) Heart rate

      (a) May decrease with onset of tachycardia or increase with onset of bradycardia

  (5) External cardiac factors

      (a) Intrathoracic pressure: elevations in intrathoracic pressure (positive-pressure ventilation) increase CVP; decreases in intrathoracic pressure decrease CVP

      (b) Intrapericardial pressure
- Cardiac tamponade
- Congenital pericardial herniation
- Ventricular filling is decreased or eliminated

      (c) Body position: primarily a factor in large animal species due to hydrostatic pressure (CVP may increase 10 to 15 cm H_2O when a horse is taken from standing to lateral recumbency)

e. Clinical approach to low CVP

  (1) Reduced effective circulating blood volume

  (2) Patients with relative or absolute hypovolemia should receive appropriate IV fluid until the CVP approaches the upper limit of normal range

   f. Clinical approach to elevated CVP
     (1) Generally indicates hypervolemia or myocardial depression/heart failure
       (a) Decrease or stop IV fluid administration
       (b) Administer drugs to improve cardiac function (dobutamine)
   g. Hazards of CVP measurement
     (1) Air embolism
     (2) Septicemia
     (3) Thrombophlebitis
   h. Equipment
     (1) IV catheter of sufficient length to reach the great veins in the chest (preferably the right atrium)
     (2) CVP manometer (see Fig.16-12)
       (a) Homemade
         • Three-way stopcock
         • Graduated cylinder or pipette
         • Connecting tubes
       (b) Commercially available
         • Baxter
         • Abbott
       (c) Appropriate fluids and a fluid administration set
   i. Procedure (see Fig. 16-12)
     (1) Thread a fluid-filled IV catheter into the jugular vein (toward the heart)
     (2) Flush the catheter with saline
     (3) Attach fluid-connecting tubes to the IV catheter
     (4) Attach a three-way stopcock and graduated cylinder
     (5) Attach the fluid administration line to the other port of the three-way stopcock
     (6) Suspend the graduated cylinder or pipette so that the three-way stopcock is below the animal's heart base; draw an imaginary line parallel to the floor between the animal's heart base and the cylinder; this marks the point of zero pressure on the cylinder
       (a) The heart base is marked by the sternum when the animal is in lateral recumbency

          (b) The heart base is marked by the point of the shoulder when the animal is standing or in dorsal recumbency

       (7) Let the fluid run through the system at the calculated flow (5 ml/lb/hr) until ready to record CVP

4. Arterial BP
   a. Noninvasive (NOTE: occluding cuffs should be one-half the width of the extremity they are placed around)
      (1) Oscillometric method (Fig. 16-13)
         (a) An air-filled occlusion cuff is placed around a peripheral limb (small animal, foal) or at the base of the tail (large animal); air is gradually released from the cuff until arterial pulsations (oscillations) are detected and electronically displayed
         (b) Advantages: easy to use; determines heart rate as well as systolic, mean, and diastolic BP

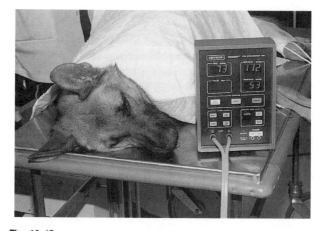

Fig. 16-13
Oscillometric peripheral pulse monitor, which is used to monitor pulse rate and blood pressure.

(c) Disadvantages: may not be absolutely accurate but should accurately reflect trends; difficult to get accurate data in animals weighing less than 8 lb (e.g., cats); accuracy depends on occluding cuff size; inaccurate at low BPs

(2) Ultrasonic Doppler apparatus (Fig. 16-14)
  (a) Doppler crystal placed over peripheral artery (e.g., dog: digital, dorsal pedal; horse: coccygeal)
  (b) Place appropriately sized inflatable cuff with pressure gauge proximal to Doppler crystal; inflate cuff until pulse sound stops, then slowly deflate until pulse is first heard; this corresponds to the systolic BP as displayed on the pressure gauge

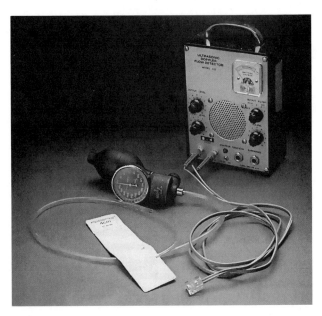

Fig. 16-14
An electronically activated Doppler crystal senses blood flow, which can be used to audibly broadcast and monitor blood pressure.

(c) Advantages: can count pulse rate and detect abnormalities in pulse rhythm

(d) Disadvantages: accuracy related to many factors; cuff size must be matched to limb circumference; measures systolic pressure only; inaccurate at low BPs

b. Invasive

(1) The technique of invasive arterial pressure monitoring provides an accurate quantitative value of the arterial pressure and a qualitative representation of the pulse waveform; BP is not an indicator of cardiac output (CO) (Figs. 16-15, 16-16)

(a) Monitoring patient's hemodynamic status

(b) Monitoring of hemodynamic effects of anesthetic drugs

(2) Physiologic significance

(a) Arterial blood pressure is expressed clinically in millimeters of mercury (mm Hg) with the zero reference at the level of the right atrium

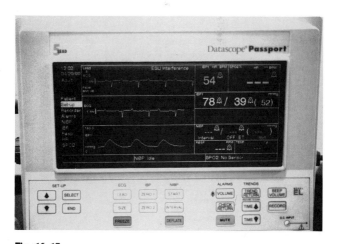

Fig. 16-15
Invasive blood pressure recording system, illustrating a pressure transducer for sensing pressure and oscilloscope for observing pressure waveforms.

(b) The mean pressure required to adequately perfuse these organs is approximately 60 mm Hg

(c) Normal arterial pressure values
- Systolic: 110 to 160 mm Hg
- Diastolic: 70 to 90 mm Hg
- Mean: 80 to 110 mm Hg
- Systolic-diastolic = pulse pressure

(d) Components of the pressure pulse (Fig. 16-17)

(e) Inotropic component: the steep ascending limb of the pressure pulse

(f) Late systole and diastole: blood pressure declines as the rate of runoff exceeds the volume input to the aorta
- Undulations in the diastolic decline are present when vascular tone is high and are caused by resonant waves in the great vessels and reflections of energy from the periphery

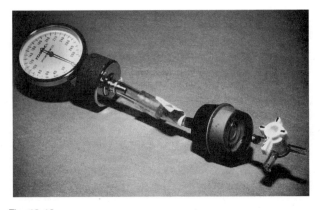

Fig. 16-16
A small blood filter attached to a three-way stopcock and then to a sphygmomanometer. This is an inexpensive method of monitoring mean arterial blood pressure.

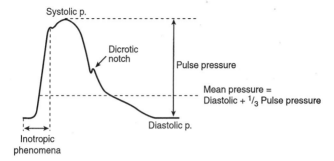

Fig. 16-17
Characteristics of the arterial pressure waveform.

(3) Primary factors affecting the arterial blood pressure
   (a) Arterial blood pressure = CO × total peripheral resistance (TPR)

$$BP = CO \times TPR$$

   - Factors increasing stroke volume or cardiac output favor an increase in arterial pressure
   - Factors increasing total peripheral resistance favor an increase in arterial pressure
   (b) CO = HR × stroke volume (SV)
   (c) Therefore:

$$\text{Arterial } BP = HR \times SV \times TPR$$

   - Indicating that decreases in HR, SV, or TPR individually or in any combination can decrease arterial blood pressure
   (d) Pulse pressure curves (Fig. 16-18)
(4) Clinical value of arterial pressure monitoring
   (a) Determine the effects of anesthetic drugs on cardiac output and peripheral resistance
   (b) Determine the adequacy of fluid therapy, drug administration (e.g., dobutamine) and ventilatory assist devices (Fig. 16-19)

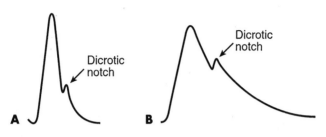

Fig. 16-18
Effects of peripheral artery vasodilation (**A**) and vasoconstriction (**B**) on the arterial blood pressure waveform.

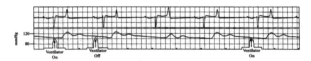

Fig. 16-19
ECG and arterial pressure waveform in an anesthetized 3-year-old horse. Note change in arterial pressure waveform during expiration.

       (c) Prevention of tissue ischemia and subsequent metabolic acidosis relies on normal mean BPs more than 60 mm Hg
- If mean BP is less than 60 mm Hg, treatment may include:
(1) Rapid IV fluid administration
(2) Decreased depth of anesthesia
(3) Initiation of positive inotrope therapy (e.g., dopamine, dobutamine)
(5) Hazards of invasive arterial pressure monitoring
       (a) Hematoma formation
       (b) Air embolization
       (c) Arterial thrombosis and occlusion (rare)
       (d) Infection (rare)
       (e) Formation of AV fistula or aneurysm (rare)

    (6) Equipment and procedure

        (a) Intraarterial catheter with three-way stop-cock

        (b) Pressure-sensing device

- Pressure transducer and oscilloscope
- Mercury manometer

        (c) Procedure

- Cannulate a peripheral artery aseptically with the arterial catheter
- Flush the catheter with heparinized saline; always aspirate first to prevent air embolism
- Attach the pressure transducer while stop-cock is closed to the artery
- Open the transducer to air to establish the baseline (zero) reference pressure with the transducer at the level of the right atrium
- Open the arterial line to the pressure transducer; pulse-pressure curve should be displayed at this point
- After removing the arterial catheter, place manual pressure on the site of cannulation for 5 minutes to prevent hematoma formation

D. Musculoskeletal system (see Chapter 12)

    1. Skeletal muscle tone

    2. Quality of elicited reflexes

    3. Peripheral nerve stimulation (see Fig.16-20; Fig. 16-21); used to assess quality of skeletal muscle responses during onset and reversal of neuromuscular blocking agents

III. Thermoregulation

A. Body temperature regulation is an integrated process involving the following body systems or organs:

    1. Central nervous system

    2. Cardiovascular system

    3. Musculoskeletal system

    4. Respiratory system

    5. Skin

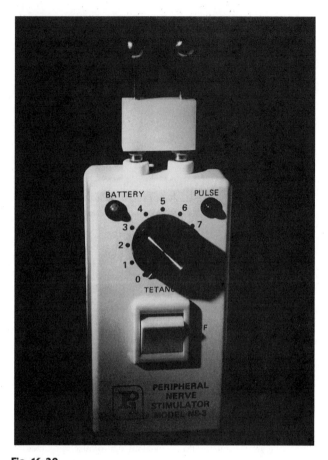

Fig. 16-20
One of a variety of peripheral nerve stimulators available to test the adequacy of neuromuscular blockade.

    B. Abnormalities of thermoregulation during anesthesia
        1. Hypothermia
           a. Heat loss in excess of production
           b. Most often encountered in small animals because of
              their larger ratio of surface area to body mass

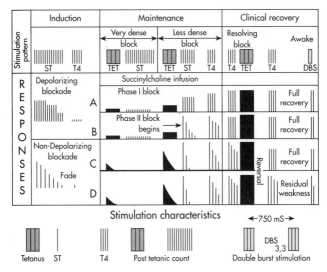

Fig. 16-21

Assessing neuromuscular function. Diagram simulates the clinical responses observed following neuromuscular stimulation. Stimulation patterns are depicted in the upper panel. (*ST,* Single twitch; *T4,* train of four; *TET,* tetanus; *DBS,* double burst-stimulation). The following four situations are demonstrated by the letters: *A,* The normal use of a succinylcholine infusion; *B,* the development of a phase II block; *C,* a nondepolarizing blockade that is reversed with full recovery; and *D,* a nondepolarizing blockade that demonstrates residual weakness.

From Barash PG, Cullen BK, Stoelting RK: *Clinical anesthesia,* ed 2, Philadelphia, 1992, JB Lippincott, p. 763.

       c. Potential causes
          (1) CNS depression
          (2) Vasodilation
          (3) Reduced heat production by skeletal muscle
          (4) Other iatrogenic causes
             (a) Cold IV fluids
             (b) Open body cavities
    2. Hyperthermia
       a. Heat production exceeding loss

b. Iatrogenically produced in response to specific drug combinations in certain species
   (1) Drugs: halothane, isoflurane, succinylcholine, and ketamine
c. Malignant hyperthermia is a genetic (autosomal recessive) defect most commonly reported in pigs; on rare occasions it is observed in dogs and other species
3. Monitoring body temperature during the anesthesia and postoperative periods should be considered an integrated response involving the specific species, drugs, and each of the body systems listed (Fig. 16-22)

IV. Integrated responses (see Table 16-2)
   A. Observed responses represent the outcome of a series of events involving simultaneous input and output of many systems, leading to combined autonomic endocrine and somatic responses (see Fig. 16-1)
   B. Integrated responses to diseases, surgical stress, and anesthetic-induced depression of certain functions are modulated by the autonomic nervous system and the adrenal medulla

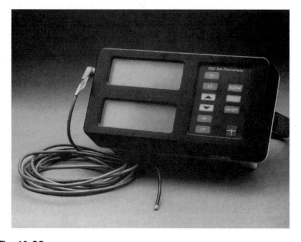

Fig. 16-22
Digital-display temperature monitoring device.

1. Sympathetic tone mediates "fight-or-flight" responses to any type of stress
   a. Causes of increased sympathetic tone
      (1) Pain
      (2) Hypotension
      (3) Hypoxemia
      (4) Hypercarbia
      (5) Ischemia
2. Parasympathetic tone may change as part of an integrated reflex
   a. Vagovagal
   b. Vagophrenic
   c. Vagal efferent (baroreceptor)

C. Correct interpretation of isolated responses requires an understanding of integration and the ability to work backwards from the observation to its cause

D. Acute intervention should be justified on the basis of the following:
   1. A set of monitored observations
   2. Rational selection of therapies to achieve desired physiologic goals
   3. The anticipated patient response

CHAPTER SEVENTEEN

Acid-Base Balance and Blood Gases

"The management of a balance of power is a permanent undertaking, not an exertion that has a foreseeable end."

HENRY KISSINGER

OVERVIEW

Traditionally, the diagnosis of acid-base disorders has hinged on the interpretation of changes in blood pH, PCO_2, and HCO_3^- concentration. Changes in pH signal either an increase (acidosis) or decrease (alkalosis) in hydrogen ions. The associated changes in carbon dioxide and bicarbonate concentration help determine the precise cause for the pH change. Alternatively, the diagnosis of acid-base disorders may be determined by changes in independent variables, which include PCO_2, strong ion concentration (e.g., Na^+, K^+, Cl^-), unmeasured anions, and total protein, which are responsible for determining the values of pH, PCO_2, and HCO_3^- (dependent variables). From a clinical standpoint, both approaches work, although the latter is usually more revealing when mixed acid-base disorders exist. Evaluation of a patient's acid-base status is useful in the diagnosis of disease processes and the formulation of therapy. Electrolyte abnormalities are frequently associated with, and may be responsible for, acid-base disorders, further emphasizing the importance of a basic understanding of pH, PCO_2, and electrolyte abnormalities.

GENERAL CONSIDERATIONS

I. Definitions

Acid: A substance that can donate a hydrogen ion (H^+)

$$Ex.: H_2CO_3 \rightarrow H^+ + HCO_3^-$$

Actual bicarbonate: The amount of bicarbonate (HCO_3^-), expressed in mEq/L of plasma

Base (B): A substance that can accept a hydrogen ion (H^+)

Examples: $OH^- + H^+ \rightarrow H_2O$
$HCO_3^- + H^+ \rightarrow H_2CO_3$

Base excess (BE): The amount of base above or below the normal buffer base, expressed in mEq/L, in blood; positive values (+) reflect excess of base (or deficit of acid), and negative values reflect a deficit of base (or excess of acid)

Buffer: A mixture of substances in a solution that resists or reduces changes in hydrogen ion concentration (changes in pH); important buffers in the body include hemoglobin and bicarbonate

BUFFERS IN WHOLE BLOOD	% BUFFERING
Hemoglobin and oxyhemoglobin	35
Organic phosphate	3
Inorganic phosphate	2
Plasma proteins	7
Plasma bicarbonate	35
RBC bicarbonate	18
Total	100

Free water: Water without electrolytes (pure H_2O); increases in free water can cause dilution acidosis; decreases in free water can cause contraction alkalosis

Partial pressure: The pressure an individual gas exerts on a column of mercury; expressed in mm Hg; see the following example of gaseous components of air

GAS (mmHg)	FRACTIONAL CONTENT (%)	PARTIAL PRESSURE
Nitrogen (N_2)	78.084	593.44
Oxygen (O_2)	20.948	159.2
Argon (Ar)	0.934	7.1
Carbon dioxide (CO_2)	0.031	0.24
Others	0.003	0.02
Total	100	760 (atmospheric pressure)

pH: The negative log of the hydrogen ion (H^+) concentration; the pH is inversely proportional to the H^+ concentration (Fig. 17-1)

Examples: $(H^+) = 0.000001 = 1 \times 10^{-6}$ pH = 6.0
$(H^+) = 1 \times 10^{-7}$ pH = 7.0
$(H^+) = 1 \times 10^{-8}$ pH = 8.0

P_{tot}: Total protein; increases in P_{tot} (weak acids) can cause metabolic (nonrespiratory) acidosis; decreases in P_{tot} cause metabolic alkalosis

Strong ions: Salts that are completely dissociated in water (e.g., Na^+, K^+, Cl^-)

Strong ion difference (SID): The difference in all the positive and negative strong ions; normally ($Na^+ + K^+ - Cl^-$); increases in SID usually cause metabolic (nonrespiratory) alkalosis; decreases in SID usually cause metabolic (nonrespiratory) acidosis

Total CO_2 content: The amount of carbon dioxide gas extractable from plasma; total CO_2 consists of:

HCO_3 (95% of the total CO_2 is HCO_3)
Carbonic acid ($H_2CO_3^-$)
Carbon dioxide

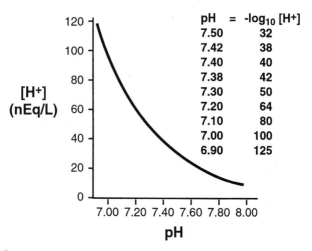

Fig. 17-1
The hydrogen ion-pH relationship.

Unmeasured anions: Strong ions (anions) that are not usually measured by chemistry machines (e.g., lactate; PO_4^{+2}, SO_4^{+2})

II. Many factors influence a patient's acid-base balance
   A. Species
   B. Diet (carnivorous versus herbivorous)
   C. Physical status
   D. Temperature
   E. Concentration of "strong" ions or salts that completely dissociate in water (e.g., Na^+, K^+, Cl^-, lactic acid)
   F. Total protein

III. Normal cellular metabolism continuously produces excess hydrogen ions, the concentration of which is regulated and eliminated by the lungs, kidneys, and gastrointestinal system to maintain an extracellular pH of approximately 7.4
   A. The kidneys eliminate hydrogen ions by excreting fixed acids
   B. The lungs reduce plasma hydrogen-ion concentration by eliminating carbon dioxide
   C. The gut participates in regulating pH by modulation of acid (HCl), base (Na^+, HCO_3^-), and water excretion

IV. Substances within the body known as *buffers* help minimize changes in pH

V. Determination of pH and blood gases is useful in determining patient acid-base status during anesthesia

VI. When interpreting the absolute values of a patient's pH and blood gases, the patient's clinical history and physical status should be considered

FORMATION AND ELIMINATION OF ACIDS AND BASES IN ANIMALS

I. The waste products of oral intake or metabolism are mostly acidic substances that release hydrogen ions
   A. Volatile acid: an acid that produces a gas
      $H_2CO_3 \rightarrow H_2O + CO_2$
   B. Nonvolatile or fixed acids: acids that cannot be converted to gas
      1. Lactate + H^+
      2. Sulfate + H^+
      3. Phosphate + H^+

II. The pathways for acid removal include the kidney, lung, and gastrointestinal tract

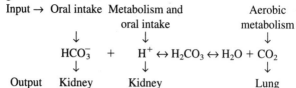

$$HCO_3^- \; + \; H^+ \leftrightarrow H_2CO_3 \leftrightarrow H_2O + CO_2$$

Input → Oral intake Metabolism and oral intake Aerobic metabolism

Output Kidney Kidney Lung

Gastrointestinal tract

This is the carbonic acid equation or CO_2 hydration equation and is the basis for explaining acid-base kinetics in the body.

A. High-protein diets (cats, dogs, pigs, humans)
  1. H^+ excess is derived from oxidation of neutral sulfur in these amino acids
    a. Methionine
    b. Cystine
    c. Cysteine
B. Diets high in plant material and grain have HCO_3^- excess from salts in:
  1. Fatty acids (acetate, propionate)
  2. Citrate (fruits)
  3. Gluconates

Example:

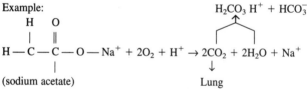

$$H-C-C-O-Na^+ + 2O_2 + H^+ \rightarrow 2CO_2 + 2H_2O + Na^+$$

(sodium acetate)   Lung

Metabolizable salts of fatty acids yield HCO_3^- after metabolism

C. Based on primary dietary intake
  1. Carnivores have acid urine or excess acid to excrete
  2. Herbivores have alkaline urine or excess base to excrete
D. Dietary and metabolic intake of acid or base equals the urinary and respiratory output, thereby maintaining the pH of the body fluids near 7.4
E. Many approaches to the diagnosis and treatment of acid-base disorders are based on the following (Henderson-Hasselbach equation):
  1. $CO_2 + H_2O \overset{CA}{\leftrightarrow} H^+ + HCO_3^-$ (carbonic anhydrase [CA])

2. $K_1 = \dfrac{[CO_2] + [H_2O]}{[H_2CO_3]}$

$K_2 = \dfrac{[H^+] + [HCO_3^-]}{[H_2CO_3]}$

3. $\dfrac{K_2}{K_1} = \dfrac{[H_+] + [HCO_3^-]}{[CO_2] + [H_2O]} = K_3$

4. Given: $[CO_2] = \alpha \times P_{CO_2}$ ($\alpha = 0.0301$ − solubility coefficient)

5. $\dfrac{K_3 \times \alpha P_{CO_2}}{[HCO_3^-]} = (H^+)$

$-\log (H^+) = pH; \quad -\log K_3 = pK$

pK is that pH at which 50% of an acid or a base is in the ionized state; The pK of the acid (pK_a) H_2CO_3 is 6.1

6. $-\log K_3 - \log \alpha P_{CO_2} + \log [HCO_3^-] = -\log [H^+]$

$pH = pK_a + \log \dfrac{[HCO_3^-]}{\alpha P_{CO_2}}$ (Henderson-Hasselbach eq)

F. In the body: pH = 7.4, pK_a = 6.1, P_{CO_2} = 40 mm Hg

1. $pH = pK_a + \log \dfrac{[HCO_3^-]}{\alpha P_{CO_2}}$

2. $7.4 = 6.1 + \log [HCO_3^-] - \log \alpha P_{CO_2}$

3. $1.3 = \log [HCO_3^-] - \log \alpha P_{CO_2}$

4. Antilog $1.3 = \dfrac{[HCO_3^-]}{0.0301 \times 40}$ antilog 1.3 = 20

$(HCO_3^-) = 20 \times 0.0301 \times 40 = 24$ mEq/L

ARTERIAL OXYGENATION

I. Normal gas partial pressures (expressed mm Hg) during inspiration in ambient air, conducting airways, terminal alveoli, and arterial and mixed venous blood*

	AMBIENT AIR	CONDUCTING AIRWAYS	TERMINAL ALVEOLI	ARTERIAL BLOOD	MIXED VENOUS BLOOD
P_{O_2}	156	149	100	95	40
P_{CO_2}	0	0	40	40	46
P_{H_2O}	15†	47	47	47	47
P_{N_2}	589	564	573	573	573
P total	760	760	760	755	706

*From Murray JF: *The normal lung,* ed 2, Philadelphia, WB Saunders, 1986.
†P_{H_2O} varies according to humidity and has a proportionate effect on P_{O_2} and P_{N_2}.

II. The inspired oxygen-arterial tension (FIO_2) relationship

    A. Relationship between FIO_2 and PaO_2

FIO$_2$%	PREDICTED IDEAL PaO$_2$ (mm Hg)
20	95 to 100
30	150
40	200
50	250
80	400
100	500

    B. The alveolar gas equation

$$P_{AO_2} = P_{IO_2} - \frac{P_{aCO_2}}{0.8}$$

III. Causes of arterial hypoxia (a reduction in PaO_2) and their effect on alveolar-arterial $P(A-a)O_2$ differences ([A-a]O_2D)

CAUSE	EFFECT ON ARTERIAL PO$_2$	EFFECT ON (A-a) O$_2$D
Hypoventilation	Decreased	No change
Diffusion abnormality	No change or decreased*	No change or decreased*
Ventilation perfusion imbalance	Decreased	Increased
Right-to-left shunt	Decreased	Increased
Reduction in inspired PO$_2$	Decreased	No change

IV. Oxygenation

    A. Efficiency of oxygenation

        1. P[A-a]O_2D

        2. PaO_2/PAO_2

---

*Effects of diffusion abnormalities are infrequently encountered at rest and are more likely to be evident during exercise.

3. Right-to-left shunt (when breathing 100% O_2)

$$Qs = \frac{(P_{AO_2} - Pa_{O_2})\,(0.003)}{4 + (P_{AO_2} - Pa_{O_2})\,(0.003)}$$

B. Adequacy of tissue oxygenation Pv_{O_2}

DELIVERY OF O_2 TO TISSUES

I. Dissolved
   A. Henry's law: Amount of O_2 dissolved is proportional to P_{O_2}; for each 1 mm Hg of P_{O_2}, there is 0.003 ml O_2/100 ml of plasma; content = solubility partial pressure
   B. Dissolved O_2 is not adequate to meet the animal's oxygen needs
II. Hemoglobin
   A. Conjugated protein of iron and porphyrin joined to the protein globin; globin has two alpha and two beta chains made of differing amino acid sequences
      1. Hemoglobin A: adult
      2. Hemoglobin F: fetal
      3. Hemoglobin S: sickle (valine-glutamic acid); poor oxygen-carrying capability
   B. Hemoglobin A is transferred from a ferrous to a ferric ion by oxidation (methemoglobin), which is not useful in O_2 carriage
      1. Nitrites
      2. Sulfonamides
      3. Benzocaine

O_2 DISSOCIATION CURVE (Fig. 17-2)

I. $O_2 + Hb = HbO_2$ (oxyhemoglobin); O_2 capacity is the amount of O_2 that can be combined with Hb; for example, 1 g Hb can combine with 1.39 ml of O_2; if there are 15 g Hb, then $1.39 \times 15 = 20.8$ ml O_2/100 ml at 100% saturation
II. O_2 saturation

$$\frac{O_2 \text{ combined with Hb} \times 100}{O_2 \text{ capacity}}$$

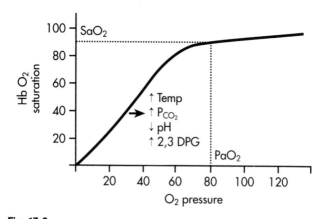

Fig. 17-2
The oxyhemoglobin dissociation curve. The effects of pH, PCO_2, temperature, and 2,3-diphosphoglycerate on hemoglobin saturation with O_2 are noteworthy, as is the effect of anemia (low Hb) on O_2 content.

III. O_2 content is the amount of O_2 present as dissolved O_2 and combined with Hb. Example: What is the O_2 content of blood if the hemoglobin concentration is 12 g/dl and the hemoglobin saturation is 96% when the PaO_2 is 100 mm Hg?

$$1.39 \text{ ml } O_2 \times 12 \text{ g (Hb)} \times 96\% = 16$$

$$100 \text{ mmHg} \times 0.003 \text{ ml/mmHg} = \frac{0.3}{16.3 \text{ ml } O_2/100 \text{ ml}}$$

IV. O_2 dissociation curve shape (see Fig. 17-2)
   A. Upper portion: PO_2 (partial pressure of oxygen) can fall slightly without affecting O_2 loading of Hb
   B. Lower portion: peripheral tissues can withdraw large amounts of O_2 with only small changes in PO_2; 5 g of reduced Hb can cause cyanosis (blue or purple discoloration of the mucous membranes)
V. Shifts in the O_2 dissociation curve are most commonly caused by changes in pH, PCO_2, and temperature
   A. Increasing temperature and PCO_2 and decreasing pH shifts the O_2 dissociation curve to the right; reverse changes have the opposite effect

B. 2,3-diphosphoglycerate (DPG) increases within red blood cells (RBC) in chronic hypoxia and shifts the O_2 dissociation curve to the right

C. Rightward shifts mean more unloading of O_2 at a given PO_2; normal PCO_2 at 50% O_2 saturation is approximately 26 mm Hg in a capillary

D. Deoxygenated Hb can carry more CO_2

CARBON DIOXIDE

I. Transport
   A. Dissolved in blood
      1. In plasma (as HCO_3^-)
      2. In RBCs as carbamino compounds
      3. Carried in physical solution
   B. The measurement of end-expired CO_2 ($ETCO_2$) and $PaCO_2$ permits the calculation of dead space ventilation (VD)

$$VD = \frac{PaCO_2 - ETCO_2}{PaCO_2}$$

CARBON MONOXIDE

I. $Hb + CO \rightarrow COHb$ (carboxyhemoglobin)
II. Carbon monoxide has about 210 times the affinity for Hb as O_2
   A. Small amounts of CO can tie up large amounts of Hb, making it unavailable for O_2 carriage
   B. PaO_2 is normal, but O_2 content is grossly reduced
   C. The oxyhemoglobin curve is shifted to the left, impairing O_2 unloading in tissues

NORMAL pH AND BLOOD GAS VALUES

I. pH = 7.40; range 7.35 to 7.45
II. PaO_2 = 95 mm Hg; range 80 to 110 mm Hg
III. PvO_2 = 40 mm Hg; range 35 to 45 mm Hg
IV. $PaCO_2$ = 40 mm Hg; range 35 to 45 mm Hg
V. $PvCO_2$ = 45 mm Hg; range 40 to 48 mm Hg

VI. $HCO_3^- = 24$ mEq/L; range 22 to 27 mEq/L (a little higher in horses and ruminants)

VII. The $PaCO_2$/pH/HCO_3^- relationship

PaCO₂ (mmHg) (ACUTE CHANGE)	pH	HCO₃⁻ (mEq/L) (EFFECT)
80	7.2	28
60	7.3	26
40	7.4	24
30	7.5	22
20	7.6	20

VIII. Nomenclature

   A. Acidemia: pH less than 7.35 (acid blood)

   1. Metabolic or nonrespiratory acidosis: an abnormal physiologic process characterized by a primary gain of acid (H^+) or primary loss of base (HCO_3^-) from the extracellular fluid

   2. Respiratory acidosis: an abnormal process in which there is a primary reduction in alveolar ventilation relative to CO_2 production ($PaCO_2$ increase)

   B. Alkalemia: pH greater than 7.45 (alkaline blood)

   1. Metabolic alkalosis or nonrespiratory: an abnormal physiologic process characterized by a primary gain in base (HCO_3^-) or loss of acid (H^+) from the extracellular fluid

   2. Respiratory alkalosis: an abnormal physiologic process in which there is a primary increase in alveolar ventilation relative to the rate of CO_2 production ($PaCO_2$ decrease)

   C. Compensation: an abnormal pH is returned toward normal by altering the component not primarily affected; for example, if the $PaCO_2$ is elevated, the HCO_3^- should be elevated (retained) to compensate

   1. If the $PaCO_2$ or HCO_3^- values are outside normal limits, but the pH is within the normal range, then the patient is fully compensated

   2. Because it takes time for the process of compensation to return the pH to within normal limits, a compensatory process implies a degree of chronicity

PRIMARY pH AND BLOOD GAS CLASSIFICATION

CLASSIFICATION	Paco₂	pH	HCO₃⁻	BE
Acute ventilatory failure	↑	↓	N	N
Chronic ventilatory failure	↑	N	↑	↑
Acute alveolar hyperventilation	↓	↑	N	N
Chronic alveolar hyperventilation	↓	N	↓	↓
Uncompensated metabolic acidosis	N	↓	↓	↓
Compensated metabolic acidosis	↓	N	↓	↓
Uncompensated metabolic alkalosis	N	↑	↑	↑
Compensated metabolic alkalosis	↑	N	↑	↑

↓, Decreased; ↑, increased; N, normal.

I. Mixed respiratory and metabolic conditions can coexist; when this occurs, look at the individual values (pH, PCO_2, HCO_3^-) to determine the severity

RAPID QUALITATIVE INTERPRETATION OF pH AND BLOOD GASES

I. Determine pH: acidemia or alkalemia; the pH is the most important value in determining the animal's acid-base status; match subsequent values to it

II. Determine PCO_2
   A. Respiratory alkalosis: less than 35 mm Hg
   B. Respiratory acidosis: greater than 50 mm Hg

III. Determine BE or HCO_3^-
   A. Metabolic alkalosis: BE > +5 mEq/L (HCO_3^- > 28 mEq/L)
   B. Metabolic acidosis: BE < −5 mEq/L (HCO_3^- < 20 mEq/L)

IV. Determine the primary problem by matching either the PCO_2 or BE or both with the pH; determine if compensation exists (pH near normal)

V. Look more closely at BE
   A. BE can be influenced by four things:
      1. Free water (use $[Na^+]$ as the measure): Na, K, and Cl are examples of strong ions
      2. $[Cl^-]$
      3. Protein concentration (A_{tot})
      4. Unidentified anion concentrations (e.g., lactic acid)

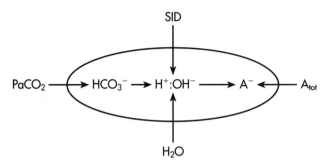

Fig. 17-3
Factors that affect acid-base balance.

   B. Abnormalities in all four can exist simultaneously (Fig.
      17-3); they can have opposite effects and therefore can off-
      set and mask each other; for example, severe lactic acido-
      sis from shock can be offset by a severe hyperchloremic al-
      kalosis from sustained vomiting; the net (observed) BE
      could be zero
VI. Determine PaO_2
   A. If PaO_2 is less than 80 mm Hg, suspect hypoxemia
   B. 5 g/dl of reduced Hb results in cyanosis in patients with
      more than 5 g/dl of Hb

PRINCIPLES OF PRACTICE

   I. The HCO_3^- concentration rises about 1 to 2 mEq/L for each
      acute 10 mm Hg increase in $PaCO_2$ above 40; maximum com-
      pensatory change in HCO_3^- is about 4 mEq/L
  II. The HCO_3^- concentration falls 1 to 2 mEq/L for each acute
      10 mm Hg decrease in $PaCO_2$ below 40; maximum compen-
      satory change in HCO_3^- is about 6 mEq/L
 III. Acute respiratory and nonrespiratory disorders can be distin-
      guished by their $PaCO_2$ and HCO_3^- values; HCO_3^- above 30
      or below 15 mEq/L implies a nonrespiratory (metabolic) com-
      ponent
  IV. During chronic elevation of the $PaCO_2$ (hypercapnea), each
      10 mm Hg increase in $PaCO_2$ causes a 4 mEq/L increase in
      HCO_3^- concentration

    V. An acute 10 mm Hg increase in $PaCO_2$ results in a 0.05 unit decrease in pH; an acute 10 mm Hg decrease in $PaCO_2$ results in a 0.10 unit increase in pH

   VI. Rapid determination of the predicted respiratory pH

      A. Determine the difference between the measured $PaCO_2$ and 40 mm Hg (the respiratory component)

      B. If the $PaCO_2$ is greater than 40, subtract half the value from 7.40

      C. If the $PaCO_2$ is less than 40, move the decimal two places to the left and add the value to 7.40

      D. Examples

         1. pH = 7.01; $PaCO_2$ = 75 ($PaCO_2$ > 40 mm Hg)
$$75 - 40 = 35; 0.35 \times 0.5 = 0.175$$
$$7.40 - 0.18 = 7.22$$

         2. pH = 7.43; $PaCO_2$ = 23 ($PaCO_2$ <40 mm Hg)
$$40 - 23 = 17$$
$$7.40 + 0.17 = 7.57$$

  VII. Rapid determination of the metabolic (nonrespiratory) component

      A. A 10 mEq/L change in HCO_3^- concentration changes pH by 0.15 units; if the pH decimal is moved two places to the right, then a 10:15 or two-thirds relationship exists

      B. The absolute difference between the measured pH and the predicted respiratory pH is the metabolic component of the pH change; moving the decimal point two places to the right and multiplying by 2/3 yields an estimate of the mEq/L variation of the buffer baseline (usually assumed as the HCO_3^- concentration change)

 VIII. Rapid quantitative clinical determination of acid-base changes

      A. Determine the predicted respiratory component of the pH change

      B. Estimate BE or deficit

      C. Examples:

         1. pH = 7.02; $PaCO_2$ = 75
Predicted respiratory pH:
$$75 - 40 = 35; 0.35 \times 0.5 = 0.175$$
$$7.40 - 0.18 = 7.22$$
Metabolic (nonrespiratory) component:
$$7.22 - 7.02 = 20 \times 2/3 = 13.3 \text{ mEq/L, or } 13.3$$
mEq/L base deficit

TABLE 17-1
QUANTITATIVE ANALYSIS OF NONRESPIRATORY ACID-BASE RATIO STATE

Free water abnormalities:	$0.3\,([Na^+] - 140)$	=	_____
Chloride abnormalities:	$102 - [Cl^-]corr$	=	_____
Hypoproteinemia:	$3(6.5 - [P_{tot}])$	=	_____
Unmeasured anions make up the balance:		=	_____
Total, or the observed (reported) BE:		=	_____

$[Cl^-]corr = [Cl^-]obs \times 140/[Na^+]$.
For [Alb] instead of $[P_{tot}]$, use $3.7\,(4.5 - [Alb])$.

  2. pH = 7.64; $PaCO_2 = 25$
      Predicted respiratory pH:
          40 − 25 = 0.15
          7.40 + 0.15 = 7.55
      Metabolic component:
          7.64 − 7.55 = 9 × 2/3 = 6 mEq/L, or 6.0 mEq/L BE

IX. Quantitative analysis of metabolic or nonrespiratory acid-base ratio state*

  A. Enter the observed BE at the bottom of Table 17-1
  B. Calculate and enter the expected contributions to BE caused by the following:
      1. Any free water abnormality
      2. Abnormalities in the corrected $[Cl^-]$
      3. Abnormalities in protein concentrations; be careful about signs (+ or −)
  C. Algebraically sum the values in "B" to determine if there are unmeasured anions; be careful about sign (+ or −)
  D. Compare "A" and "C"; the observed BE should never be greater than the summed values in "C"; if the observed BE is less, the presence of unmeasured anions (UA^-) equal in magnitude to the difference of the summed values in B and BE can be inferred

---

*Modified from Leith DE: Proceedings of the Ninth ACVIM Forum, New Orleans, May 1991.

X. Example

If:

   $pH = 7.250$, $Na^+ = 135$

   $PCO_2 = 75$, $Cl^- = 79$

   $BE = 2$; $P_{tot} + 8.4$

Then:

   Free water abnormality $= -1.5$

   Chloride abnormality $= +20$

   Hyperproteinemia $= -5.7$

   Observed BE $= 2$

Therefore:

   $UA^- = 14.8$

   $[(12.8) + (2) = 14.8]$

This patient has considerable unmeasured ions (14.8 mEg/L), which suggests a severe nonrespiratory acidosis

XI. Summary of acid-base disorders

   A. All acid-base disturbances are caused by changes in $PaCO_2$, SID, and P_{tot}

   B. Since protein concentration is not manipulated clinically, all acid-base disturbances are corrected by changes in $PaCO_2$ and SID

XII. Therapy

   A. Base deficits of less than 10 mEq/L are not routinely treated

   B. pH above 7.20 is not routinely treated unless there is evidence of shock

   C. Since extracellular water is approximately 25% to 30% body weight, base deficits $\times$ body weight (kg) 25% = amount of HCO_3^- needed as replacement, or

$$\frac{\text{Base deficit} \times \text{wt (kg)}}{4} = \text{mEq } HCO_3^- \text{ required}$$

COMMON CAUSES OF ACID-BASE IMBALANCE

I. Respiratory acidosis

   A. Anesthesia or respiratory depressant drugs

   B. Obesity

   C. Pulmonary disease

   D. Rib or thoracic disease; trauma

   E. Brain damage

  II. Respiratory alkalosis
      A. Anxiety, fear
      B. Fever
      C. Endotoxemia
      D. Pneumonia, pulmonary embolus
      E. Hypoxemia
      F. Left-to-right shunts
      G. Heart failure
 III. Metabolic acidosis
      A. Renal disease (uremia)
      B. Chronic vomiting
      C. Diarrhea
      D. Exercise fatigue, hypoxia, ischemia, shock, trauma
      E. Diabetes
  IV. Metabolic alkalosis
      A. Acute vomiting
      B. Hypokalemia
      C. Excessive use of diuretics

ACID-BASE AND ELECTROLYTE INTERRELATIONSHIPS

   I. Most CO_2 entering the blood passes into RBCs, where the majority of CO_2 enters into a reversible formation with HCO_3^-

$$CO_2 + H_2O \leftrightarrow\ ^{CA} H_2CO_3^- \leftrightarrow H^+ + HCO_3^-$$

The HCO_3^- formed by this reaction diffuses out of RBCs; this movement sets up an electrostatic difference across the cell membrane, which is neutralized by the movement of Cl^- from plasma into the RBC (chloride shift)

  II. The location and absolute numbers of positively and negatively charged ions (strong ions) and their difference in combination with CO_2 production, the resultant PCO_2, and the total protein determine pH (H^+) and (HCO_3^-) changes in the body; the principal strong ions are Na^+, K^+, and Cl^-; SID = (Na^+) + (K^+) − (Cl^-) (see Fig. 17-3)

 III. Changes in strong ions in various body fluids result in changes in SID, which provide the major mechanism for acid-base interactions

  IV. To maintain electrical neutrality, electrolyte shifts generally occur simultaneously with acid (H^+) or base (HCO_3^-) shifts; the most important electrolyte shift occurring with acid-base changes is K^+; for example, when HCO_3^- is added to the extracellular fluid, hydrogen ions (H^+) leave cells, causing K^+ to move intracellularly to maintain electrical equilibrium; therefore:

A. In metabolic alkalosis, suspect hypokalemia
B. In metabolic acidosis, suspect hyperkalemia

CHAPTER EIGHTEEN

Pain

"Dying is nothing, but pain is a very serious matter."
HENRY JACOB BIGELOW, 1871

OVERVIEW

The definition, recognition, quantitation, and treatment of pain has become a central issue in veterinary practice. Providing pain relief is as important as choosing the proper sedative, muscle relaxant, and injectable or inhalant anesthetic. This is particularly true for pain in the perioperative period. Apprehension and stress, produced by fear, can initiate a variety of potentially deleterious neurohumoral reactions (stress response) and can sensitize both the peripheral and central nervous systems to noxious stimuli, which heightens pain awareness. Understanding pain pathways and the mechanisms of action of analgesic therapies helps veterinarians treat pain before it occurs. This practice is called *preemptive analgesia*. The best way to treat pain is to preempt it.

GENERAL CONSIDERATIONS

I. Definitions

Allodynia: A change in the sensitivity to pain in which a stimulus produces pain when it ordinarily would not

Analgesia: Absence of sensibility to pain

Analgesic: Any method or drug that relieves pain

Analgia: Painlessness

Central sensitization: A change (prolonged response) in the excitability of neurons in the spinal cord to nociceptive afferent input

Deep pain: Originates in tendons, joints, muscles, and periosteum; it is not unusual for deep pain to cause a drop in blood pressure, a slowing of the pulse, nausea, vomiting, and sweating; can cause reflex cramping of nearby skeletal muscles

Distress: A state in which the animal is unable to adapt to an altered environment or altered stimuli

Field or production surgery: Any surgery performed on farm or free-ranging wild animals residing in their natural or production habitat

Hyperalgesia: An error in pain perception in which there is an excessive sensitivity to pain; secondary hyperalgesia is present when hypersensitivity to pain spreads to uninjured tissue

Institutional Animal Care and Use Committee: A committee whose existence is required by the United States Department of Agriculture and the Department of Health and Human Services at institutions conducting research on animals; consists of veterinarians, practicing scientists, nonscientists, and individuals not affiliated with the institution; responsible for evaluating the institutional animal care and use programs and making recommendations to the administration of the institution; ultimately responsible for approving or disapproving the use of animals in research at the institution on a case-by-case basis

Major surgery: Any surgical intervention that penetrates and exposes a body cavity; any procedure that has the potential for inducing permanent physical or physiologic impairment; any procedure associated with orthopedics or extensive tissue dissection or transection

Minor surgery: Any surgical intervention that produces minimal impairment of physical or physiologic function (e.g., laparoscopy, superficial vascular cutdown, and percutaneous biopsy)

Neuralgia: Pain exhibiting periodic intensification, which extends along the course of one or more nerves

Nonsurvival/nonrecovery surgery: A surgical procedure performed under general anesthesia at the conclusion of which the animal is euthanized without regaining consciousness

Pain: Perception of an unpleasant sensory or emotional experience that results from potential or actual tissue damage

Perioperative: All events associated with a surgical procedure

Preemptive analgesia: The administration of an analgesic before pain develops

Projected pain: An error in the localization of pain; occurs with superficial pain, which is normally quite accurately located; injury to a nerve containing pain pathways causes a phantom pain to be projected into the uninjured area at the origin of the pain fibers

Referred pain: Pain originating in one part of the body but perceived as occurring in another; occurs as the result of the synapses in the spinal cord of visceral pain fibers with pain fibers from the skin

Stoic: Indifferent to pain or pleasure

Stress: The effect induced by external (e.g., physical or environmental) events or internal (e.g., physiologic or psychologic) factors, referred to as *stressors,* that induce alteration in an animal's biologic equilibrium

Superficial or cutaneous pain: Originating on an outer surface (skin) and well localized; it may be sharp or acute or it may be chronic, burning, or aching; may cause an increase in the pulse rate and blood pressure

Surgery: The act of incising living tissue; an operative procedure; the room or facility where an operative procedure is done

Surgical facility: A group of interrelated rooms specifically designed for the conduct of surgery as well as for preoperative and postoperative functions associated with the conduct of surgery in animals

Survival/recovery surgery: A surgical procedure from which animals recover from the effects of general anesthesia and become conscious

Perception of pain: Only humans report and demand treatment of pain; pain in animals must be inferred by the observation of deviations from normal behavior; pain may manifest itself as a limp or altered gait; withdrawal of an injured part; awkward, abnormal postures; a worried or distressed expression; looking at, licking, scratching, or kicking at the site of perceived pain; these and similar signs are the only clues a veterinarian can use to diagnose the presence and magnitude of pain; it seems likely that the presence of pain in animals is underdiagnosed, and, when diagnosed, that its magnitude is underestimated

Visceral pain: Originating from internal organs, visceral pain is poorly localized; small injuries may not cause severe pain, but diffuse foci can produce extremely severe pain; pulling and twisting of viscera, mesenteries, and ligaments can cause pain in an anesthetized patient; visceral pain can be perceived as a pain on the body surface; this error in pain localization is called *referred pain;* if the visceral involvement results in an inflammation that extends to an area of parietal peritoneum, pleura, or pericardium, pain fibers from these areas are also stimulated; pain fibers in the parietal peritoneum or pleura are innervated like the skin and are capable of sensing acute, highly localized pain referring to the corresponding area on the surface of the body; visceral pain can also produce skeletal muscle spasm of the abdominal wall over the affected area; usually involves the parietal peritoneum

II. Physiology of pain and pain pathways
  A. Peripheral pain receptors
    1. Mechanosensitive
      a. Stress, stretching
      b. Compression, crushing
    2. Thermosensitive; involves temperature change
      a. Heat
      b. Cold
    3. Chemosensitive
      a. Neurotransmitters (Ach)
      b. Prostaglandins (PGE_2)
      c. Autocoids
        (1) Bradykinin
        (2) 5-hydroxytryptamine (5HT)
        (3) Histamine
        (4) Potassium
        (5) Proteolytic enzymes
      d. Acids (e.g., lactic acid)
      e. Cytokines
        (1) Tumor necrosis factor
        (2) Interleukin-1,6,8
        (3) Calcitonin gene-related peptide
  B. Peripheral nerves
    1. Myelinated A-δ nerve fibers transmit acute, accurately localized, (epicritic) sharp pain
    2. Nonmyelinated C nerve fibers transmit chronic, diffuse (protopathic), dull, burning, and aching pain

C. Spinal cord pathways
   1. Peripheral nerves enter the spinal cord through the dorsal roots and then ascend or descend one or two segments in Lissauer's tract
   2. Peripheral nerves terminate in the dorsal horn gray matter (substantia gelatinosa)
   3. Peripheral nerves synapse with nerves of the spinothalamic tract and are carried centrally to the following:
      a. Thalamus: somatosensory cortex
      b. Reticular activating system, which is important in activating the autonomic nervous system, limbic system, amygdala, and locus coeruleus; the following conditions can result:
         (1) Sleep arousal
         (2) Cardiopulmonary changes
         (3) Aversion reaction
         (4) Stress response
   4. Spinal cord pain receptors
      a. Facilitatory
         (1) Substance P receptors (neurokinin-1; NK-1 type)
         (2) Glutamate receptors (N-methyl-D-aspartate [NMDA type])
         (3) Prostaglandin receptors
      b. Inhibitory
         (1) Gamma-aminobutyric acid-B receptors
         (2) Opioid receptors (μ, κ, others)
         (3) α_2 receptors
         (4) Adenosine receptors (A_1-type)
   5. Central perception
      a. Pain is inferred by observation of deviations from normal behavior and physiologic responses
         (1) Altered gait
         (2) Increased locomotion
         (3) Reluctance to move
         (4) Abnormal posture
         (5) Licking, scratching
         (6) Self-mutilation
         (7) Aversion
         (8) Vocalization

        (9) Aggression

        (10) Tachycardia, tachypnea

   b. Pain in anesthetized animals is inferred by changes in response to manipulation (surgical or otherwise)

        (1) Movement

        (2) Trembling

        (3) Increased heart rate or respiratory rate

        (4) Increased arterial blood pressure

   c. Pain or stress is inferred by increases in circulating "stress" substances

        (1) Adrenocorticotrophic hormone

        (2) Glucose

        (3) Catecholamines (dopamine, epinephrine, norepinephrine)

        (4) Beta-endorphin

        (5) Leu-enkephalin

        (6) Lactic acid

        (7) Free fatty acids

III. Response to tissue injury

  A. Classification of pain

    1. Physiologic pain, which is experienced in everyday life and serves a protective role from noxious stimuli (e.g., heat, cold, pressure)

      a. Well localized

      b. Transient

      c. High threshold

    2. Clinical pain is composed of inflammatory pain and neuropathic pain

      a. Inflammatory pain is caused by peripheral tissue damage (e.g., crushing, burning, surgery)

        (1) Low threshold to pain (allodynia)

        (2) Exaggerated response to noxious stimuli (hyperalgesia)

        (3) Poorly localized (secondary hyperalgesia)

        (4) Initiates peripheral and central sensitization

      b. Neuropathic pain is caused by damage to the nervous system; characteristics are similar to those of inflammatory pain

    3. Clinical pain differs from physiologic pain because of the presence of pathologic hypersensitivity

B. Peripheral and central hypersensitization
   1. Peripheral sensitization causes a decrease in pain threshold
      a. At the site of injury
      b. In surrounding tissue
   2. Central sensitization
      a. Activity-dependent increase in the excitability of spinal neurons termed *spinal facilitation* or *windup*
         (1) Evokes progressively greater responses in dorsal-horn, wide dynamic-range neurons
         (2) Increases the size of peripheral receptive fields
         (3) Demonstrates continual changes (field plasticity) in spatial, temporal, and threshold qualities that parallel post injury hyperalgesia
      b. Central sensitization includes "windup" and a prolonged phase of hyperalgesia; mediated by substance P (NK-1) and glutamate (NMDA) receptors
   3. Differences between peripheral and central sensitization
      a. Peripheral sensitization is produced by low-intensity stimuli activating A-δ and C nociceptors
      b. Central sensitization is produced by normal, low-threshold A-β sensory fibers because of changes in central processing from neural inputs
C. Implications for pain therapy
   1. Complete analgesia is required intraoperatively, regardless of whether the patient is conscious; intraoperative analgesia can be produced by general anesthesia, local anesthetics, and a variety of analgesic drugs (Table 18-1)
      a. Inhalation anesthetics (halothane, isoflurane, sevoflurane)
      b. Hypnotics (barbiturates, etomidate, propofol)
      c. Dissociogenic drugs (ketamine, tiletamine)
      d. Local anesthetics (lidocaine, mepivacaine)
      e. Opioids (morphine, meperidine, oxymorphone, butorphanol)
      f. α₂-agonists (xylazine, detomidine, medetomidine, romifidine)
      g. Nonsteroidal antiinflammatory drugs (NSAIDs); aspirin, phenylbutazone, ketoprofen, carprofen, etodolac

TABLE **18-1**

INJECTABLE ANALGESIC DRUGS AND THEIR MECHANISM OF ACTION

DRUG	MECHANISM OF ACTION
Opioids (morphine, meperidine, oxymorphone)	Combine with opioid receptors to produce sedation, analgesia, and euphoria
α_2 agonists (xylazine, detomidine, medetomidine, romifidine)	Combine with α_2 receptors to produce sedation, muscle relaxation, and analgesia
Nonsteroidal, antiinflammatory drugs: flunixin meglumine, phenylbutazone, aspirin, carprofen, ketoprofen	Act centrally (CNS) on the hypothalamus; antiinflammatory and analgesic activity mediated by peripheral inhibition of prostaglandins
Local anesthetics (lidocaine, bupivacaine)	Block nerve transmission of electrical impulses

CNS, Central nervous system.

2. Converting clinical pain to physiologic pain may be sufficient before and after surgery; best accomplished with behavioral modifiers and antiinflammatory drugs
   a. Opioids
   b. α_2-agonists
   c. NSAIDs
3. Prevent the establishment of pain and central sensitization (Table 18-2)
   a. Preemptive analgesia; drug combinations (opioids-tranquilizers) may be needed
   b. Dose and routes of drug administration can produce select effects; intravenous, intramuscular, subcutaneous, and oral versus epidural, intrathecal, and site-specific administration

TABLE 18-2
ANALGESIC DRUGS AND DOSAGES*

DRUG	DOSE (mg/kg) DOGS	DOSE (mg/kg) CATS	ROUTES	DOSE INTERVAL (HR)
Local anesthetics				
Epidural drugs†				
Lidocaine	2.0	2.0	—	1-3
Bupivacaine	0.5	0.5	—	4-6
Ropivacaine	0.5	0.5	—	4-12
Morphine	0.1	0.1	—	>10
Oxymorphone	0.05	0.05	—	>10
Butorphanol	0.25	0.25	—	2-4
Medetomidine	0.01	0.01	—	4
Opioids				
Agonists				
Morphine	0.2-2.0	0.05-0.2 0.1-0.3 mg/kg/hr	IV, IM IV	1-4 12-48
Meperidine	1.0-4.0	Not Used	IM	0.5-1

Drug			Route	Onset/Duration (hr)
Oxymorphone	0.2-1.0	0.05-0.1	IV, IM	2-4
Fentanyl	0.01	0.01	IV	0.2-0.5
		0.001-0.003 mg/kg/hr	IV	12-72
	0.005	0.005	Transdermal patch	10-12 onset of effect; >120 hr duration
Agonist-Antagonist				
Butorphanol	0.2-0.4	0.2-0.4	IV, IM	1-2
		0.1-0.3 mg/kg/hr	IV	6-12
Pentazocine	1.0-3.0	1.0-2.0	IV, IM	2-4
Nalbuphine	0.5-1.5	0.5-1.5	IV, IM	1-4
α_2-Agonists				
Medetomidine	0.005-0.01	0.005-0.01	IV, IM	1-4
Xylazine	0.01-0.2	0.01-0.2	IV, SO	1-3
Romifidine	0.04-0.08	0.08-0.2	IM, SQ	2-4

*Refer to the text for description of local, regional, intercostal, and intrapleural nerve blocks (bupivacaine and ropivacaine 1-3 mg/kg, for selective nerve blocks). Lidocaine can be administered by infusion (2-3 ml/kg/hr [50 μg/kg/min]; IV) as a adjunct to analgesia.

†Drug is diluted in 1 ml of 0.9% saline/5 kg; epidural opioids and local anesthetics are frequently combined (0.1 mg/kg of oxymorphone diluted in 0.75% bupivacaine to a volume of 1 ml/5 kg) to produce longer-acting analgesic effects.

NOTE: Morphine (0.1 mg/kg) has been administered intraarticularly for added analgesia following stifle joint surgery in dogs.
Magnesium Sulfate 6-8 mg/kg/hr or 5-15 mEq/L/hr can be administered as an adjunct to analgesia.

Continued

TABLE 18-2
ANALGESIC DRUGS AND DOSAGES*—cont'd

DRUG	DOSE (mg/kg) DOGS	DOSE (mg/kg) CATS	ROUTES	DOSE INTERVAL (HR)
Nonsteroidal antiinflammatory drugs				
Salicylates				
Aspirin	10-25	10-15	PO	8-12 (dogs); 24-48 (cats)
Propionic acids				
Carprofen	1.0-2.0	Not used	PO	12
Ibuprofen	5.0-10.0	Not used	PO	24-48
Naproxen	1.0-2.0	Not used	PO	24
Ketoprofen	0.5-1.0	0.5-1.0	PO	24
Etodolac	10-15	Not used	PO	24
Fenamates				
Flunixin meglumine	0.5-1.0	Not used	IV, IM	24; do not repeat
Meclofenamic acid	1.0-2.0	Not used	PO	24

Pyrazoles				
Phenylbutazone	10-25	10-15	PO	8-12
Oxicams				
Piroxicam	0.2-0.4	Not used	PO	48
Phenacetin Derivatives				
Acetaminophen	10-15	Not used	PO	12

Schedule I: Substances in this schedule have no accepted medical use in the United States and have a high abuse potential (e.g., heroin, marijuana, LSD, methaqualone)

Schedule II: Substances in this schedule have high abuse potential with severe psychic or physical dependence liability (e.g., morphine, oxymorphone, meperidine, fentanyl, amphetamine, pentobarbital, phencyclidane, Innovar-Vet); records for Schedule II drugs must be maintained separately from those in Schedules III and IV

Schedule III: Less abuse potential than Schedule II; no examples in veterinary medicine

Schedule IV: Less abuse potential than Schedule III (e.g., chloral hydrate, diazepam, pentazocine)

Schedule V: Limited abuse potential (e.g., some drugs for antitussive and antidiarrheal use)

PO, By mouth; *IV*, intravenous; *IM*, intramuscular; *GI*, gastrointestinal.

CHAPTER NINETEEN

Anesthetic Procedures and Techniques in Dogs and Cats

"Come now let us reason together."
LYNDON BAINES JOHNSON

OVERVIEW

Anesthetic procedures and techniques developed for small animals are designed to produce the desired result safely, effectively, and economically. Previous techniques using single drugs have largely been abandoned. Rather, techniques producing chemical restraint and anesthesia by combining different types of drugs in reduced dosages are used, reducing unwanted side effects and toxicity. The advantage of combination drug therapy over single-drug therapy is a more ideal anesthetic state including hypnosis, analgesia, and muscle relaxation. Combination drug therapy requires a comprehensive knowledge of the pharmacology of anesthetic drugs, their interactions, and potential side effects.

GENERAL CONSIDERATIONS

I. A variety of anesthetic procedures and techniques can be used to safely produce chemical restraint and anesthesia in dogs and cats

II. The choice of anesthetic regimen is influenced by the following characteristics:
   A. Breed
   B. Temperament
   C. Health and physical condition
   D. The purpose of chemical restraint and anesthesia
   E. The familiarity of personnel with the drugs being used

   F. Concurrent medication
   G. The amount of available assistance
III. Whenever possible, drugs that are reversible should be used
IV. If unconsciousness occurs, endotracheal intubation should always be performed to ensure a patent airway
 V. Careful monitoring is mandatory to recognize and compensate for effects
VI. Food and water should be withheld for approximately 6 hours before surgery, except in very small, very young, or diseased patients

PREANESTHETIC EVALUATION (SEE CHAPTER 2)

  I. Review patient history
 II. Perform a physical examination
III. Review available laboratory data
IV. Formulate a specific anesthetic plan (Fig. 19-1)
   A. Determine whether additional preoperative tests are needed
   B. Choose drugs appropriate to patient needs
 V. Gather appropriate equipment and supplies
   A. Endotracheal tube
     1. Select diameter based on patient size
     2. If using a cuffed tube, check cuff for leaks by injecting air
     3. Use a stylet for small-diameter, flimsy tubes (Fig. 19-2)
     4. Use a Cole catheter in neonates, rodents, birds, and reptiles (Fig. 19-3)
     5. Use a small amount of sterile lubricant
   B. Laryngoscope (see Fig. 19-4)
     1. Aids intubation by allowing visualization, illumination, and manipulation of tongue and laryngeal structures
     2. May be optional, depending on species, anatomy, and patient size
   C. Anesthetic machine and breathing system
     1. Size and type of system determined by patient size
       a. For patients weighing less than 400 lb, use the small-animal anesthetic machine (adult human anesthetic system)
         (1) Use the circle system for patients weighing more than 10 lb

PREANESTHETIC EVALUATION

ANESTHETIST: _____
DATE: _____
CLINICIAN: _____
WARD/CAGE OR STALL #: _____

PROCEDURE: ....

BODY WEIGHT: .... **AGE:** ....

TEMPERAMENT:

OBJECTIVE FINDINGS	CBC
Temp _____ Pulse _____ Resp. _____	WBC _____ TP _____ PCV _____
Cardiac auscultation _____	Fibrinogen _____
Pulse quality _____	SERUM CHEMISTRIES
Mucous membrane color _____	BUN _____ GLUCOSE _____
Capillary refill time _____	AST(SGOT) _____
Respiratory auscultation _____	ALT(SGPT) _____
	URINE SPECIFIC GRAVITY _____
ASSESSMENT: Physical status I II III IV V E	OTHER RESULTS _____
Reasons:	PRIOR ANESTHESIA _____

COMPLICATIONS ANTICIPATED   pre op, intra op, post op: consider age , body wt., breed, position, surgical procedure, physical status.

Plan   Anesthesia regimen (include <u>reasons</u> as related to <u>this animal</u>)
(Include premeds, induction agent, inhalation agent, O$_2$ flow rate, post op analgesics)

DRUG	ROUTE	DOSE/#	MG	ML	REASONS OR JUSTIFICATION

MONITORING: Esophageal stethoscope, Doppler, ECG, Temp. Probe, Blood gas, Arterial Line, Other _____

IV FLUID TYPE _____ Dose: MLS/HR _____ DROPS/MIN _____

ADMINISTRATION SET: MINI DRIP (60 drops/ml)   MAXI DRIP (10 drops/ml)

Approved _____

Fig. 19-1
Anesthetic plan sheet.

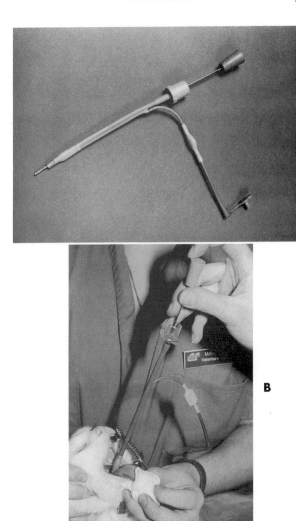

Fig. 19-2
A stylet can be used to stiffen small endotracheal tubes to facilitate tracheal intubation.

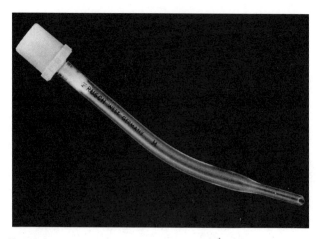

Fig. 19-3
A Cole catheter facilitates intubation of neonates, rodents, birds, and reptiles.

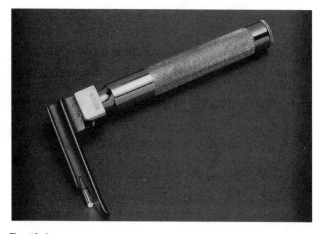

Fig. 19-4
A laryngoscope facilitates visualization and illumination for intubation.

       (2) Use the non-rebreathing system for patients weighing less than 10 lb

  2. Rebreathing bag should be approximately five times the tidal volume. Tidal volume is 5 to 7 ml/lb (5×5 ml/lb = 25 ml/lb)

  3. Refill carbon dioxide absorbent canister if material is exhausted

  4. Evaluate anesthetic system for possible malfunctions (see Chapter 14)

    a. Fill vaporizer and check operation

    b. Turn on flowmeters and check for free movement of indicator balls or slides

    c. Close pop-off valve and pressurize the system to 40 cm water using oxygen flush valve; check for leaks (Fig. 19-5)

  5. Connect waste gas scavenging system to the anesthetic machine

D. Fresh gases

  1. Oxygen

    a. Connect to "house" system, if available

    b. Attach smaller tanks to machine; change oxygen tank if pressure gauge reads less than 500 psi

  2. Nitrous oxide

    a. Optional

    b. Change tank if pressure gauge reads less than 750 psi

E. Intravenous administration supplies

  1. Intravenous catheter

  2. Appropriate intravenous fluids

  3. Solution administration set (mini-drip; 60 drops/ml)

  4. Fluid infusion pump (Fig. 19-6)

F. Drugs

  1. Calculate appropriate drug dosage and volume

  2. Withdraw drugs into labeled syringes

G. Ancillary supplies

  1. 4×4-inch gauze sponges

  2. Adhesive tape

  3. Roll gauze

  4. Esophageal stethoscope catheter and earpiece or Doppler

  5. Additional monitoring equipment (BP, capnograph, pulse oximeter) if required

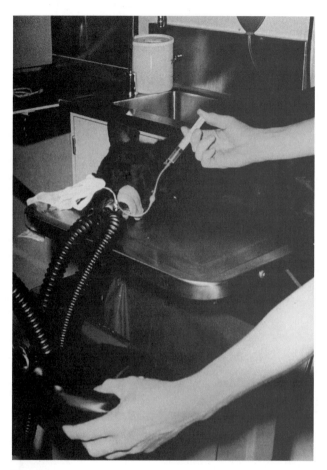

Fig. 19-5
Escape of gas from around the endotracheal tube can be eliminated by inflating the endotracheal tube cuff (right hand) until no gas escapes from the mouth during rebreathing bag compression (left hand) to 30 cm H_2O.

PREANESTHETIC MEDICATION

I. Choice of drug determined by the patient's preoperative condition and any other special considerations pertinent to the procedure

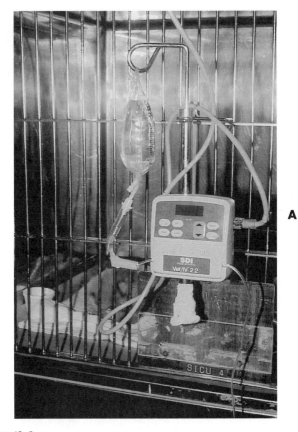

Fig. 19-6

Examples of infusion pumps. **A,** Infusion pump that uses a fluid administration set. *Continued*

   II. Drugs to be given intramuscularly (IM) or subcutaneously (SQ) should be administered 10 to 30 minutes before catheterization and induction

  III. Drugs used as premedications

     A. Anticholinergics

       1. Atropine 0.1 mg/lb IM or IV

       2. Glycopyrrolate 0.005 mg/lb IM or IV

     B. Acepromazine 0.1 mg/lb IM, maximum total dose 4 mg

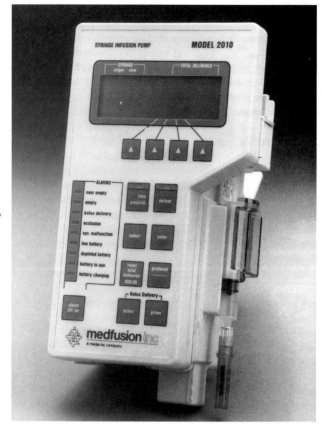

Fig. 19-6, cont'd
B, Infusion pump that uses a syringe.

    C. Diazepam 0.1 mg/lb IV, maximum total dose 5 mg; use midazolam as an alternative, same dose; diazepam or midazolam are usually administered in conjunction with opioids

    D. Opioids

       1. Morphine 0.1 to 0.3 mg/lb IM (dogs), 0.05 to 0.1 mg/lb IM (cats)

       2. Oxymorphone 0.05 to 0.15 mg/lb IM

       3. Meperidine 0.5 to 3 mg/lb IM

E. Xylazine 0.1 to 0.5 mg/lb IM
F. Medetomidine 5 to 10 mg/lb IM
G. Ketamine (cats) 3 to 5 mg/lb IM
H. Telazol 1 to 3 mg/lb IM

INDUCTION

I. Intravenous
  A. Catheterize vein(s) (generally the cephalic vein)
  B. Start IV fluid administration to ensure catheter patency
    1. Lower fluid bag or bottle below patient's thorax to allow blood to siphon back into catheter; this confirms catheter placement within the vein
  C. Inject induction drug(s) at appropriate rate(s), allowing time for patient equilibration before administering further increments
  D. Specific IV induction drugs (see Chapter 9)
    1. Ultrashort-acting barbiturates
      a. Thiopental 2% to 5%; 3 to 5 mg/lb
      b. Methohexital 2%
    2. Pentobarbital
    3. Etomidate (0.5 to 1 mg/lb IV)
    4. Propofol (1 to 2 mg/lb IV)
    5. Combinations
      a. Diazepam 0.1 mg/lb IV; lidocaine 2 mg/lb IV; thiopental 2 mg/lb IV (dogs only)
        (1) Useful in animals with CNS depression
        (2) Stabilizes myocardium
        (3) Reduces thiobarbiturate dosage
      b. Diazepam-ketamine: simultaneous administration of diazepam (0.125 mg/lb IV) and ketamine (2.5 mg/lb IV)
        (1) Mix equal parts of diazepam (5 mg/ml in stock vial) and ketamine (100 mg/ml in stock vial) to yield a mixture that is 2.5 mg/ml diazepam and 50 mg/ml ketamine
        (2) Use 1 ml of mixture per 20 pounds; add opioid or α_2-agonist for added analgesia
      c. Diazepam, opioid, etomidate, or propofol

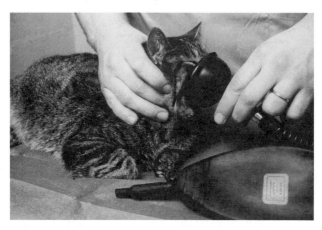

Fig. 19-7
A face mask is often used to induce cats and small dogs to anesthesia.

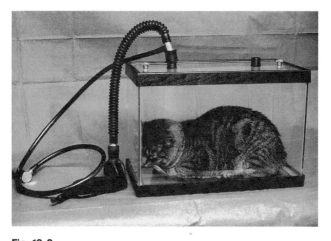

Fig. 19-8
An induction chamber is used to confine cats and small animals for induction to general anesthesia with an inhaled anesthetic.

II. Inhalant
  A. Face mask (Fig. 19-7)
    1. Be aware of potential for vomiting and possible aspiration
    2. Ensure adequate patient restraint
    3. Environmental pollution is significant
  B. Induction chamber (Fig. 19-8)
    1. For cats, small dogs, rodents, birds, and snakes
    2. Use high, fresh-gas flow rates
    3. Monitor patient closely for loss of righting reflex, then remove from box
    4. Atmospheric pollution with anesthetic gases is significant

ENDOTRACHEAL INTUBATION

  I. Open the patient's mouth and manipulate the tongue to the side with the endotracheal tube; grasp the tongue with a gauze sponge, and retract the tongue between the lower canine teeth to hold the mandible open (Fig. 19-9, *A*)
  II. Locate the larynx and insert the endotracheal tube
  A. Direct visualization
  B. Use a laryngoscope to facilitate visualization of the larynx (Fig. 19-9, *B, C*)
  C. Potential difficulties
    1. Laryngospasm (0.1 ml lidocaine sprayed into the glottis reduces spasms)
      a. Patient too light
      b. Larynx sensitized
    2. Soft-palate displacement prevents rostroventral movement of the epiglottis; push the soft palate dorsally with the endotracheal tube to release epiglottis
  D. Turn on oxygen
  E. Connect the breathing system to the endotracheal tube, and secure the tube to the patient
  F. Monitor respirations and pulse
    1. If pulses are present, turn on the vaporizer and nitrous oxide if desired

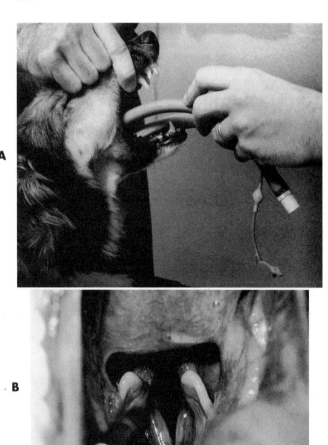

Fig. 19-9
A, Most dogs and cats are easily intubated without a laryngoscope. **B,** A laryngoscope is used to facilitate visualization of the larynx.

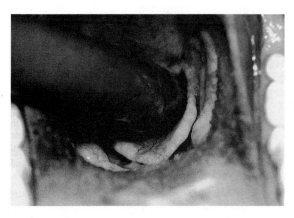

Fig. 19-9, cont'd
C, Placement of the endotracheal tube.

2. If pulses are absent, leave oxygen on and diagnose the cause of the absent or weak pulses; do not start inhalation drugs (see Chapter 28)
3. Spontaneous ventilation (assist ventilation if required)
4. Apnea, dyspnea
   a. Anesthetic induction drugs may depress the patient's ventilatory drive; begin mechanical ventilation using the breathing system
   b. Endotracheal tube may be obstructed or kinked
   c. If bronchial intubation has occurred, withdraw the tube into the trachea
   d. Pneumothorax or pneumomediastinum
      (1) Relieve intrathoracic pressure by percutaneous needle insertion
      (2) Evaluate hemodynamic status
G. Set the vaporizer to a maintenance concentration determined by monitoring patient responses
H. Connect monitors (ECG; pulse oximeter)

MAINTENANCE OF ANESTHESIA

    I. Monitoring (see Chapter 16)

   II. Record concentrations, doses, and time administered for anesthetic drugs given; readjust dosages according to patient response, depth of anesthesia, and amount of analgesia needed

  III. Check patency of airway frequently
     A. Blocked or kinked tube
     B. Overinflation of cuff
     C. Tube impinging at bifurcation of trachea

  IV. Maintain the endotracheal tube, head, and neck in a natural, slightly curved position to prevent kinking of the tube; position the patient to avoid excessive flexion of neck, abduction of limbs, and pressure on thorax

   V. Calculate IV fluids needed and adjust fluid flow rate; record all fluids (total volumes), electrolytes, and other drugs administered

  VI. Complete anesthetic record (Fig. 19-10)
     A. Note the start and end of the anesthetic period
     B. Note the start and end of the surgical period
     C. Note all major surgical events
     D. Note all changes in patient status, cardiorespiratory variables, and anesthetic technique
     E. Note all laboratory results during anesthesia (e.g., blood gases)

 VII. Nitrous oxide: turn off N_2O 5 to 10 minutes before the end of the surgical period; methoxyflurane: reduce concentration as surgery nears completion, and turn off 5 to 10 minutes before the end

VIII. Turn off the inhalant anesthetic at the end of surgery or earlier, depending on the depth of anesthesia

  IX. Oxygen: deliver (10 ml/lb or more) into the recovery period; empty the rebreathing bag to dump anesthetic gases and hasten recovery

THE RECOVERY PERIOD

    I. Deflate the endotracheal tube cuff; extubate it when the animal is swallowing

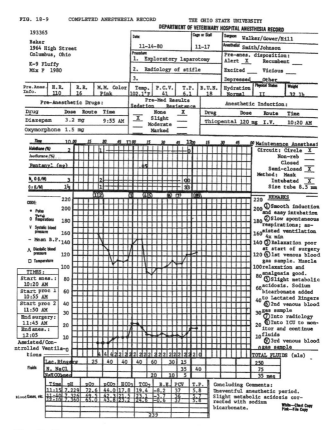

Fig. 19-10
Completed anesthesia record.

II. Administer oxygen as necessary (endotracheal tube, mask, oxygen cage) to maintain oxygenation

III. Position the animal in sternal recumbency with its head extended

IV. Observe the animal until it can maintain sternal recumbency

V. Keep the airway free of secretions (use postural drainage, sponges, and suction tubes)

    VI. Check temperature; raise and maintain body temperature using towels, heating pads, heat lamps, or warm air blankets

   VII. Change the animal's positions frequently, and stimulate it by rubbing its body and flexing and extending its limbs

 VIII. Tranquilizers and analgesics may be needed if the animal becomes excited or is in pain during recovery

    IX. Maintain IV fluids as needed

     X. Periodically monitor the patient until it is able to maintain a sternal position or stand unsupported

   XI. Consider drug antagonists if necessary

       A. Opioids: naloxone

       B. α_2-agonists: yohimbine, tolazoline, and atipamazole

       C. Benzodiazepines: flumazenil

       D. Respiratory depression: doxapram

       E. Bradycardia: atropine, glycopyrrolate

CHAPTER TWENTY

Anesthetic Procedures and Techniques in Horses

"The little neglect may breed mischief . . . for want of a nail the shoe was lost; for want of a shoe the horse was lost; and for want of a horse the rider was lost."

BENJAMIN FRANKLIN

OVERVIEW

Injectable and inhalant anesthetic techniques are popular for producing general anesthesia in horses. The ability to predict drug effects and drug actions is the single most important asset of a good equine anesthetist. Patient temperament varies and has considerable influence on the amount of drug required and anesthetic technique. Both bolus and infusions of anesthetic drugs (total intravenous anesthesia [TIVA]) are combined with physical restraint and used to induce and maintain general anesthesia in horses. Anesthetic techniques are designed to produce rapid and safe induction to and recovery from lateral recumbency and to maximize muscle relaxation and analgesia while maintaining normal cardiopulmonary status. Horses frequently benefit from assistance to regain and maintain a standing position following general anesthesia.

GENERAL CONSIDERATIONS

I. Preparation of the equine surgical patient
   A. Withhold food for approximately 4 to 8 hours before surgery; do not withhold water
   B. Pull or pad all shoes to prevent injury; clip the surgical site before the induction to anesthesia (if possible)

    C. Groom the horse and wipe it with a moist cloth to remove dander; place an intravenous catheter before induction

    D. Perform a complete physical examination with emphasis on cardiorespiratory function

    E. Weigh each animal and note body type (e.g., lean/racing, conditioned, draft)

    F. Give each animal preanesthetic medication approximately 5 to 20 minutes before induction of anesthesia

    G. Rinse the mouth with water before induction

    H. Clean the feet before induction

  II. All horses develop some degree of acid-base disturbance under anesthesia, particularly respiratory acidosis

 III. Proper positioning and appropriate padding of the head, shoulder, and hip minimize cardiopulmonary compromise and the development of neuropathies and myopathies

 IV. Assisted or controlled ventilation is required to maintain normal arterial carbon dioxide concentrations during prolonged anesthesia in the horse

  V. Prevention of hypotension and hypoxemia helps avoid postoperative complications, including myopathy

 VI. Horses should be watched closely during the recovery period and, if needed, assisted to a standing position

    A. Nasotracheal intubation may be required in horses that snore or demonstrate signs of upper airway obstruction

PREANESTHETIC EVALUATION

  I. Review patient history

 II. Conduct a physical evaluation

    A. Determine age, weight, sex

    B. Judge the temperament of the horse

    C. Perform a physical examination; emphasize the cardiopulmonary system; check for subclinical respiratory disease

    D. Determine the degree of lameness or ataxia

    E. Review the concurrent or previous drug history

    F. Assess the procedure to be performed

    G. Prepare an anesthetic care plan

 III. Conduct a laboratory evaluation

    A. Routine evaluation

      1. Complete blood count (HCT, Hb)

2. Total protein
3. Fibrinogen
B. Suggested further evaluation
1. Serum electrolytes
2. Serum chemistry

PREANESTHETIC MEDICATIONS

I. Xylazine (used to produce sedation, analgesia, and muscle relaxation)
  A. Dose: 0.5 to 1 mg/lb IM
     0.2 to 0.5 mg/lb IV
  B. Onset of action: within 2 to 3 minutes after intravenous administration and within 10 to 15 minutes after intramuscular administration
  C. Duration: 30 minutes after intravenous administration and 60 minutes after intramuscular administration
  D. Sinus bradycardia and first- and second-degree heart block may occur
II. Detomidine (similar to xylazine)
  A. Dose: 5 to 10 ug/lb IV
     10 to 20 ug/lb IM
  B. Longer duration of action than xylazine
III. Acepromazine (used to produce a calming effect)
  A. Dose: 10 to 40 mg/1000 lb IM; 5 to 20 mg/1000 lb IV
  B. Onset of action: within 10 to 20 minutes
  C. Duration: 2 to 3 hours
  D. Hypotensive effect may last for 12 hours
IV. Chloral hydrate (used to produce or enhance sedation); 10 to 50 mg/lb

ANESTHETIC EQUIPMENT

I. Collect the necessary equipment
  A. Endotracheal tubes
    1. Choose the largest tube possible (30, 26, 20, or 15 mm); most tube size designations are related to inside diameter
    2. Check the endotracheal tube cuff for leaks
    3. Use lubricating jelly for the endotracheal tube

      4. Use 25- and 60-cc syringe to inflate the endotracheal tube cuff

      5. Cotton mouth gag or speculum (2-inch polyvinylchloride plumber's pipe)

B. Intravenous catheter for intravenous anesthetic drug or fluid administration (Fig. 20-1)

      1. Commercially available 10-, 12-, and 14-gauge catheters

      2. Tubing for an adult patient 500 to 1000 lb

         a. 240 polyethylene tubing or commercial catheter

         b. 10-gauge, 2-inch venapuncture needle

         c. 14-gauge disposable needle

         d. Three-way stopcock

         e. 12-ml syringe with heparinized saline solution

C. Pressure bag for administration of intravenous drugs (e.g., guaifenesin)

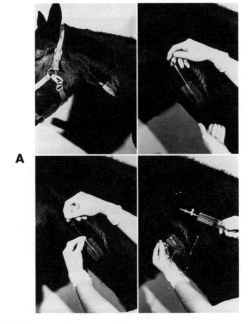

Fig. 20-1
A, Placement of intravenous catheter.

D. Chest rope for restraining front legs (Fig. 20-2)
E. Proper padding (Fig. 20-2)
F. Monitoring equipment (see Chapter 16)
    1. ECG monitor
    2. Blood pressure recording device
    3. Stethoscope

II. Before induction of general anesthesia
    A. The anesthetic machine should be examined to be sure the vaporizer has an adequate anesthetic level; the circle system should be tested for leaks
        1. The anesthetic system can be checked for leaks by occluding the Y piece that connects to the endotracheal tube, closing the pop-off valve, and flushing oxygen through the system; if pressure is maintained, the system is not leaking

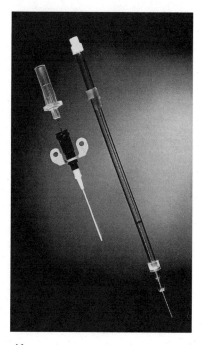

B

Fig. 20-1, cont'd
B, Types of intravenous catheters.

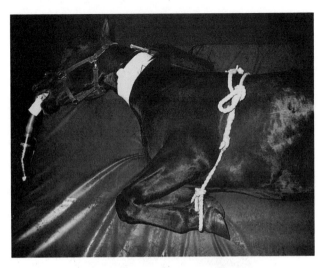

Fig. 20-2
During general anesthesia, horses are usually positioned on large foam rubber pads or on air or water mattresses with their front legs restrained. Once the horse is properly positioned, the halter should be removed.

    2. The circle system should be capable of maintaining a pressure of approximately 40 cm of water
B. Check gas pressures in the tanks
    1. Oxygen should be 2500 psi
C. Fresh carbon dioxide absorbent should be placed in the canister after approximately 6 hours of use
D. Fresh gas flow rate
    1. Oxygen: 1 L/250 lb; minimum of 3 L/1000 lb; high flow rates, up to 1 L/100 lb, are used during induction and recovery to denitrogenate and remove anesthetic vapors, respectively

INDUCTION

I. Ketamine
    A. Dose: 0.7 to 1 mg/lb IV after xylazine, detomidine, romifidine, or guaifenesin

    B. Usually administered with diazepam, but after an α_2-agonist

    C. 10% contains 100 mg/ml

    D. Short-acting (10 to 15 minutes)

    E. Causes apneustic breathing pattern

II. Guaifenesin: centrally acting skeletal muscle relaxant

    A. Dose: 50 mg/lb to produce recumbency; 25 mg/lb to produce ataxia and relaxation

    B. 5% or 10% solution (50 or 100 mg/ml)

    C. Administered before or in solution with thiopental sodium or ketamine

    D. Duration: 10 to 20 minutes

    E. Causes minimal analgesia and sedation by itself

    F. Toxic signs include the following:

        1. Apneustic breathing pattern or apnea

        2. Muscle rigidity

        3. Hypotension

III. Diazepam (muscle relaxant)

    A. Dose: 0.02 to 0.05 mg/lb

    B. Administered before thiopental or with ketamine

    C. Duration: 5 to 15 minutes

    D. No analgesia, minimal sedation

IV. Thiopental sodium

    A. Dose: without guaifenesin 4 to 7 mg/lb; with guaifenesin 2 to 4 mg/lb

    B. Ultrashort-acting (5 to 10 minutes)

    C. Causes cardiovascular depression and may cause transient apnea (dose dependent)

V. Telazol (tiletamine/zolazepam)

    A. Dose: 0.25 to 0.5 mg/lb

    B. Similar to ketamine and used in the same manner

    C. Greater muscle relaxation

    D. Longer duration of action

    E. Greater respiratory depression

VI. Halothane, isoflurane, sevoflurane: 3% to 5% concentration and high oxygen flow can be used for induction in foals using a nasotracheal tube or mask

ENDOTRACHEAL INTUBATION

I. Endotracheal intubation (Fig. 20-3)
  A. Intubation is performed blindly
   1. Place a bite block between the incisors
   2. Extend the head and neck
   3. Advance the tube over the base of the tongue into the pharynx
   4. Rotate the tube as it is advanced into the trachea
   5. Repeat if unsuccessful
  B. If the tube appears too small, choose a larger one
  C. Do not advance the tip past the thoracic inlet
  D. Secure the tube with gauze, if necessary
  E. Nasal intubation can be performed in adult horses and foals (Fig. 20-4)
  F. Two clean endotracheal tubes and a speculum or mouth gag should be available for induction
  G. Connect the endotracheal tube to the anesthetic system; the rebreathing bag size should be at least five times the tidal volume; 15-L or 30-L bags are standard

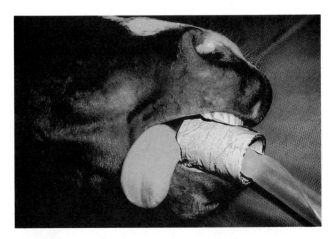

Fig. 20-3
Endotracheal intubation is performed blindly in horses and foals.

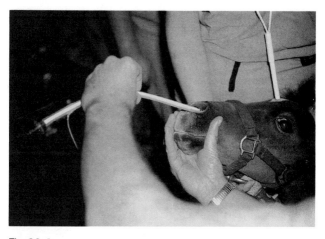

Fig. 20-4
Nasal intubation is easily performed in adult horses and foals.

    H. Inflate the endotracheal tube cuff, and check to see that it does not leak by squeezing the rebreathing bag, thereby expanding the animal's lungs
      1. 15 to 20 cm water or 10 to 15 mm Hg pressure is sufficient
      2. Do not overinflate the cuff; generally, 50 to 75 ml is adequate to inflate the cuff of an endotracheal tube in a 1000-lb patient (Fig. 20-5)

MAINTENANCE OF ANESTHESIA

    I. Total intravenous anesthesia (TIVA): a mixture of 500 ml of 5% guaifenesin, 500 mg of ketamine, and 250 to 500 mg of xylazine mixed together and delivered to effect (Table 20-1)
    II. Inhalation anesthesia
      A. Halothane: 1% to 3%
      B. Isoflurane: 1% to 3%
      C. Sevoflurane: 2% to 4%
    III. Monitoring (see Chapter 16)
      A. Body temperature
        1. Changes very little but usually decreases in large animals during anesthesia

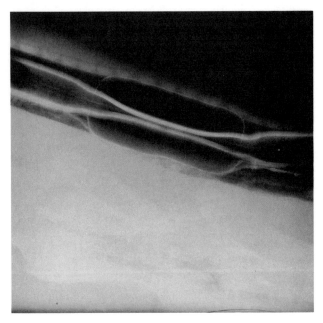

Fig. 20-5
Accidental overinflation of the endotracheal tube cuff can result in tube occlusion.

   2. May decrease in foals
   3. May increase if muscle relaxation is inadequate
   B. Chart all anesthetic and surgical events and the animal's response (see Fig. 19-10)
   C. Monitor all vital signs (i.e., cardiovascular, respiratory) and the depth of anesthesia (i.e., unconsciousness, eye signs)
   D. Measure and maintain arterial blood pressure (especially important) greater than 60 mm of Hg
      1. Administer fluids
      2. Reduce anesthetic delivery if possible
      3. Administer dobutamine (1 to 3 μg/kg/min)
IV. Administration of fluids (see Chapter 26)

TABLE **20-1**

TOTAL INTRAVENOUS ANESTHESIA (TIVA) TECHNIQUE IN HORSES

DRUG COMBINATIONS	CONCENTRATION (mg/ml)	INFUSION DOSE
Xylazine	1	1-2 ml/lb/hr to effect
Guaifenesin	100	
Ketamine*	2	
Detomidine	0.02	1-2 ml/lb/hr to effect
Guaifenesin	100	
Ketamine*	2	
Medetomidine	0.02	1-2 ml/lb/hr to effect
Guaifenesin	100	
Ketamine*	2	
Romifidine	0.06	1-2 ml/lb/hr to effect
Guaifenesin	100	
Ketamine*	2	

Butorphanol (0.01 mg/lb) may be added to enhance analgesia.
Ketamine is generally infused at rates of 25-75 μg/lb/min following adequate muscle relaxation.
*4 mg/ml ketamine reduces infusion to 0.4 ml/lb/h.

THE RECOVERY PERIOD

I. Turn off the vaporizer before the oxygen
II. Administer oxygen until the patient is swallowing, if possible; then extubate
III. Oxygen is routinely administered by the following:
    A. O_2 humidifier (minimum flow rate 15 L/min)
    B. O_2 demand valve
IV. Keep tranquilizers, ropes, and emergency drugs available in case of rough recoveries
    A. Make sure the cuff on the endotracheal tube is deflated
    B. Keep the animal's head and muzzle down to allow drainage
    C. Assist the animal to a standing position, if necessary
    D. Administer sedative (50 mg xylazine) to adult horses if they demonstrate any of the following:
        1. Excessive nystagmus or oculogyric activity
        2. Excessive muscle tremors
        3. Disorientation and loss of equilibrium

COMMON ANESTHETIC PROBLEMS

    I. Hypotension (mean arterial blood pressure less than 50 mm Hg)

    II. Hypoventilation ($PaCO_2$ greater than 55 mm Hg)

    III. Hypoxemia (PaO_2 less than 60 mm Hg)

        A. PaO_2 should be greater than 250 mm Hg when breathing 100% O_2

    IV. Bradycardia (heart rate less than 30 bpm)

    V. Difficulty maintaining adequate anesthetic depth

    VI. Nonrespiratory (metabolic) acidosis

    VII. Underhydration or overhydration

    VIII. Nasal edema and/or upper airway obstruction

    IX. Poor or prolonged recovery

    X. Neuropathy and/or myopathy

CHAPTER TWENTY-ONE

Anesthetic Procedures and Techniques in Ruminants

"You've got to stop and eat the roses along the way."

ANONYMOUS PHILOSOPHER

OVERVIEW

Physical restraint and local anesthetic techniques are frequently used in ruminants to provide immobility and analgesia. General anesthesia techniques are similar to those for dogs, cats, or horses. Regurgitation of rumen contents and bloat (distention of the rumen) are potential hazards not usually encountered in dogs, cats, or horses. Close observation and monitoring of palpebral and ocular reflexes, eyeball position, and pupil size can be used to monitor the depth of anesthesia in ruminants. Recovery from anesthesia is generally quiet and uneventful and does not routinely require assistance.

GENERAL CONSIDERATIONS

I. Preparation of the ruminant for anesthesia and surgery
   A. The most important factor in decreasing the risk of regurgitation is to decrease rumen size and pressure before anesthesia
      1. Withhold food for 12 to 36 hours in large ruminants
      2. Withhold water for 8 to 12 hours in large ruminants
      3. Withhold food for 12 to 24 hours in sheep and goats; there is no need to withhold water
      4. Withhold food for 2 to 4 hours in calves, lambs, and young kids; when these animals are less than 1 month of age, they are essentially monogastric and are less prone to regurgitation during anesthesia

B. Side effects of withholding food are minimal
   1. Mild metabolic alkalosis is observed in healthy animals
   2. Bradycardia in adult cattle results from increased vagal tone
C. Endotracheal and rumen tubes can be placed, when appropriate, to avoid bloat and aspiration of rumen contents

II. Most surgical techniques in cattle can be performed using local or regional anesthesia (see Chapter 5)

III. General anesthesia is required if local or regional anesthetic techniques are inadequate; light stages of anesthesia may predispose the animal to stress, which may result in tachycardia and hypertension

PREANESTHETIC EVALUATION

I. Preanesthetic evaluation is very similar to that in horses
   A. Physical examination
   B. Basic laboratory tests
      1. PCV or Hb
      2. Plasma total protein

PREANESTHETIC MEDICATION

I. Preanesthetic drugs are used to calm or sedate ruminants or to decrease the dose of a more potent intravenous or inhalation anesthetic

II. Tranquilizers are not approved for use in food animals; drug residues in milk and meat products are problematic

III. Popular preanesthetic medications include the following drugs:
   A. Xylazine
      1. One tenth the intravenous dose used in horses: 0.05 mg/lb or less IV; 0.1 to 0.3 IM mg/lb IM
      2. Only low-concentration xylazine is recommended (20 mg/ml)
      3. A moderate dose of 0.01 to 0.05 mg/lb IV generally induces recumbency and depresses or abolishes pharyngeal and laryngeal reflexes, thus allowing easy intubation and inhalation anesthesia without additional medication

4. Side effects
   a. Cardiovascular depression
   b. Respiratory depression
   c. Rumen atony with bloat
   d. Hyperglycemia from decreased plasma insulin
   e. Diuresis
   f. Decreased hematocrit
   g. Premature delivery in late pregnancy
5. Antagonists
   a. Nonspecific antagonists:
      (1) Doxapram 0.1 mg/lb IV can be used as a respiratory stimulant
   b. Specific antagonists:
      (1) Atipamezole 5 μg/lb IV
      (2) Yohimbine
      (3) Tolazoline

B. Detomidine or medetomidine
   1. Dose is similar to other species: 5 to 10 μg/lb IM
   2. Effects are similar to xylazine
   3. Antagonists: see section on xylazine on p. 344
C. Acepromazine (to produce a calming effect)
   1. Not frequently used because of prolonged elimination
   2. Dose: 20 to 40 mg/1000 lb IM; 5 to 10 mg/1000 lb IV
   3. Onset of tranquilization is within 10 to 20 minutes
   4. Duration of tranquilization is 2 to 4 hours
D. Ketamine or Telazol
   1. Dose: ketamine, up to 1 mg/lb IV or 1 to 3 mg/lb IM; Telazol, 0.5 mg/lb IV or 2 mg/lb IM
   2. Prior administration of xylazine (0.1 mg/lb IM) decreases ketamine or Telazol dosage by one half
   3. Ocular, pharyngeal, and laryngeal reflexes are depressed
   4. Compatible with inhalation anesthetics
   5. Side effects
      a. Respiratory depression
      b. Hypotension
E. Atropine, glycopyrrolate
   1. Not frequently used
   2. Saliva flow is best controlled by pointing the animal's head downward and placing an endotracheal tube with an inflatable cuff

3. Anticholinergics increase the viscosity of the saliva (without significantly decreasing the volume of saliva)
4. Atropine sulfate, 2 mg/100 lb IM or SQ, may be useful in preventing bradycardia and hypotension during manipulation of viscera
5. The duration of action of atropine in ruminants is short
6. Anticholinergics increase the incidence of bloat because of a decrease in intestinal motility and an accumulation of gas from bacterial fermentation

INDUCTION

I. Barbiturates
   A. Thiopental sodium (Pentothal) is an ultrashort-acting (10 to 15 minutes) barbiturate with predictable effects
      1. Doses of 3 to 5 mg/lb of thiopental will achieve light surgical anesthesia within 12 to 15 seconds
      2. Less barbiturate is needed if the animal is premedicated or induced with guaifenesin
      3. Barbiturates should be used with caution in animals less than 3 months of age
      4. Barbiturates rapidly cross the placental barrier and depress fetal respiration
II. Guaifenesin
   A. Dose: 25 mg/lb IV in small increments until effective, followed by thiobarbiturates or ketamine
   B. 5% solution (50 mg/ml) in water or with 5% dextrose; more concentrated solutions (more than 7%) may cause hemolysis
   C. Can be used in combination with xylazine, thiopental, ketamine, or Telazol
III. Xylazine-ketamine combination
   A. Dose: 0.02 mg/lb xylazine and 1 mg/lb ketamine IV
      1. Both drugs can be administered in the same syringe
      2. When given intravenously, immobilization occurs in approximately 45 to 90 seconds, supplying anesthesia for 20 to 30 minutes; standing recovery occurs 2 hours or more after the initial injection
      3. When given intramuscularly, induction time is 3 to 10 minutes; anesthesia and recovery times are increased

4. Decreases heart rate, respiratory rate, and temperature; an apneustic respiratory pattern and salivation are seen in ruminants

IV. Xylazine-ketamine-guaifenesin combination ("triple drip")

   A. Dose: 30 to 50 mg xylazine + 500 mg ketamine in 500 ml of 5% guaifenesin given in small increments to effect, approximately 0.5 to 1 ml IV; anesthesia can be continued at a rate of 1 ml/lb/hr

      1. All three drugs are soluble in water

      2. Induction is gradual and generally uneventful but may require some physical restraint

      3. Anesthesia is adequate for periods of 30 to 90 minutes; respiration may need to be assisted

      4. Drug overdose causes apnea and hypotension

      5. Only ketamine (500 mg) and guaifenesin (500 ml of 5%) are used in calm animals

V. Ketamine

   A. Ketamine (1 ml;100 mg/ml) mixed 50:50 with diazepam (1 ml; 5 mg/ml) 1 ml 21 to 40 lb is used in small ruminants

VI. Telazol

   A. 0.025 to 0.5 mg/lb IV; 1 to 3 mg/lb IM

      1. Produces excellent, short-term (20 to 30 minutes) surgical anesthesia

      2. May produce respiratory depression

VII. Masking down with an inhalation anesthetic: animals under 150 lb can be induced using a mask induction technique with 3% to 4% halothane, 3% isoflurane, or 4% to 6% sevoflurane; the animal is intubated and maintained at 1% to 2%

ENDOTRACHEAL INTUBATION

I. Intubation should immediately follow the induction of anesthesia

II. Several techniques are useful

   A. A dental speculum or mouth gag can be placed in the mouth

   B. Method 1: insert an arm into the oral cavity of the adult cow, reflect the epiglottis forward manually, and guide the endotracheal tube into the larynx

   C. Method 2: extend the patient's head and neck, and gently advance the tube into the trachea during inspiration

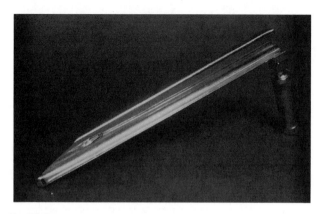

Fig. 21-1
Endotracheal intubation in cattle, sheep, and goats can be facilitated with a long-blade laryngoscope.

    D. Intubation may be facilitated by a laryngoscope and endoscopic light (Fig. 21-1)

    E. In small ruminants, a long, small-diameter dowel made of wood, steel, or plastic may be placed into the trachea first; the endotracheal tube can then be passed over it (Fig. 21-2)

    F. Intubation should be done quickly to avoid regurgitation and aspiration of fluid

    G. A tracheostomy may be performed if necessary

MAINTENANCE OF ANESTHESIA

    I. Total intravenous anesthesia (TIVA) (see Table 20-1)
        A. Triple drip (see p. 347)

    II. Inhalation anesthetic drugs produce general anesthesia very effectively, particularly for prolonged surgical procedures

    III. Induction is completed with 3% to 5% halothane, 2% to 4% isoflurane, or 4 to 6% sevoflurane

    IV. A surgical plane of anesthesia may be maintained at 0.5% to 2% halothane, 1% to 2% isoflurane, or 3% to 4% sevoflurane

    V. If surgical procedures last longer than 1 hour or blood carbon dioxide concentrations are greater than 60 mm Hg, ventilate ruminants to minimize respiratory acidosis

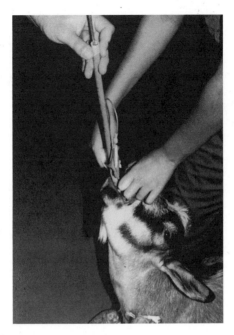

Fig. 21-2
To facilitate intubation in small ruminants, a steel dowel can be placed in the trachea and the endotracheal tube slid over it.

MONITORING

I. The position of the eyeball provides a useful guide to anesthetic depth

A. Ocular reflexes are good indicators of anesthetic depth; the corneal reflex should be present throughout anesthesia and the palpebral reflex depressed by inhalation anesthesia

B. The eyeball often rotates medioventrally when the patient is in a light surgical plane of anesthesia (Fig. 21-3)

C. The iris and pupil are centered when the patient is in a deep surgical plane of anesthesia or awake; dilated pupils are a sign of anesthetic overdose when using inhalation anesthesia

D. The auricular artery, located on the dorsal surface of the ear, can be cannulated to monitor arterial blood pressure

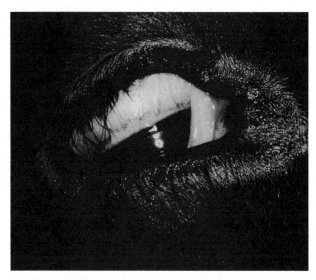

Fig. 21-3
The bovine eye rotates ventromedially during light planes of anesthesia.

   II. See "Monitoring Equipment," Chapter 16
  III. Administration of fluids (see Chapter 26)

THE RECOVERY PERIOD

   I. Ruminants are allowed to breathe 100% oxygen for several
       minutes before being disconnected from the anesthetic ma-
       chine
  II. Leave the endotracheal tube in place with the cuff partially in-
       flated until the laryngeal reflex returns to prevent aspiration of
       regurgitated material
 III. Position the patient's head to allow drainage before the endo-
       tracheal tube is pulled
  IV. Leave the cuff inflated while the endotracheal tube is removed
   V. Pass a stomach tube before removing the endotracheal tube to
       decompress the rumen if the animal has bloated
  VI. To avoid regurgitation, position ruminants on their right side
       or in sternal recumbency once the tube is pulled

VII. Cattle do not usually require assistance during inhalation anesthesia recovery

COMMON ANESTHETIC PROBLEMS

I. The most frequently encountered problems associated with sedation and general anesthesia include the following:
   A. Regurgitation
   B. Bloat
   C. Inadequate oxygenation
   D. Injury
   E. Respiratory depression and apnea
   F. Pulmonary aspiration

II. Regurgitation is caused by a vagal effect on reticular contractions and parasympathetic effects on pharyngoesophageal and gastroesophageal sphincters
   A. Anesthetic drugs increase the risk of regurgitation in the following ways:
      1. By relaxing the pharyngoesophageal sphincter
      2. By relaxing the gastroesophageal sphincter
      3. By depressing the swallow reflex
   B. Recumbency also increases the risk of regurgitation

CHAPTER TWENTY-TWO

Anesthetic Procedures and Techniques in Pigs

"It is a bad plan that admits of no modification."
PUBLILIUS SYRUS

OVERVIEW

Swine anesthesia is a unique challenge. Swine have few superficial veins that are easily accessible, other than those on the dorsal surface of the ear. Ear veins may be difficult to use because of previous identification and tagging procedures; therefore, most chemical restraining drugs are administered intramuscularly (IM). Pigs are difficult to intubate because of their small oral cavity, large tongue, and the presence of a pharyngeal diverticulum. Respiratory depression and elevations of body temperature are frequently associated with chemical restraint and general anesthesia. Respiratory depression may be caused by the combined respiratory-depressant effects of chemical restraining drugs and the limited expansion of the chest wall because of abnormal body positioning and body fat. Elevation in body temperature occurs because of the low body surface area to body mass ratio, the relative absence of sweat glands, and inefficient thermoregulatory mechanisms. Hyperpyrexia and malignant hyperthermia have been reported in genetically predisposed pigs and can be triggered by a variety of intravenous and inhalation anesthetics. Physical restraint combined with sedatives, tranquilizers, and local anesthetic techniques are the usual methods for simple surgical procedures in pigs. General anesthesia using inhalation anesthetics provides excellent, stable anesthesia for prolonged or complicated surgical procedures.

GENERAL CONSIDERATIONS

I. Surgical preparation of the pig
   A. Obtain a complete history and do a complete physical examination; pay particular attention to the respiratory system
   B. Withhold food for 8 to 12 hours in adults, 1 to 3 hours in neonates
   C. Do not withhold water
   D. Avoid stressing the pig by leaving it with other pigs until it is tranquilized
II. The preanesthetic evaluation
   A. Physical examination
   B. Basic laboratory tests, including a complete blood count

ANESTHETIC PROCEDURES

I. Telazol-ketamine-xylazine (TKX) combination
   A. Formulation: reconstitute 500 mg of Telazol powder with 2.5 ml of xylazine (100 mg/ml) and 2.5 ml of ketamine (100 mg/ml)
   B. Administer the combination intramuscularly at 0.5 to 1 ml/50 lb body weight
   C. Provides useful restraint and short-term anesthesia
   D. Endotracheal intubation can be performed
   E. Compatible with inhalant agents
   F. Duration of action is 20 to 30 minutes; recovery occurs in 60 to 90 minutes
II. Lumbosacral epidural or spinal anesthesia are commonly used local anesthetic techniques in pigs (see Chapter 5)
   A. The major advantages are minimal systemic effects and the minimal effect on the fetuses during cesarean section
   B. Disadvantages include lack of unconsciousness, necessitating physical restraint of the forelimbs
   C. A 3- to 5-inch, 18-gauge spinal needle is used to facilitate administration of 2% lidocaine hydrochloride
      1. The dose varies from 0.2 to 0.5 ml/10 lb, with the higher dosage providing anesthesia cranially to the paralumbar fossa; spinal doses are one half of epidural doses

III. Intratesticular injection

    A. Large boars can be castrated by using physical restraint and the injection of 15 to 30 mg/kg of sodium pentobarbital into each testicle

    B. Anesthesia occurs in approximately 5 minutes

    C. As soon as the testicles are removed, the source of anesthetic is removed

IV. Atropine-acepromazine-ketamine combination

    A. Dosage: 0.02 mg/lb atropine and 0.05 to 0.2 mg/lb acepromazine IM, followed in 20 minutes by 5 mg/lb IM ketamine

    B. Useful for minor surgical or medical procedures, such as detusking or castration of large boars

    C. Advantages

        1. Ease of administration

        2. Some analgesia and muscle relaxation within 5 minutes; lasts 10 to 15 minutes

    D. Disadvantages

        1. Additional analgesia is required with a local anesthetic

        2. A 20-minute waiting period between administration of drugs is necessary

        3. Hypotension

V. Atropine-xylazine-ketamine combination

    A. Dosage: 0.02 mg/lb atropine and 1 to 3 mg/lb xylazine IM, followed in 10 minutes with 5 mg/lb IM ketamine

    B. Advantages

        1. Ease of administration

        2. Some analgesia and muscle relaxation within 5 minutes; lasts 10 to 15 minutes

    C. Disadvantages

        1. Xylazine has a short duration of action because it is rapidly metabolized

        2. Muscle movement is involuntary during the anesthetic period

VI. Xylazine-ketamine-guaifenesin combination

    A. Dosage: 500 mg xylazine + 500 mg ketamine mixed in 500 ml 5% guaifenesin; given intravenously in small increments until effective, approximately 1 to 2 ml/lb IV

    B. Advantages

        1. Gradual induction

      2. Stable hemodynamics

      3. Good muscle relaxation

   C. Disadvantages

      1. Respiratory depression may require assisted ventilation

VII. Xylazine-Telazol

   A. Dosage: xylazine 0.1 to 0.5 mg/lb IM followed in 5 minutes by Telazol 1 to 3 mg/lb IM

   B. Advantages

      1. Ease of administration

      2. Good analgesia and muscle relaxation

      3. Minimal cardiovascular depression

   C. Disadvantages

      1. Occasional respiratory depression

      2. Light plane of anesthesia

      3. Short duration of action; may need to be supplemented

      4. Pigs may remain drowsy for 24 hours

      5. Increased salivation

VIII. Inhalation anesthesia

   A. The inhalation anesthetics, halothane, isoflurane, or sevoflurane, are administered

      1. For induction (by mask) to anesthesia

      2. For maintenance of anesthesia after the pig is induced with other drugs

   B. Inhalation drugs (Fig. 22-1) can be administered in the following ways:

      1. Through a face mask

      2. Through nasal tubes, which are made from human nasal tube adapters and small-animal endotracheal tubes (6 to 8 mm)

      3. Through endotracheal intubation, which is preferred; laryngoscope or long, rigid dowel rods can be used to pass the endotracheal tube

   C. Advantages

      1. Good control of anesthesia

      2. Excellent muscle relaxation

      3. Ease of administration

   D. Disadvantages

      1. Expensive equipment required

      2. Not generally suited for field conditions

      3. Halothane can induce hyperthermia in pigs

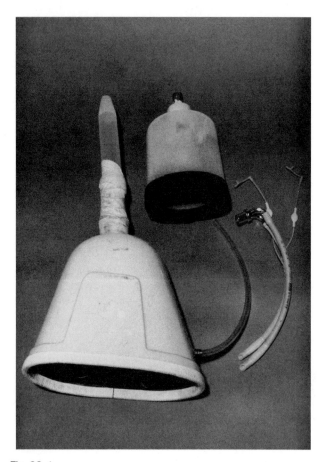

Fig. 22-1
Face masks and nasal endotracheal tubes can be used as an alternative to endotracheal intubation in pigs.

MONITORING

I. Monitoring anesthesia in pigs is similar to that for other species (see Chapter 16); the auricular artery, located on the dorsal surface of the ear, can be cannulated to monitor arterial blood pressure

  II. Signs of malignant hyperthermia
    A. Extreme muscle rigidity
    B. Increased temperature (more than 107° F); hot to the touch
    C. Tachycardia
    D. Tachypnea
    E. Metabolic acidosis
III. Treatment of hyperthermia in pigs
    A. Dantrolene: 1 to 3 mg/lb IV; 10 mg/lb per os
    B. Supportive treatment
      1. Fluids
      2. Bicarbonate
      3. Steroids
      4. Oxygen
      5. Body cooling

THE RECOVERY PERIOD

  I. Administer oxygen and/or assist ventilation if necessary
  II. Position the pig in sternal recumbency
III. Place the pig in a well-ventilated, cool, and quiet environment
IV. Assess vital signs periodically

COMMON ANESTHETIC PROBLEMS

  I. Respiratory depression is a frequent sequela to the administration of depressant drugs in pigs
    A. Estimate the size of the pig's trachea before drug administration; it may be very narrow
      1. Use a laryngoscope and pre-place a stiff polyethylene stylet
    B. Be prepared for respiratory emergencies
      1. Have a variety of endotracheal tube sizes available
      2. Be prepared to do a tracheotomy
        a. No. 10 blade and scalpel
        b. Hemostat
        c. Cuffed tracheostomy tube
        d. Respiratory stimulants, such as doxapram, may be necessary

II. Increases in body temperature are frequently associated with inhalation anesthesia in pigs

    A. The pig has a low body surface area relative to body mass

    B. The pig has relatively poor thermoregulatory mechanisms and relatively few sweat glands

    C. Depolarizing neuromuscular blocking agents and inhalation anesthetics can trigger malignant hyperthermia

        1. Several strains of pigs (e.g., Landrace, Poland China) are genetically predisposed to malignant hyperthermia

        2. Dantrolene (1 mg/lb IV) is the only truly effective therapy for malignant hyperthermia

CHAPTER TWENTY-THREE

Anesthesia for Cesarean Section

"The hand that rocks the cradle is the hand that rules the world."

WILLIAM ROSS WALLACE

OVERVIEW

Anesthetic drugs used in pregnant animals affect the fetus. Generally, the effects of anesthetic drugs are more pronounced and longer-lasting in the fetus than in the mother. Drugs that cross the placental barrier slowly, or not at all, are preferred. Anesthetic drugs may induce or inhibit parturition by altering uterine function. This chapter describes the changes that occur in maternal physiology during advanced pregnancy and the effects of anesthetic drugs in pregnant animals.

GENERAL CONSIDERATIONS

I. Pregnancy, especially the immediate preparturient period, causes significant alterations in maternal physiology
   A. Altered pharmacokinetics and pharmacodynamics
   B. Changes in hemodynamics
      1. Increased heart rate
      2. Increased cardiac output
      3. Increased blood volume
      4. The weight of the gravid uterus causes aortocaval compression during dorsal recumbency; cardiac reserve is decreased because of increased cardiac output and aortocaval compression

5. Central venous pressure and systemic blood pressure remain relatively unchanged but may increase during labor

C. Changes in respiration
    1. Increased breathing rate
    2. Decreased functional residual capacity (FRC)
    3. The gravid uterus may restrict breathing by cranially displacing the diaphragm

II. Anesthetic drug and technique considerations
    A. Providing optimal analgesia for surgery
    B. Preventing maternal hypoxemia or hypotension
    C. Minimizing fetal depression
    D. Minimizing postoperative maternal depression
    E. Neither inducing nor preventing uterine contractions

CHANGES IN MATERNAL PHYSIOLOGY IN ADVANCED PREGNANCY

I. Central nervous system (CNS)
    A. Increased progesterone concentration decreases inhalation anesthetic requirement
    B. Vascular engorgement decreases the size of the epidural space; decreased volume of local anesthetic is required for epidural anesthesia

II. Respiratory system
    A. Alveolar ventilation is increased because of increased respiratory center sensitivity to CO_2, which is progesterone-induced; increased alveolar ventilation and decreased FRC result in a more rapid alveolar rate of rise in inhalation anesthetics
    B. FRC is decreased because of anterior displacement of diaphragm
        1. Relative anemia refers to the pregnant patient not tolerating blood loss as well as the nonpregnant patient
        2. Patients with a history of heart disease may decompensate
    C. Small airways constrict at higher lung volumes; airway closure and decreased FRC cause greater ventilation perfusion mismatches, which may result in decreased oxygenation

III. Cardiovascular system
  A. Maternal blood volume is increased by approximately 30%
  B. Packed cell volume and plasma-protein concentration are decreased
  C. Cardiac output is increased 30% to 50% because of increases in stroke volume and heart rate
IV. Gastrointestinal system
  A. Placental gastric secretion increases gastric acidity
    1. Increases the chance of regurgitation and aspiration pneumonia
    2. Increases the need for a properly fitting cuffed endotracheal tube
  B. The stomach is displaced cranially, and the tone to the lower esophageal sphincter is altered
V. Other changes: decreased plasma cholinesterase (pseudo-cholinesterase)
  A. Prolonged duration of action of succinylcholine
  B. Prolonged duration of action of ester local anesthetics

DRUG TRANSFER ACROSS THE PLACENTA

I. Factors influencing drug transfer
  A. Surface area and diffusion characteristics of the placenta; the surface area of the placenta is large, and diffusion distance is small in all species
  B. Diffusion properties of drugs
    1. High lipid solubility, which increases diffusibility
    2. Lower molecular weight, which increases diffusibility
    3. Decreased degree of ionization and protein binding, which increases diffusibility
  C. Relative maternal and fetal drug concentrations
    1. Discrete bolus doses of drugs result in rapid transfer of drug to the fetus, initially and rapidly declining maternal concentrations
    2. Continuous-infusion, repeated bolus administration, and the administration of inhalation anesthetics result in continuously high maternal drug concentration and continual drug transfer to the fetus

UTEROPLACENTAL CIRCULATION AND FETAL VIABILITY

I. Conditions that decrease circulating maternal blood volume can decrease placental perfusion, resulting in fetal hypoxia and acidosis; this includes maternal dehydration, hemorrhage (shock), and drug-induced hypotension
  A. Dehydration
    1. Prolonged labor
    2. Concurrent disease
  B. Hemorrhage and shock
    1. Prolonged labor
    2. Supine positioning: decreases venous return
    3. Anesthetic drugs
    4. Surgically related hemorrhage
    5. Hemorrhagic or endotoxic shock
  C. Drugs: anesthetic drugs cause peripheral vasodilation and hypotension

MATERNAL AND FETAL EFFECTS FROM ANESTHETIC DRUGS USED FOR CESAREAN SECTION

  I. Anticholinergics—drug effects
    A. Both atropine and scopolamine pass placental barriers rapidly
      1. Fetal tachycardia noted within 10 to 15 minutes
      2. Fetal disorientation or excitement may be caused by central action of atropine or scopolamine
      3. Fetal effects may vary, depending on the amount of drug absorbed
    B. Glycopyrrolate does not cross the placenta in significant quantities because of its large molecular size and charge
    C. Anticholinergics can reduce placental activity
  II. Local anesthetic drugs
    A. Drug effects
      1. Local anesthetic drugs administered by any route cross the placental barrier
        a. Drug effects depend on the total dose, the interval between final dose and delivery, and whether epinephrine is used

       b. Doses of local anesthetics used clinically usually do not produce significant depression in the fetus

B. Lidocaine

   1. Lidocaine is the preferred local anesthetic for cesarean section because of clinical experience and relatively low toxicity

   2. Appears in umbilical venous blood of the fetus within 2 to 3 minutes

   3. No correlation has been found between the degree of neonatal depression and the umbilical venous concentration of lidocaine

III. Preanesthetic (sedatives, tranquilizers, opioids) drug effects

A. Drug effects: preanesthetic drugs reduce the amount of potentially more dangerous anesthetic drugs

   1. Phenothiazines (acepromazine)

      a. Rapidly appear in fetal blood

      b. Produce little to no apparent effect on the newborn when used in clinical dosages

      c. α-Adrenergic blockade may produce hypotension in stressed animals, resulting in decreased uterine blood flow and fetal hypoxia

      d. Decrease uterine tone

   2. Benzodiazepines (diazepam, midazolam)

      a. Concentrations higher in fetal blood than in maternal blood

      b. Produce minimal respiratory and cardiovascular depression

      c. Duration of action depends on redistribution away from the CNS

   3. α_2-Agonists (xylazine, detomidine, medetomidine, romifidine)

      a. Respiratory depression may be severe in both the mother and fetus

      b. Use in low doses and be prepared to administer an antagonist (yohimbine, tolazoline, atipamazole)

      c. α_2-Agonists increase uterine pressure in cattle; may be abortifacients; effects in other species is unknown

   4. Opioids

      a. Frequently used as preanesthetic medication for sedation and analgesia or administered epidurally

364 DRUGS USED FOR CESAREAN SECTION

        b. Readily cross the placenta
        c. Concentrations may be higher in the fetus than in the mother because of a lower fetal pH
        d. Moderate maternal doses do not produce serious CNS depression in neonates; the effect can be reversed by opioid antagonists (naloxone)
        e. Since naloxone has a shorter duration of action than most opioids, neonates should be observed for several hours and re-dosed as needed
        f. Specific opioid drugs
            (1) Meperidine (Demerol)
                (a) Reaches the fetal circulation rapidly
                (b) No significant depression is apparent if birth is within the first hour
            (2) Morphine
                (a) Causes observable clinical CNS depression in the newborn
                (b) Has a direct vasoconstrictor effect on placental vessels
            (3) Oxymorphone (Numorphan)
                (a) Better analgesia and sedation than meperidine or morphine but has a shorter duration of effect
                (b) Can produce neonatal depression
            (4) Fentanyl (Sublimaze); 100 times more potent as an analgesic than morphine, with respiratory depression of shorter duration
IV. Injectable anesthetic drugs
    A. Dissociogenic agents (ketamine, tiletamine)
        1. Produce restraint and analgesia
        2. Produce poor muscle relaxation
        3. Rapidly cross the placenta, producing fetal depression within 5 to 10 minutes
        4. Specific dissociogenic drugs
            a. Ketamine
                (1) Good restraint in queens with minimal fetal depression when used intravenously (IV) or intramuscularly (IM) in low dosages (1 mg/lb IV; 5 mg/lb IM)

        (2) Poor muscle relaxation and questionable ability to block deep pain

        (3) May increase uterine tone and decrease uterine blood flow, leading to fetal hypoxia

        (4) Fetal blood levels reach 70% of those in the mother

        (5) Minimal clinical CNS depression is evident in the neonate

    b. Telazol (tiletamine-zolazepam)

        (1) Similar to ketamine but produces better muscle relaxation

        (2) Greater respiratory depression

B. Propofol

  1. Used for induction of anesthesia in parturients

    a. Single bolus (1 to 3 mg/lb IV) followed by inhalant anesthetic

  2. Crosses the placenta readily but produces short duration effects on the fetus

  3. Large volume of distribution causes plasma concentrations to fall rapidly

  4. Fetal respiratory depression is a concern

C. Barbiturates

  1. Readily crosses the placenta into fetal circulation

  2. Phenobarbital should be avoided because of prolonged fetal CNS depression and reduced fetal ability to metabolize drugs

  3. Dose of barbiturates that does not produce anesthesia in the mother can completely inhibit fetal respiratory movements

  4. Ultrashort-acting barbiturates (thiopental)

    a. Thiobarbiturates cross the placenta readily and achieve equilibrium within 5 minutes

    b. A single dose of 4 mg/lb at induction produces only modest placental transfer and does not endanger the normal fetus

        (1) Because of a dependence on redistribution for their duration of action, the use of small doses of an ultrashort-acting barbiturate has not been associated with a significant degree of fetal CNS depression

        (2) Re-dosing is discouraged

        (3) Peak drug concentrations occur in the fetus within 10 minutes

V. Peripheral muscle relaxants: neuromuscular blocking drugs include succinylcholine, pancuronium, atracurium, and vecuronium

  A. These drugs are highly ionized with a high molecular weight, resulting in minimal and poor placental transfer

  B. No analgesia is produced; used only in combination with other drugs

  C. There is no demonstrable effect on the newborn

  D. Succinylcholine metabolism is reduced because of a decrease in pseudocholinesterase

VI. Inhalation anesthetic drugs

  A. All inhalation anesthetic drugs readily cross the placenta because of their low molecular weight and lipid solubility

  B. The degree of fetal CNS depression depends on the depth and duration of maternal anesthesia

  C. Specific inhalation drugs

    1. Nitrous oxide

      a. Rapidly crosses the placenta

      b. Administration exceeding 15 minutes may result in fetal CNS depression

      c. Diffusion hypoxia, which may occur in the fetus, can be minimized with oxygen therapy

      d. When used in the mother with adequate amounts of oxygen, there is minimal effect on the neonate

    2. Halothane

      a. Quickly appears in the fetal circulation

      b. Rapid and potent uterine relaxant

        (1) Inhibits uterine involution

        (2) Increases the risk of uterine hemorrhage

      c. If used for cesarean section, the procedure should be performed as quickly as possible; neonatal CNS depression should resolve rapidly if adequate ventilation is provided at birth

    3. Isoflurane

      a. Quickly appears in fetal circulation

      b. Rapid and potent uterine relaxant

    c. If used for cesarean section, the procedure should be performed as quickly as possible

      (1) The degree of fetal CNS depression does not correlate with maternal blood concentration

      (2) Neonatal respiratory depression may be severe, requiring postparturient ventilation

    d. Rapid elimination of this agent with ventilation may be an advantage

  4. Sevoflurane and desflurane are similar to isoflurane; desflurane's rapid onset and elimination minimize the duration of maternal and fetal CNS depression

ANESTHETIC TECHNIQUES

I. General principles

  A. The choice of a particular anesthetic technique should be influenced by familiarity with the technique or drug and avoidance of excessive fetal CNS depression

  B. Intubation is desirable in all patients

  C. Use local and regional analgesic techniques when possible

  D. Presurgical preparation and oxygenation should be completed before the administration of anesthetic drugs

  E. Avoid excessive physical restraint: sedatives, tranquilizers, and other drugs that can be antagonized are preferred over excessive physical force and subsequent maternal-fetal distress

  F. Avoid dorsal recumbency, if possible; left lateral recumbency may be the safest method

II. Anesthetic techniques by species (Table 23-1)

TABLE 23-1
ANESTHETIC TECHNIQUES BY SPECIES

SPECIES	DRUG/TECHNIQUE	DOSAGE	COMMENTS
Local techniques			
Dog, cat	1. Epidural with 2% lidocaine or morphine	1 ml/7.5 lb body weight lidocaine; 0.1 mg/lb body weight morphine	Requires assistant for physical restraint; use sedative/tranquilizer in all, but extremely tractable patients
General techniques			
	2. Diazepam-ketamine induction	0.125 mg/lb diazepam plus 2.5 mg/lb ketamine IV	Single-bolus dose depresses fetus minimally
	Telazol induction	1-3 mg/lb IM	Single administration causes minimal fetal CNS depression Diazepam-ketamine good in patients who are depressed and in shock
	Maintenance		
	Halothane, isoflurane, or sevoflurane in 50% N_2O and oxygen followed by muscle relaxant (atracurium, pancuronium) if needed	See Chapters 8, 9, and 11	Administer inhalation agent as late into procedure as possible

Intractable animal

	3. Premedication		
	Dogs: acepromazine-oxymorphone	0.5 mg/lb of each maximum 4 mg of each	Controlled ventilation necessary when using relaxants
	Dogs or cats: valium-ketamine induction	1 ml of a 50:50 mixture per 10 lbs, IM	Sedative-hypnotics generally increase fetal CNS depression; therefore use sparingly
	4. Telazol	3-5 mg/lb IM	
Horse	1. Premedication: acepromazine, -xylazine, detomidine, or romifidine	Acepromazine: 0.02 mg/lb IV Xylazine: 0.1-0.3 mg/lb IV Detomidine: 5-10 µg/lb Romifidine: 40-80 µg/lb	Adjust dosage for physical condition of mother; rely on guaifenesin to produce relaxation and to allow less ketamine to be used
	Induction: guaifenesin plus ketamine	Guaifenesin: 25-50 mg/lb Ketamine: 0.7-1 mg/lb	
	Maintenance: halothane, isoflurane		

Local techniques

Cow	1. Standing paravertebral analgesia, line block, inverted L block	2% lidocaine (see Chapter 5 for techniques)	Suitable for tractable animals without a sedative Suitable for animals in good physical condition
	2. Anterior epidural	2% lidocaine, 1 ml/lb at Cx_1-Cx_2 junction	Induces recumbency and sensory block anterior to umbilicus Watch for hypotension Intubate if possible

Continued

IV, Intravenously; *IM,* intramuscularly.

TABLE 23-1

ANESTHETIC TECHNIQUES BY SPECIES—cont'd

SPECIES	DRUG/TECHNIQUE	DOSAGE	COMMENTS
General techniques			
Cow— cont'd	3. Guaifenesin-ketamine-xylazine	500 mg ketamine 25 mg xylazine 500 ml and 5% guaifenesin + 0.25-0.5 mg/lb until effective for maintenance	
Sheep, goat	1. Guaifenesin-ketamine	500 ml 5% guaifenesin containing 500 mg ketamine 0.25-1 mg/lb induction maintenance until effective	Intubate; copious salivation Moderate to poor muscle relaxation Can add 25 mg xylazine to mixture, but fetal CNS depression is greater Use for induction to gas or as IV technique Guaifenesin allows small bolus doses of ketamine
	2. Guaifenesin-ketamine induction; halothane, isoflurane	25 mg/lb guaifenesin 1 mg/lb ketamine	

3. Diazepam-ketamine	1 ml diazepam plus 1 ml ketamine Administer 1 ml/30 lbs Until effective	
4. Mask induction halothane, isoflurane, or sevoflurane		Useful in sick, toxic animals and when fetal viability is of no concern

Maintenance

Pig: Isoflurane or halothane

1. Epidural	2% lidocaine (see Chapter 4 for technique) 0.5 mg/lb 3-5 mg/lb	Restraint of sow's head and front legs necessary Good chemical restraint; however, relatively more fetal CNS depression than with epidural
2. Xylazine plus ketamine		Excellent short-term restraint
3. Xylazine 2.5 ml Ketamine 2.5 ml in Telazol	1 ml/50 lbs, IM	
4. 500 mg ketamine plus 500 mg xylazine in 500 ml 5% guaifenesin	1 ml of mixture per lb until effective for maintenance	Requires placement of IV catheter

CHAPTER TWENTY-FOUR

Anesthetic Procedures in Exotic Pets

"'The time has come,' the walrus said, 'to talk of many things.'"

LEWIS CARROLL

OVERVIEW

The number of exotic animals being maintained as pets and for profit is increasing. Anesthesia for nontraditional species is accomplished by using the same techniques and drugs used in domestic animals. Because exotic species demonstrate idiosyncrasies and widely varying sensitivities to drugs, it is frequently necessary to make modifications. This chapter is an overview of the basic information needed to successfully immobilize the exotic animals that are likely to be encountered by general practitioners.*

GENERAL CONSIDERATIONS

I. Preanesthetic considerations
  A. Discussions with owners
    1. Ensure that the client has realistic expectations
    2. Detail prognosis and risks; owners may not understand that exotic animals respond differently to immobilization than domestic animals

---

*For more detailed descriptions of chemical restraint and anesthesia in laboratory animals, including primates, refer to the following article: Flecknell PA: *Laboratory animal anesthesia: a practical introduction for research workers and technicians,* ed 2, San Diego, 1996, Academic Press.

3. Determine the aftercare provider; owners may not be able to administer treatments to exotic pets
4. Discuss costs

B. Reduce the animal's stress; exotic animals have high sympathetic drive; excessive stress can induce complications that include arrhythmias, hypertension, and hyperthermia, which can result in death

C. Presurgical evaluation and patient selection
1. Physical examination: contraindications to anesthesia
   a. Abnormally slow recovery rate (the amount of time an animal needs to return to normal respirations after 2 minutes of physical restraint or pursuit); a normal amount of time is less than 3 to 5 minutes
   b. Shock; septicemia; acidosis
   c. Anemia or cyanosis
   d. Prolonged clotting
   e. Cachexia; obesity
   f. Animal has not fasted (if regurgitation is likely)
   g. Severe weakness and CNS depression
   h. Dehydration
   i. Ascites
2. Laboratory evaluation: contraindications to anesthesia
   a. If packed cell volume (PCV) is low, a blood transfusion may be needed

GENUS	PCV (%)
Avian	<25
Reptile	<17 to 20
Amphibian	<20
Rodent/lagomorph	<20
Mustelid	<25
Felid	<15
Swine	<20
Camelid	<20

b. If PCV is high, fluids may be needed

GENUS	PCV (%)
Avian	>50 to 60
Reptile	>50 to 60
Amphibian	>60
Rodent/lagomorph	>55 to 60
Mustelid	>60
Felid	>50
Swine	>50
Camelid	>50

c. If total protein is less than 3 g/dl, amino acid or plasma supplementation may be needed; refractometers and colorimetric tests frequently used at diagnostic laboratories for mammalian blood often register falsely low proteins in non-mammalian species; the biuret method is the most accurate in avian species

d. If glucose is low, administer 5% dextrose or delay anesthesia

GENUS	GLUCOSE (MG/DL)
Avian	<150
Reptile	<50 to 80
Amphibian	<50
Rodent/lagomorph	<80 to 100
Mustelid	<80 to 100
Felid	<80
Swine	<60
Camelid	<60

e. If calcium is less than 8 mg/dl, correct the level

f. If potassium is less than 3.5 mg/dl, correct the level

3. Further evaluation

a. Oral/fecal gram stains in non-mammalians

b. Culture and sensitivity

c. Fecal/urinalysis

d. Complete hemogram/serum profile

e. Radiographs/ultrasound

f. Clotting profile

g. Electrocardiogram (ECG)/echocardiography

II. Preanesthetic fasting

	TIME (HOURS)
Avian <100 g	0
Large psittacine	1 to 2
Raptor, ratite, fowl, waterfowl	12 to 24
Carnivorous reptile ingesting whole prey	> 5 days
Reptile < 200 g	2 to 4
Reptile 200 to 500 g	12
Reptile >500 g	24+
Amphibian	24
Fish	24
Rodent <200 g	2
Rodent >200 g/lagomorph	>6
Mustelid	12
	<2 h in ferrets with insulinoma
Felid	24
Swine	24
Camelid	24 to 48

III. Maintenance of homoiothermy
   A. Hypothermia depresses the respiratory control system
      1. Small animals are predisposed to hypothermia; they lose heat rapidly secondary to high surface area-to-volume ratios
      2. Ectotherms (reptiles, fish, and amphibians) do not generate their own heat; they require external heat sources to maintain their body temperature; hypothermia depresses the immune system and slows healing
      3. Hypothermia can result in brain damage, shock, electrolyte imbalances, and disseminated intravascular coagulation
         a. Well-insulated small animals such as rabbits, chinchillas, water birds, and birds in winter plumage are susceptible to hyperthermia
         b. Ungulates are prone to malignant hyperthermia; stress, high ambient temperature, and high relative humidity during immobilization increase the likelihood of hyperthermia
   B. Methods of monitoring core body temperature (skin temperature is not reliable)

      1. Esophageal thermometer

      2. Rectal/cloacal thermometer

  C. Heat sources

      1. To avoid iatrogenic burns and hyperthermia, always monitor heat sources

        a. Skin temperature

        b. Surface temperature where the patient's body contacts

        c. Ambient temperature in incubators

      2. Water-circulating heating pad

        a. Very safe

        b. High maintenance cost if punctured

      3. Electric heating pads

        a. Likely to cause iatrogenic burns

        b. Inexpensive

        c. Should never be set on high

      4. Incubators

        a. Must be preheated

        b. Useful before and after anesthesia

        c. Must be escape-proof

      5. Hot-water bottles

        a. Very safe

        b. Act as a heat sink after they are cool

      6. Warm air blankets (Bair Hugger; made by Augustine Medical)

        a. Very safe

        b. Blankets warm immediate surroundings

        c. Patient temperature must be monitored

IV. Fluids

  A. Preheat to 80° F to 95° F for animals weighing less than 1 kg and for all ectotherms

      1. Incubator

        a. Even, reliable temperature must be maintained

        b. Microbial growth may occur

      2. Warm water bath

        a. Even, reliable temperature must be maintained

        b. Water must be kept warm

      3. Microwave fluids

        a. Frequently have hot spots

        b. Should be well mixed

4. Placing intravenous tubing in warm water bath
   a. Quick method to warm fluids in emergency
   b. Effluent temperature must be carefully monitored
5. Fluid heating devices (Hotline, Level 1)
   a. Warms intravenous fluids to above 40° C

B. Administration (route)
1. Intravenous or intraosseous administration is best; the humerus in all birds and the femur in many birds are pneumatic bones; placing intraosseous catheters in these bones causes iatrogenic drowning
2. Subcutaneous fluids (usually 5% to 10% of body weight) are given before induction of anesthesia to allow absorption and volume expansion
3. Intraperitoneal fluids
   a. More rapidly absorbed than subcutaneous fluids
   b. Could cause peritonitis
   c. Must be warmed to body temperature
   d. Not in birds
   e. Not in pregnant animals
   f. Bladder should be expressed before administration
4. Colonic fluids
   a. Isotonic, warmed solution may be given as an enema
   b. Fluids are often absorbed more rapidly across the mucosa of the colon than from the subcutaneous space

C. Fluid rates
1. Standard maintenance: 40 to 100 ml/kg/24 hr; the higher end of the range is used for neonates, birds, and animals with high metabolism rates
2. Intraoperative: 10 to 20 ml/kg/hr
3. Shock: 30 to 80 ml/kg in 20 minutes

D. Fluid rate control
1. Rates less than 10 ml/hr require an intravenous fluid infusion pump to ensure accuracy
2. Rates of 10 to 50 ml/hr are accurately measured with in-line flow controls or burette fluid chambers
3. Rates greater than 50 ml/hr are accurately measured off of most fluid containers

E. Fluid choice (see Chapter 25)

F. Blood transfusion (see Chapter 25)
1. Ethylenediamine tetra-acetic acid should not be used in small patients to avoid hypocalcemia

2. Heparin is the anticoagulant of choice for birds
3. Birds can receive one interspecies or genera transfusion if a donor of the same species is not available, but survival of RBC over 24 hours is limited; intraspecific or at least intragenera transfusions are preferred
   a. Pigeons are the most common donors
   b. Transfusions should not be repeated for at least 3 weeks

G. Blood substitutes
   1. Oxyglobin (Biopure Corp.) can be used in most species as a blood substitute (10 to 30 ml/kg)

V. Premedication

A. If necessary, administer antibiotics to achieve adequate serum levels before induction of anesthesia

B. Select appropriate preanesthetic medication (Tables 24-1, 24-2)

C. Avian
   1. Atropine is not indicated in the presence of respiratory secretions, because it makes them more viscous
   2. Preanesthetics are rarely indicated if the bird is small enough to be manually restrained
      a. Most are overridden
      b. They may delay recovery

TABLE **24-1**

SEDATIVE AND ANALGESIC DRUGS FOR USE IN BIRDS

DRUG	DOSE
Alphaxalone/alphadolone	10-14 mg/kg IV
Buprenorphine	0.01-0.05 mg/kg IM
Butorphanol	2-4 mg/kg IM
Equithesin	2.5 ml/kg IM
Flunixin	1-10 mg/kg IM
Ketamine >1 kg	15-20 mg/kg IM
<1 kg	30-40 mg/kg IM
Ketamine/midazolam	20-40 mg/kg IM+
	4 mg/kg IM
Ketamine/xylazine	10-30 mg/kg IM+
	2-6 mg/kg IM
Ketoprofen	2 mg/kg SQ
Metomidate	10-20 mg/kg IM

      c. They may depress respirations

      d. Overall, diazepam/midazolam is the most efficacious and safe— 0.5 to 1 mg/kg intramuscularly (see Tables 24-2, 24-5)

   3. Because their long legs are susceptible to trauma, ratites, storks, and long-legged wading birds weighing more than 30 lb may benefit from sedation before capture and/or restraint

      a. Xylazine: 0.2 to 0.4 mg/kg IM

      b. Tiletamine-zolazepam (Telazol): 2 to 5 mg/kg IM

D. Reptile

   1. Atropine is not indicated in the presence of respiratory secretions, because it makes them more viscous

   2. Preanesthetics are rarely indicated, except in large, aggressive, and/or venomous reptiles

E. Amphibian: preanesthetics are not routinely used

F. Fish: preanesthetics are not routinely used

TABLE 24-2
AVIAN ANESTHESIA

SPECIES	DRUG	IM DOSAGE
Birds >250 g	Ketamine	10 mg/kg
	Ketamine	20-40 mg/kg
	Diazepam	1-1.5 mg/kg
Birds <250 g	Ketamine	30 mg/kg
Parakeet	Ketamine	30 mg/kg
	Xylazine	6.5 mg/kg
Cockatiel	Ketamine	25 mg/kg
	Xylazine	2.5 mg/kg
Amazon	Ketamine	10-20 mg/kg
	Xylazine	1-2 mg/kg
African Grey	Ketamine	15-20 mg/kg
	Xylazine	1.5 mg/kg
Cockatoo	Ketamine	20-30 mg/kg
	Xylazine	2.5-3.5 mg/kg
Macaw	Ketamine	15 mg/kg
	Xylazine	1.5-2 mg/kg
Hawks, falcons	Ketamine	25-30 mg/kg
	Xylazine	2 mg/kg
Owls	Ketamine	10-15 mg/kg
	Xylazine	2 mg/kg

   G. Rodent
1. Atropine is useful for decreasing airway secretions
   a. 0.04 mg/kg IM, subcutaneously (SQ) (rat, mouse, hamster, gerbil)
   b. 0.2 mg/kg IM, SQ (guinea pig, chinchilla)
   c. 0.2 to 1 mg/kg IM, SQ (rabbit)
2. One third of rabbits possess atropinase, therefore making it of questionable value
3. Acepromazine and diazepam are effective preanesthetics
   a. Acepromazine: 1 to 2 mg/kg IM
   b. Diazepam: 3 to 5 mg/kg IM; 0.4 to 3 mg/kg IM for guinea pigs
4. Acepromazine is not recommended in gerbils, because it may potentiate seizures

   H. Mustelid (ferrets)
1. Preanesthetics are usually not necessary
2. Atropine: 0.04 mg/kg IM, SQ
3. Acepromazine and diazepam are effective preanesthetics
   a. Acepromazine: 0.1 to 0.5 mg/kg IM
   b. Diazepam: 1 to 2 mg/kg IM

   I. Felid
1. Preanesthetics are not routinely used
2. Atropine can be used at standard domestic cat doses
   a. Atropine: 0.045 mg/kg SQ, IM, IV
   b. Glycopyrrolate: 0.01 mg/kg SQ, IM, IV

   J. Swine (see Chapter 22)

   K. Camelid
1. Medetomidine 20 μg/kg IM

VI. Monitoring plane of anesthesia
   A. Generalities
1. Pulse rate and character: a decrease in the heart rate to less than 80% of the stabilized rate after induction indicates that anesthesia should be lightened
2. Respiratory rate, volume, and character (e.g., apneustic)
   a. A decreasing pulse rate or apneustic/erratic patterns indicate that anesthesia should be lightened
   b. Ectotherms normally develop apnea at surgical planes of anesthesia; plan to administer positive

pressure ventilation at least four to six times per minute

B. Equipment
  1. ECG modifications
     a. To protect delicate skin or to penetrate thick skin, attach clips to steel sutures or metal hubbed needles placed through the skin at lead sites
     b. Attach clips to alcohol-soaked pads placed at the usual lead sites
     c. Wings are used for forelimb lead sites in birds
     d. Place one clip cranial and one caudal to the heart in legless animals
  2. Doppler placement
     a. Over the heart in small animals
     b. Over the peripheral artery
        (1) Avian: medial metatarsal, brachial
        (2) Reptile: tail artery
        (3) Rodent/lagomorph: ear, femoral, saphenous, foot pad
        (4) Mustelid: tail, foot pad, saphenous
  3. Pulse oximeter
     a. Measures oxygenation in addition to heart rate
     b. Placement: tongue, esophageal
        (1) Measures across any nonpigmented capillary bed
        (2) Mucous membranes are excellent sampling sites: oral or nasal mucosa, cloaca, vulva
        (3) Measures through nonpigmented skin: ear, wing web, thin skin of flank or abdomen
  4. Respiratory monitor must be sensitive enough to detect small tidal volumes

AVIAN ANESTHESIA (LESS THAN 30 LB)

I. Attainment of surgical anesthesia
  A. Toe, tail, and cloacal pinches should induce slow withdrawal
  B. Most birds have a slow third-eyelid response; the loss of this response in birds indicates that anesthesia should be lightened
  C. See Tables 24-1, 24-2

II. Anesthetic agent recommendations

    A. Inhalation anesthesia is preferred over injectable anesthesia

        1. The safety and efficacy of injectable anesthetics vary among species and individual animals

        2. It is extremely difficult to titrate the dose of injectable anesthetics; therefore, inhalants are preferred

    B. Oxygen flow rates

        1. Greater than 100 ml/min in small birds

        2. 0.5 to 2 L/min/kg; maximum dose is 3 to 4 L

    C. Use a non-rebreathing system for all birds weighing less than 15 lb

        1. Restrain the bird by hand or use toweling

        2. Place the bird's head inside a clear plastic bag taped to the end of the Y- or T-piece while oxygen and anesthetic gas are flowing

        3. Hold the bird until it is relaxed and then maintain anesthesia with a mask or intubation

    D. Intubate all birds weighing more than 100 g

        1. Birds weighing less than 100 g should be intubated for procedures longer than 30 minutes or for procedures involving the coelomic cavity; small face masks are commercially available or can be fashioned from 35- to 60-cc syringe cases and rubber gloves

        2. The glottis is easily visualized at the base of the tongue

            a. The trachea is composed of nonexpansible, complete tracheal rings; cuffs are not recommended

            b. Tissue swelling secondary to tube-induced tracheitis can occlude the trachea in birds weighing less than 100 g

            c. Small endotracheal tubes can be fashioned from catheters, the hub end of butterfly catheters, or red rubber feeding tubes; the hubs of these items fit into adapters made for commercially available 3.5- to 4.5-mm endotracheal tubes

            d. Making the tubes just long enough to ensure secure placement can minimize dead space

            e. Tubes should be taped securely to the bird's beak to avoid the sensitive cere

      f. Tubes should be monitored for occlusion; mucous plugs and kinking are common; always have a replacement tube immediately available

  3. If the trachea is occluded, the caudal thoracic air sacs can be cannulated at the site usually used for surgical sexing with a red rubber feeding tube cut to 2 to 5 cm in length; suture the tube in place; use the tube in the same fashion as an endotracheal tube; use aseptic technique to prevent life-threatening air sacculitis

  4. Birds do not tolerate apnea

      a. Positive pressure ventilation is required at least two times per minute to assist self-ventilating birds; ventilate 10 to 15 times per minute in apneic birds; tidal volume is approximately 15 ml/kg

      b. Birds have no pulmonary reserve; air is stored in the air sacs, which have no gas exchange capability

E. Isoflurane and sevoflurane are the anesthetics of choice in birds

  1. Induce isoflurane 3% to 4%; sevoflurane 4% to 5%

  2. Maintain isoflurane 0.5% to 2.5%; sevoflurane 3% to 4%

  3. Induction usually takes less than 5 minutes

      a. Induction is more rapid in birds than in mammals because of the cross-current system of the blood and air capillaries in addition to the greater proportional surface area of the lung; this makes the gas exchange in birds more efficient than in mammals

      b. Small changes in the vaporizer setting can cause rapid and dramatic changes in the plane of anesthesia; monitoring the level of anesthesia is critical

      c. Recovery is rapid (usually less than 5 minutes for a procedure less than 45 minutes); hold the bird in a towel until it is able to walk

      d. Apnea is an important signal to lighten anesthesia immediately; cardiac arrest often follows within 2 to 5 minutes of onset of apnea; the endotracheal tube should always be checked for occlusion

F. Halothane is an acceptable anesthetic in birds

  1. Induce at 2.5% to 3.5%

  2. Maintain at 1% to 2%

    3. Induction usually takes 5 to 10 minutes

    4. Peracute cardiac arrest with no warning is a recognized risk of using halothane as an anesthetic in birds

    5. Recovery usually takes 5 to 15 minutes for a 45-minute procedure

G. Methoxyflurane has been used successfully in birds but is associated with higher mortality rates than isoflurane or halothane

H. Injectable anesthetics

    1. Accurate body weight in grams is critical

    2. Effects of injectable anesthetics vary significantly among species and individual birds

    3. Recommended dosages are only guidelines

    4. Administer intramuscular injections in the pectoral muscles only

    5. Use of ketamine alone produces poor relaxation and turbulent recoveries; ketamine does not produce acceptable anesthesia in most fowl

    6. Xylazine causes excellent muscle relaxation and produces calm recoveries, but it is a significant respiratory depressant; avoid using it in ill birds

    7. Benzodiazepines have significantly variable effects; when they are not overridden, they produce safe sedation and muscle relaxation

    8. The combination of ketamine with xylazine or a benzodiazepine given intramuscularly usually produces adequate anesthesia for minor procedures

       a. Diazepam: 0.5 to 1 mg/kg; ketamine: 10 to 50 mg/kg IM; use higher doses for smaller birds

       b. Xylazine and ketamine: see Table 24-1

       c. Tiletamine/zolazepam: 4 to 25 mg/kg IM

          (1) Parakeet: 15 to 20 mg/kg IM

          (2) Duck: 5 to 10 mg/kg IM

       d. If a deeper plane of anesthesia is needed

          (1) After waiting 10 minutes, readminister one fourth to one half of the ketamine dose

       e. If the plane of anesthesia is still inadequate, postpone the procedure for 24 hours before attempting anesthesia again

9. Recovery from injectable anesthetics is variable, but it usually takes more than 45 minutes after a 45-minute procedure
   a. Wrap the bird in a towel to control its wings
   b. Place the bird in a warm, dark, and quiet recovery area
   c. If the bird panics, hold it until it completely recovers
10. Use one fourth to one half of the intramuscular dose if administering drugs intravenously

I. Anesthetic emergencies
   1. Apnea
      a. Positive-pressure ventilation; if no endotracheal tube is available, lift and compress the sternum
      b. Flush system free of anesthetic gas; administer 100% O_2
      c. Doxapram: intravenously, intraosseously (IO), or intramuscularly 5 mg/kg
      d. To reverse xylazine: yohimbine 1 mg/kg IV, IO; atipamazole 5 to 10 μg/kg IV
   2. Cardiac arrest
      a. Epinephrine 5 to 10 μg/kg IV, IO, or intratracheally (IT)
      b. Lift and compress sternum
      c. Perform a laparotomy and use fingertips or cotton-tipped applicators to perform internal cardiac massage
      d. See Chapters 27 and 28 for additional information on treating anesthetic emergencies

J. Recovery
   1. Continue monitoring the patient until it has recovered
   2. Provide warmth
   3. Monitor hydration and energy needs
   4. Reduce the incidence and severity of self-induced trauma

K. Analgesia
   1. Butorphanol: 0.5 to 2.0 mg/kg IM

AVIAN ANESTHESIA (MORE THAN 30 LB; LONG-LEGGED)

I. The same general principles apply as for smaller birds
II. Unless they are very weak, these birds are large enough to require chemical sedation before induction of inhalant anesthesia

   A. Large ratites (ostriches) are extremely dangerous; they should never be approached from the front; a forward kick can disembowel a person

   B. Using large sheets of wood as shields, herd large ratites into a corner or chute from the sides and rear (head first)

   C. Long-billed birds, such as storks and herons, strike swiftly with their beaks; it is *imperative* that eye protection be worn; first restrain these birds from over the back by their wings and neck; a second person should then grasp and protect the legs; if the likelihood of hyperthermia is low, the beak may be taped partially shut by placing padding between and over the upper and lower tips of the beak

   D. If the head can be reached safely, hood it with soft material to help calm and restrain the bird; ensure that the mouth and nares are open to the air to decrease the likelihood of hyperthermia

   E. Capture myopathy, compartmentalization syndrome, hyperthermia, and leg fractures resulting from violent recoveries are complications associated with anesthesia in large, long-legged birds

      1. Adequate padding, maintenance of blood pressure, and oxygenation during these procedures is critical (see Chapter 20)

      2. Reduce the handling needed to administer sedatives to a minimum; keep the induction and recovery areas as quiet and dark as possible

      3. Well-padded induction and recovery areas are desirable; a recovery stall slightly larger than a recumbent bird often makes it feel secure; after the bird has completely recovered, the hood can be removed and the crate opened for the bird's release; give it time to stand on its own; if a bird becomes agitated before it is fully recovered, inject it with 0.1 to 0.2 mg/kg of diazepam

F. If the bird has not fasted, inflate the cuff on the endotracheal tube to prevent aspiration; regurgitation is common in birds that have not fasted

III. Injectable anesthetics are useful for short procedures and for induction of inhalant anesthesia

    A. Intravenous injections can be administered in the brachial veins in standing animals (e.g., ostriches and emus); some calm birds tolerate jugular injections; rheas have poor brachial veins but are small enough to be manually restrained for inhalant anesthesia after an intramuscular sedative

    B. Brachial, jugular, and medial metatarsal veins are excellent sites for indwelling intravenous catheters

    C. Ratites (ostriches, emus, moas, kiwis)

        1. Xylazine: 0.5 to 1 mg/kg IM, followed by ketamine, 2 to 4 mg/kg IV after 15 minutes

        2. Xylazine: 0.25 mg/kg and ketamine, 2.2 mg/kg IV

        3. Tiletamine/zolazepam: 4 to 10 mg/kg IM

        4. Tiletamine/zolazepam: 2 to 6 mg/kg IV

        5. Diazepam: 0.2 to 0.3 mg/kg and ketamine, 2.2 mg/kg IV

REPTILE ANESTHESIA

I. Never use hypothermia

    A. It depresses bodily functions, including the immune system, and delays healing

    B. It does not provide analgesia

    C. It delays recovery from anesthesia

II. Induction of anesthesia

    A. Excitement is followed by loss of motor control; loss of the righting reflex is followed by muscle relaxation; surgical anesthesia is attained when toe, tail, and vent pinches do not elicit a withdrawal

    B. Most reptiles with third eyelids retain this reflex; a decrease in heart rate to less than 80% of the stabilized rate indicates that anesthesia should be lightened; heart rate is often the only reliable indicator of a reptile's level of anesthesia; it should be carefully monitored

    C. Most reptiles (less than 500 g) can be induced by a mask or chamber at 2% to 4% isoflurane; use intravenous or intraosseous propofol to induce anesthesia in larger reptiles; follow this with isoflurane gas anesthesia

1. Watch for apnea
2. Chelonians, aquatic squamates, and crocodilians can hold their breath for long periods of time; it can be difficult to extract a chelonian's head from its shell and open its beak; injectable sedatives are often required to allow intubation and positive-pressure respiration to maintain inhalant anesthesia; venomous or large, aggressive reptiles may require injectable anesthetics for safe restraint
   a. Propofol: 5 to 7 mg/kg in colubrid snakes; 10 to 12 mg/kg in birds; 12 to 15 mg/kg in chelonians; 5 to 14 mg/kg in lizards
   b. Ketamine: 20 to 60 mg/kg IM
   c. Ketamine: 5 to 15 mg/kg IV, IO
   d. Tiletamine/zolazepam: 10 to 40 mg/kg IM (squamates); 5 to 15 mg/kg IM (chelonians, crocodilians)
   e. Succinylcholine: *for intubation only*
      (1) No analgesia
      (2) Paralyzes muscles, including muscles of respiration
      (3) Intubate and assist respiration for approximately 1 hour after injection, sometimes longer
      (4) Do not repeat within 24 hours
      (5) 0.25 to 1.5 mg/kg IM (chelonians, crocodilians) in front half of animal
D. Intubation (similar to birds)
   1. Glottis is located at the base of the tongue
   2. Glottis is harder to see in chelonians
   3. Crocodilians possess a pharyngeal membrane that allows them to breathe with a mouth full of food or water; this membrane must be pushed aside to see the glottis
   4. In some crocodilians the trachea is bent in on itself; therefore, the endotracheal tube does not advance as far as expected
   5. The tracheal rings are complete in chelonians and crocodilians; the trachea bifurcates cranially; to avoid intubation of only one bronchus, very short endotracheal tubes should be used

6. All reptiles attaining surgical levels of anesthesia must be intubated; exceptional care is needed for reptiles weighing less than 100 g to prevent tube-induced tracheitis

E. Maintenance
  1. Isoflurane (1% to 2%) or sevoflurane (2% to 4%) are the anesthetics of choice
  2. Oxygen flow rates: 1 L/0.3 to 1 kg; 1 L/5 to 10 kg for larger reptiles
  3. Ventilate the animal at least three to six times per minute
  4. Halothane has been used successfully
  5. Methoxyflurane has been associated with death in snakes
  6. Maintaining body temperature is essential

F. Recovery
  1. Recovery with isoflurane usually takes less than 20 minutes for procedures lasting less than 1 hour
  2. Recovery may take hours to days with injectable anesthetics
  3. Positive-pressure ventilation must be continued until the animal is breathing regularly on its own
     a. Some reptiles breathe when stimulated, but not on their own
     b. During recovery, reduce ventilation to twice per minute; room air or exhaled air may be used to increase the carbon dioxide concentration to stimulate respirations; be careful not to induce anoxia
  4. Heat and fluids accelerate recovery times

G. Emergencies
  1. Respiratory arrest
     a. Apnea is frequent; if the animal is stable, administer positive-pressure ventilation
     b. In turtles, extending and retracting the front legs can temporarily facilitate respirations while an endotracheal tube is being placed
     c. To reverse xylazine: yohimbine 1 mg/kg IV
     d. Doxapram: 5 mg/kg IV, IO, IM
  2. Cardiac arrest
     a. Administer 100% oxygen
     b. Use chest compressions in reptiles without shells

    c. Perform a laparotomy and manually compress the heart

    d. Epinephrine: 5 to 10 mg/kg IV, IO, IC, IT

    e. See Chapters 27 and 28 for further information

AMPHIBIAN ANESTHESIA

  I. Indications

    A. Any painful procedure

    B. Diagnostic imaging

  II. Preanesthetic considerations

    A. See general considerations on p. 372

    B. Withhold food from the animal 24 hours before anesthesia

    C. Significant respiration occurs across moist skin

      1. Do not allow skin to completely dry out

      2. Handle the animal with wet latex gloves or wet hands

    D. Preanesthetic medications are not commonly used

    E. Ectotherm

      1. Maintain adequate body temperature with external heat sources

      2. Hypothermia prolongs recovery and depresses the immune system

    F. Animals weighing more than 100 g should be intubated (see avian anesthesia earlier in this chapter)

 III. Stages of anesthesia

    A. Similar to mammals

    B. Erythema of ventral abdomen during induction

    C. Abdominal respirations cease with heavy sedation, but pharyngeal (gular) respirations continue

    D. Corneal reflex is lost before loss of the withdrawal reflex

 IV. Anesthetic agents

    A. Tricaine methane sulfonate (3-aminobenzoic acid ethyl ester; ethyl m-aminobenzoate, MS222; Finquel)

      1. Routes

        a. Immersion baths; keep tank of untreated water for recovery tank

        b. Parenteral—IM or SQ; use sterile solution

      2. Dose is species dependent

        a. Immersion bath: 50 to 100 mg/L

        b. 100 mg/kg SQ or IM (0.1 ml/10 g body weight with a 1% solution)

    3. Induction takes 5 to 20 minutes
    4. Recovery takes 10 to 30 minutes; keep skin moist with untreated water and maintain normal temperature
    5. Wide margin of safety
    6. Suppliers
       a. Argent Chemical Laboratories
          8702 152nd Ave NE
          Redmond, WA 98052
          1-800-426-6258
       b. Crescent Research Chemicals
          5301 N 37th Place
          Paradise Valley, AZ 85253

B. Isoflurane
    1. Intubate and ventilate after masking the animal
    2. Induce at 3% to 4% for 5 to 15 minutes
    3. Maintain at 1% to 2.5%
    4. Keep skin moist and maintain normal temperature
    5. Isoflurane is irritating to amphibian skin
    6. Isoflurane is a respiratory depressant; use intermittent positive-pressure ventilation
    7. Recovery takes 10 to 30 minutes; keep the animal warm and moist

C. Ketamine
    1. Good for diagnostics, but not surgery
    2. 100 to 200 mg/kg SQ or IM
    3. Reflexes remain intact
    4. Induction takes 10 to 20 minutes
    5. Recovery takes 20 to 60 minutes

FISH ANESTHESIA

I. Indications
    A. Any painful procedure
    B. Sedation during shipping
    C. Diagnostic imaging
    D. Stripping milt (eggs)
II. Preanesthetic considerations
    A. See previous general considerations, p. 372
    B. Obligate water breathers
       1. Require oxygenated water moving over gills to oxygenate blood

2. Normal water flow pattern is through the mouth, over the gills, and out the operculum
3. Provide water flow during anesthesia by using frequent immersion or a small recirculating pump and airstone; a pump tube should be placed in the fish's mouth so that water flow is maintained across the gills

C. Exterior mucus layer is an important part of the integument
1. Use the least amount of restraint possible
2. Use wet latex gloves when handling the fish to minimize disruption to the mucus layer

D. Withhold food 24 hours before anesthesia

E. Have a recovery tank ready with water identical to the fish's preanesthetic conditions

F. Preanesthetic medications are not commonly used

G. Ectotherms
1. Maintain adequate body temperature with external heat sources
2. Hypothermia prolongs recovery and depresses the immune system

III. Stages of anesthesia

STAGE	PLANE	CATEGORY	FISH RESPONSES
0		Normal	Normal
I	1	Light sedation	Decreased response to visual stimuli
I	2	Deep sedation	Voluntary swimming stopped, normal posture, no response to external stimuli
II	1	Light narcosis	Excitement, loss of balance
II	2	Deep narcosis	Equilibrium lost, normal respiratory rate responds to pain
III	1	Light anesthesia	Decreased respiratory rate, deep pain present
III	2	Surgical anesthesia	Low respiratory rate, low heart rate, no deep pain
IV		Medullary collapse	Cardiac and respiratory arrest

IV. Anesthetic agents
A. Tricaine methane sulfonate (3-aminobenzoic acid ethyl ester; ethyl m-aminobenzoate, MS222; Finquel)

1. The only anesthetic licensed for use in fish
2. Commonly used as an immersion bath; keep tank of untreated water for recovery bath
3. Dose is species dependent; sedation is generally achieved at 20 to 50 mg/L, anesthesia at 50 to 100 mg/L; the depth of anesthesia is controlled by switching from a water bath that contains an anesthetic to an untreated water bath
4. Acidic solution: buffer with imidazole or sodium hydroxide to normal tank pH
5. Rapid induction takes 1 to 5 minutes
6. Rapid recovery takes 10 to 15 minutes; to prevent hypoxia, keep water moving over the fish's gills
7. Wide margin of safety
8. Suppliers
   a. Argent Chemical Laboratories
      8702 152nd Ave NE
      Redmond, WA 98052
      1-800-426-6258
   b. Crescent Research Chemicals
      5301 N 37th Place
      Paradise Valley, AZ 85253
B. Halothane
   1. 0.5 to 40 mg/L of water; liquid halothane added to water
   2. Narrow margin of safety
   3. Not a preferred anesthetic agent
C. Isoflurane
   1. Not a preferred anesthetic agent
   2. Liquid isoflurane can be added to water
V. Treatment of anesthetic overdose
   A. Move the fish to untreated, oxygenated water
   B. Increase gentle water flow over the gills
   C. If spontaneous respirations do not occur in 2 minutes, assist respirations
      1. Move the fish gently through the water
      2. Slowly pump oxygenated water into the fish's mouth and across its gills

RABBIT AND RODENT ANESTHESIA

I. Generalities
   A. Rabbits, guinea pigs, and chinchillas frequently hold their breath and then take deep, rapid breaths when being masked down or induced in a chamber; this behavior can result in death if the concentration of anesthetic gases is high; to reduce risk, do the following:
      1. Use preanesthetics (diazepam or midazolam)
      2. Use nitrous oxide followed by an anesthetic agent
      3. Use a low induction setting
   B. Levels of anesthesia
      1. Excitement phase
      2. Loss of coordination
      3. Muscle relaxation
      4. Surgical anesthesia is attained when toe, ear, and tail pinches do not elicit a withdrawal
      5. Loss of corneal reflexes varies significantly among individual animals and anesthetic agents; a loss of these reflexes in an animal that previously had them indicates that anesthesia should be lightened
      6. A decreasing respiratory or heart rate or abnormal breathing patterns are also indications to lighten anesthesia

II. Intubation (Table 24-3)
   A. It is difficult to intubate rodents and lagomorphs because of their small size and long, thin oral cavities
   B. Masks are effective for short procedures
   C. Intubation techniques and considerations
      1. Small endotracheal tubes clog and kink easily
         a. Check tube patency with positive-pressure ventilation at least every 2 minutes
         b. Have a replacement tube handy
         c. If a tube is clogged, try to reposition or suction it; if the tube does not become patent, maintain anesthesia by mask or injectables or place a new tube
      2. Be careful not to create iatrogenic tracheitis
      3. Prolonged, oral, or thoracic procedures require intubation
      4. Oxygen flow
         a. 500 ml/min minimum
         b. 0.5 to 2 L/min/kg; 3 to 4 L/min maximum
         c. 1 L every 5 to 10 kg

TABLE **24-3**
ENDOTRACHEAL INTUBATION: EQUIPMENT REQUIRED

SPECIES	BODY WEIGHT	ENDOTRACHEAL TUBE DIAMETER
Rabbit	1-3 kg	2-3 mm O/D
	3-7 kg	3-6 mm O/D
Rat	200-400 g	18-12 gauge plastic cannula
Mouse	25-35 g	1.0 mm
Guinea pig	400-1000 g	16-12 gauge plastic cannula
Hamster	120 g	1.5 mm
Primate	<0.5 kg	Not reported
	0.5-20 kg	2-8 mm O/D
Pig	1-10 kg	2-6 mm O/D
	0.5-20 kg	6-15 mm O/D

D. Oral intubation: requires practice and luck (Fig. 24-1)
 1. Dorsal, lateral, or ventral recumbency
 2. Extend the head and neck
 3. Keep straight
 4. Grasp the animal's tongue and pull it forward
 5. Stylet or tube is bounced off the roof of the mouth and into the larynx
 6. A laryngoscope is helpful in larger animals (Fig. 24-2)
 7. In large rabbits, a small, rigid arthroscope can be introduced into the mouth to allow visualization of the glottis; however, damage to the instrument by the animal's molars is possible
 8. Use of topical lidocaine can suppress laryngospasm
 9. Repeated attempts at intubation can cause life-threatening hemorrhage and swelling

E. Retrograde technique (Fig. 24-3)
 1. Aseptically prepare the ventral neck
 2. Pass an over-the-needle catheter into the trachea
 3. Retrograde it through the larynx
 4. Use the catheter as a stylet for the endotracheal tube
 5. Remove the catheter
 6. In animals with fat necks, a "cut down" to the trachea is required

F. Induction
 1. Isoflurane: 2% to 3%
 2. Halothane: 2% to 4%
 3. Sevoflurane: 3% to 5%

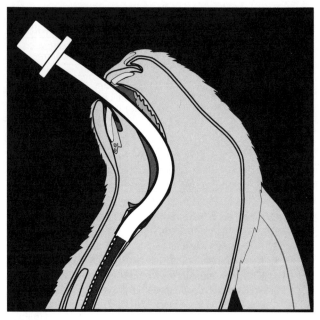

Fig. 24-1
Rodent/lagomorph endotracheal intubation. Extend the head and neck. Bounce the endotracheal tube off the roof of the mouth and into the larynx.

    G. Maintenance
        1. Isoflurane: 0.25% to 2%
        2. Halothane: 0.25% to 2%
        3. Sevoflurane: 2% to 3%
        4. Methoxyflurane: not recommended
        5. Use of nitrous oxide is similar to use in other domestic mammals
    H. Recovery
        1. Isoflurane or sevoflurane takes 5 to 15 minutes for surgeries that last less than an hour
        2. Halothane takes 10 to 20 minutes for surgeries that last less than an hour
        3. Keep the animal warm
        4. Watch the animal's hydration and energy needs

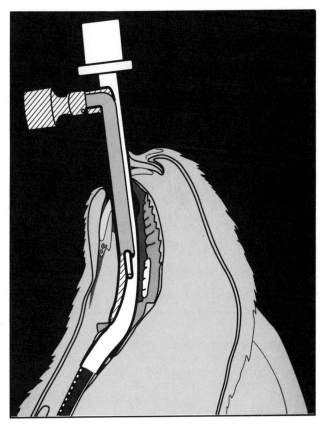

Fig. 24-2
Rodent/lagomorph endotracheal intubation with laryngoscope. Extend the head and neck. Depress the tongue with a laryngoscope. Bounce the endotracheal tube off of the roof of the mouth and into the larynx.

I. Analgesia (Table 24-4)
   1. Butorphanol
      a. Rabbits: 5 to 10 mg/kg SQ
      b. Guinea pigs: 2 mg/kg SQ
      c. Other rodents: 1 to 5 mg/kg SQ

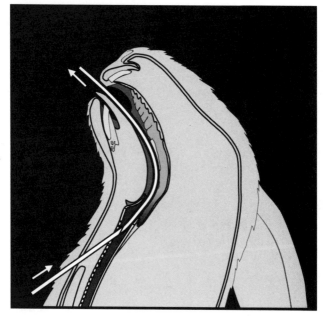

Fig. 24-3
A, Rodent/lagomorph endotracheal intubation, retrograde technique. Aseptically prepare ventral neck. Locate the trachea (may require a cut down). Insert a through-the-needle catheter into the trachea as if performing a tracheal wash, but direct the catheter proximally.

J. Injectables (Table 24-5)
  1. Results vary significantly among individual animals
  2. Poor muscle relaxation and poor analgesia are the most frequent problems
  3. Injectable anesthetics are most useful for diagnostics or minor procedures
  4. Dosages listed are only guidelines (see Tables 24-4 and 24-5)
  5. Barbiturates produce excellent muscle relaxation
     a. Their margin of safety is very low
     b. They are not recommended for use in pets

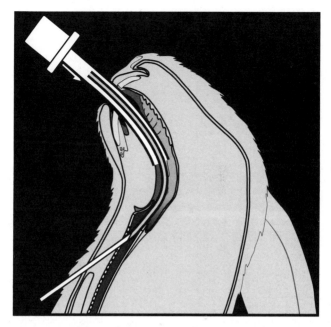

Fig. 24-3 cont'd
B, Use the catheter as a stylet to direct the endotracheal tube into the larynx. Once the endotracheal tube is correctly positioned, remove the catheter.

    c. Barbiturates are useful for euthanasia
    d. Pentobarbital: dilute to less than 10 mg/ml

Rat	25 to 40 mg/kg IP, IV
Mouse	40 to 80 mg/kg IP, IV
Guinea pig	30 to 40 mg/kg IP, IV
Chinchilla	35 to 40 mg/kg IP
Rabbit	25 to 40 mg/kg IV
Hamster	50 to 90 mg/kg IP
Gerbil	40 to 60 mg/kg IP

K. Emergencies (see Chapters 25 and 26)

TABLE 24-4
ANALGESIC DRUGS FOR RABBITS AND RODENTS

DRUG	RABBIT	RAT	MOUSE	GUINEA PIG
Aspirin	100 mg/kg PO	100 mg/kg PO	120 mg/kg PO	87 mg/kg PO
Carprofen	1.5 mg/kg PO b.i.d.	5 mg/kg SQ	—	—
Flunixin	1.1 mg/kg SQ, IM q 12 hours	2.5 mg/kg SQ, IM q 12 hours	2.5 mg/kg SQ, IM q 12 hours	—
Ketoprofen	3 mg/kg IM	—	—	—
Buprenorphine	0.01-0.05 mg/kg SQ, IV 8-12 hourly	0.01-0.05 mg/kg SQ, IV or 0.1-0.25 mg/kg PO 8-12 hourly	0.05-0.1 mg/kg SQ 12 hourly	0.05 mg/kg SQ 8-12 hourly
Butorphanol	0.1-0.5 mg/kg IV 4 hourly	2 mg/kg SQ 4 hourly	1-5 mg/kg SQ 4 hourly	—
Morphine	2-5 mg/kg SQ, IM 2-4 hourly	2.5 mg/kg SQ 2-4 hourly	2.5 mg/kg SQ 2-4 hourly	2-5 mg/kg SQ, IM 4 hourly

Note that considerable individual and strain variation in response may be encountered; therefore, it is essential to assess the analgesic effect in each animal.

TABLE 24-5
RABBIT AND RODENT ANESTHESIA

SPECIES	DRUG	DOSAGE
Rat, mouse, hamster, chinchilla, gerbil	Diazepam	Sedation only 3-5 mg/kg IM
Guinea pig	Diazepam	Sedation only 0.5-3 mg/kg IM
Rabbit	Diazepam	Sedation only 1-4 mg/kg IM
	Midazolam	1-2 mg/kg IM
	Medetomidine	0.1-0.4 mg/kg IM
All but gerbils	Acepromazine	Sedation only 1-2 mg/kg IM
Rat, mouse	Ketamine	60-80 mg/kg IM
	Xylazine	7-15 mg/kg IM
Rabbit, guinea pig, chinchilla	Ketamine	30-40 mg/kg IM
	Xylazine	5-8 mg/kg IM
Hamster, gerbil	Ketamine	50 mg/kg IP
	Xylazine	2-5 mg/kg IP
Rabbit, guinea pig	Ketamine	35-40 mg/kg IM
	Xylazine	4-6 mg/kg IM
Rat, mouse, guinea pig	Ketamine	20-40 mg/kg IM
	Acepromazine	0.75 mg/kg IM
	Xylazine	2-5 mg/kg IM

IM, Intramuscularly; *IP,* intraperitoneally.
Medetomidine (50-100 μg/kg IM, SQ) can be used in place of xylazine.

FERRET ANESTHESIA

   I. Information in Chapters 7 and 19 is applicable to ferrets
  II. Introduction (Tables 24-6, 24-7)
     A. Because they lack substantial claws, ferrets are easier to hold in a towel and mask down with isoflurane than cats
     B. Mask induction is used for very ill ferrets to eliminate the side effects associated with many injectable anesthetics and for short procedures such as diagnostics; this allows the ferret to be returned to the owner quickly
     C. Monitoring the depth of anesthesia is similar to cats
     D. Because of their small size, ferrets require a non-rebreathing system
     E. Ferrets are easily intubated
        1. 2.5- to 3-mm endotracheal tubes
        2. A laryngoscope is helpful

TABLE 24-6
ANALGESIC DRUGS FOR FERRETS

DRUG	FERRET
Aspirin	200 mg/kg PO
Flunixin	0.5-2 mg/kg SQ
	12-24 hourly
Buprenorphine	0.01-0.03 mg/kg IV, IM, SQ
	8-12 hourly
Butorphanol	0.4 mg/kg IM
	4-6 hourly
Morphine	0.5 mg/kg SQ, IM
	6 hourly
Pethidine (meperidine)	5-10 mg/kg SQ, IM
	2-4 hourly

Note that considerable individual and strain variation in response may be encountered; therefore, it is essential to assess the analgesic effect in each animal.

TABLE 24-7
ANESTHETIC DRUGS FOR FERRETS

DRUG	DOSAGE
Alphaxalone/alphadolone	8-12 mg/kg IV, 12-15 mg/kg IM
Ketamine/acepromazine	25 mg/kg IM+ 0.25 mg/kg IM
Ketamine/diazepam	25 mg/kg IM+ 2 mg/kg IM
Ketamine/medetomidine	8 mg/kg IM+ 0.1 mg/kg IM
Ketamine/xylazine	25 mg/kg IM+ 1-2 mg/kg IM
Pentobarbitone	25-30 mg/kg IV, 36 mg/kg IP
Urethane	1500 mg/kg IV

   III. Isoflurane or sevoflurane
      A. Induce at 2.5% to 4%
      B. Maintain at 1% to 3%
      C. Recovery time is similar to cats
   IV. Halothane
      A. Do not use for mask induction
      B. Maintain at 0.5% to 1.5%
      C. Recovery time is similar to cats
   V. Injectables
      A. Tiletamine/zolazepam
         1. Light sedation: 3 to 5 mg/kg IM
         2. Anesthesia: 8 to 12 mg/kg IM

      B. Ketamine: 20 to 25 mg/kg IM
         Diazepam: 2 to 3 mg/kg IM
      C. Ketamine: 25 to 35 mg/kg IM
         Acepromazine: 0.2 to 0.3 mg/kg IM
      D. Ketamine: 10 to 20 mg/kg IM
         Xylazine: 2.2 mg/kg IM
      E. Ketamine: 8 mg/kg IM
         Medetomidine: 0.1 mg/kg IM
  VI. Analgesia and anesthesia (see Tables 24-6 and 24-7)
 VII. Emergencies (see Chapters 25, 27, and 28)

EXOTIC CAT ANESTHESIA

   I. Preanesthetic considerations
      A. See the general considerations section at the beginning of this chapter
      B. Withhold food from the animal for 24 hours; withhold water for 12 hours
      C. Respect the animal's strength
      D. Remote delivery (pole syringe, darting equipment) is often needed to ensure human safety
      E. Premedication is similar to that used in domestic cats but often is not needed
      F. Higher drug doses are needed for excited animals; create a calm and quiet environment for induction to anesthesia
  II. Stages of anesthesia
      A. Similar to other mammals
      B. Sudden arousal of animals sedated with xylazine alone or medetomidine and ketamine is possible; supplementation may be needed
 III. Anesthetic agents
      A. Xylazine
         1. Rarely used alone because of the possibility of sudden arousal
         2. Significant respiratory depressant
      B. Ketamine
         1. Used alone for short procedures in small cats; 5 to 20 mg/kg IM
         2. Seizures have been reported in some species of exotic cats recovering from ketamine or ketamine-combination anesthesia; control with diazepam

C. Medetomidine/ketamine IM
   1. Medetomidine: 0.040 to 0.060 mg/kg
   2. Ketamine: 2.0 to 3.0 mg/kg
   3. Intubate and place on isoflurane or be prepared to supplement ketamine 1 to 2 mg/kg IV if procedure is longer than 20 minutes
   4. At the conclusion of the procedure or after 20 minutes (whichever comes first), reverse medetomidine with atipamazole at five times the medetomidine dose intramuscularly or intravenously
   5. Bradycardia is common with medetomidine; this is rarely a clinical problem, but animals should be supplemented with O_2; this combination may not be appropriate for severely debilitated felines
D. Ketamine/xylazine combination IV
   1. Ketamine: 8 mg/kg
   2. Xylazine: 0.6 mg/kg
   3. Intubate and place the animal on isoflurane inhalation anesthesia if the procedure takes longer than 20 minutes
E. Ketamine/diazepam combination IV
   1. Ketamine: 5 to 8 mg/kg
   2. Diazepam: 0.1 mg/kg
   3. Intubate and place the animal on isoflurane inhalation anesthesia if the procedure takes longer than 20 minutes
F. Tiletamine/zolazepam (Telazol)
   1. A 500-mg vial can be reconstituted to a final concentration of 100 to 500 mg/ml depending on the volume of diluent added for use in darting equipment
   2. Dose: 1.5 to 4 mg/kg IM for most species
      a. Sufficient for intubation
      b. Intubate and place the animal on isoflurane inhalation anesthesia if the procedure takes longer than 20 minutes
      c. Snow leopards require a higher dose
      d. Excessive salivation is seen in some species
      e. Recovery from anesthesia is smooth but prolonged compared to ketamine alone or ketamine combinations
      f. Delayed (3 to 10 days after immobilization) adverse drug reaction is seen in some Siberian and white tigers

G. Isoflurane or sevoflurane are the inhalation anesthetics of choice; halothane can be used
   1. Small cats can be anesthetized in a chamber
   2. Face mask delivery can be used to supplement other anesthetics
   3. Dose
      a. Induce at 3% to 4%
      b. Maintain at 1% to 2% isoflurane; 2% to 3% sevoflurane
      c. Oxygen flow rate is 1 to 6 L/min
   4. Intubate the animal if the procedure takes longer than 20 minutes

IV. Treatment of anesthetic overdose
   A. Treat an overdose as an anesthetic emergency in domestic cats, but be prepared for arousal of the animal
   B. Xylazine can be reversed with yohimbine (0.125 mg/kg IM or IV), although results are not as dramatic as in other species
   C. Adverse tiletamine/zolazepam reactions in tigers have been treated with diazepam and dexamethasone
   D. Medetomidine can be reversed with atipamazole at five times the medetomidine dose intramuscularly or intravenously
   E. Telazol can be partially antagonized with Mazicon (flumazenil)

CAMELID ANESTHESIA (LLAMAS, CAMELS, ALPACAS)

I. Preanesthetic considerations
   A. See the general considerations section at the beginning of this chapter
   B. Withhold food from the animal for 24 to 48 hours; withhold water for 24 hours, weather permitting
   C. Patient positioning is important to reduce regurgitation
      1. Keep the animal's head elevated above the rumen
      2. Do not roll an anesthetized animal dorsally
      3. If regurgitation occurs, position the animal's head with the muzzle below the level of the poll and ensure an open airway

    D. Intubate animals if the procedure takes longer than 20 minutes

    E. Place a jugular catheter

II. Stages of anesthesia are similar to other mammals

III. Anesthetic agents

    A. Neonates: mask with isoflurane; intubate the animal if the procedure takes longer than 20 minutes

    B. Juveniles and adults

      1. Local anesthesia

        a. See Chapter 5

        b. A line block or an inverted L block using standard agents is common

        c. Regional nerve blocks are more difficult

        d. Dosage must be tailored to animal size

    C. Sedation

      1. Xylazine: 0.1 to 0.2 mg/kg IV or IM

      2. Medetomidine: 0.01 to 0.02 mg/kg IV

                    0.02 to 0.04 mg/kg IM

      3. Butorphanol: 0.05 to 0.1 mg/kg IM

    D. Anesthesia

      1. Ketamine/xylazine

        a. Ketamine: 5 mg/kg IM

               3 to 5 mg/kg IV

        b. Xylazine: 0.4 mg/kg IM

               0.25 mg/kg IV

      2. Medetomidine/ketamine

        a. Ketamine: 2 to 4 mg/kg IM or IV

        b. Medetomidine: 0.04 to 0.08 mg/kg IM or IV

      3. Telazol: 0.75 to 1.5 mg/kg IM

      4. Propofol: 1 to 3 mg/kg IV

IV. Analgesics

    A. Phenylbutazone: 2 to 4 mg/kg PO SID; may consider administration of cimetidine: 2.2 mg/kg concurrently

    B. Flunixin meglumine: 1.1 mg/kg IV SID

      1. Avoid intra-arterial injection

      2. Ulcerogenic: administer cimetidine concurrently

    C. Aspirin: 25 to 50 mg/kg PO BID

V. Treatment of anesthetic overdose

    A. Treat as anesthetic emergency as in other mammals

    B. Xylazine can be reversed with yohimbine 0.25 mg/kg IV

C. Atipamazole is used to antagonize medetomidine at five times the medetomidine dose intramuscularly or intravenously

POT-BELLIED PIG ANESTHESIA

I. Preanesthetic considerations
   A. See the general considerations section at the beginning of this chapter
   B. Withhold food from the animal for 24 hours
   C. Warn the owner and the hospital staff that the pig may squeal when restrained
   D. Premedication is not generally needed
   E. Endotracheal intubation can be challenging (see Chapter 22)
   F. Watch for hyperthermia, although it is less of a problem in pot-bellied pigs than in other pigs
II. Stages of anesthesia are similar to other mammals
III. Anesthetic agents
   A. Isoflurane or sevoflurane
      1. Can be used as the sole anesthetic agent in small animals
      2. Agent of choice for inhalation anesthesia
      3. Deliver from a precision vaporizer with a face mask or an endotracheal tube
         a. Induction: 3% to 4% isoflurane; 3% to 5% sevoflurane
         b. Maintenance: 1% to 2% isoflurane; 2% to 4% sevoflurane
         c. Oxygen flow rate: 2 to 3 L/min
   B. Tiletamine/zolazepam/ketamine/xylazine injectable combination
      1. Reconstitute a 500-mg vial of Telazol with 2.5 ml of 10% ketamine and 2.5 ml of 10% xylazine
      2. Each milliliter of resultant mixture contains the following:
         a. 50 mg tiletamine
         b. 50 mg ketamine
         c. 50 mg zolazepam
         d. 50 mg xylazine

    3. Dose
       a. Sedation: 0.006 to 0.012 ml/kg IM
       b. Surgical anesthesia and intubation: 0.018 to 0.024 ml/kg IM
       c. Requires 20 to 40 minutes to take effect
       d. Can be supplemented with 0.1- to 0.5-ml bolus in the auricular vein

C. Midazolam/medetomidine/butorphanol
    1. Midazolam: 0.3 mg/kg IM
    2. Medetomidine: 0.07 to 0.08 mg/kg IM
    3. Butorphanol: 0.3 mg/kg IM
    4. Supplementation
       a. Intubate and maintain on isoflurane
       b. Propofol: 1 mg/kg IV
       c. Ketamine: 1 mg/kg IV
    5. Antagonists
       a. Atipamazole: 0.08 mg/kg IM or IV
       b. Naltrexone: 0.05 to 0.1 mg/kg IM or IV
       c. Restrain the animal until it is coordinated

D. Telazol/medetomidine/butorphanol
    1. Telazol: 0.5 mg/kg IM
    2. Medetomidine: 0.07 to 0.08 mg/kg IM
    3. Butorphanol: 0.3 mg/kg IM
    4. Supplementation (see section C4 above)
    5. Antagonists (see section C5 above)

E. Provide supplemental oxygen to all immobilized pigs via nasal tube at 5 L/min

VI. Treatment of anesthetic overdose
    A. If using isoflurane, turn vaporizer off and flush system
    B. Administer oxygen
    C. If xylazine has been given, reverse with yohimbine 0.125 mg/kg IV
    D. If medetomidine has been given, antagonize with atipamazole at five times the medetomidine dose
    E. If a narcotic has been given, antagonize with naltrexone 0.1 mg/kg IM or IV
    F. Perform cardiopulmonary resuscitation as for other mammals

CHAPTER TWENTY-FIVE

Fluid Administration during Anesthesia

"One can drink too much, but one never drinks enough."

GOTTHOLD EPHRAIM LESSING

OVERVIEW

Fluid therapy is a vital adjunct to any anesthetic plan. Almost all drugs used to produce chemical restraint and anesthesia decrease the force of cardiac contraction and relax blood vessels, increasing intravascular volume. These actions decrease cardiac output (blood flow) and arterial blood pressure. The routine administration of fluids during anesthesia helps to maintain an adequate and effective circulating blood volume and near-normal cardiac output. Choices for acute fluid therapy include balanced electrolyte solutions (crystalloids), colloids, cell-free blood substitutes, and blood.

GENERAL CONSIDERATIONS (TABLE 25-1)

I. Anesthesia, surgery, and many of the diseases for which surgical intervention is required interfere with water and acid-base balance and decrease the effective circulating blood volume

   A. Disease produces changes in fluid, electrolyte, and acid-base balance (Table 25-2)

   B. Imbalances caused by anesthesia

      1. Inhalation and intravenous (IV) anesthetic agents

         a. Depress myocardial contractility and therefore decrease cardiac output and tissue perfusion; metabolic acidosis may ensue

         b. Induce generalized vasodilation; relative hypovolemia and hypotension may result

TABLE 25-1
NORMAL ELECTROLYTE COMPOSITION OF SERUM (mEq/L)

	NA$^+$	K$^+$	CA^{++}	MG^{++}	HPO$_4^-$	CL$^-$	HCO$_3^-$
Dog	145-155	4.0-5.4	9.8-12.8	1.8-2.4	2.5-7.3	104-117	18-25
Cat	150-170	3.7-6	9.1-12.3	—	2.8-8.7	111-128	18-22
Horse	137-143	3.2-4.5	11.6-13.4	2.2-2.8	1.5-5.1	98-105	23-31
Cow	137-148	3.1-5.1	8.9-11.6	2.2-3.4	4.5-8.2	84-102	23-31

TABLE 25-2
COMMON DISEASES AND EXPECTED ELECTROLYTE ABNORMALITIES

DISEASE SYNDROME	WATER	NA+	K+	CA++	MG++	HPO4-	CL-	HCO3-
Gastric loss, vomiting	Loss	↓	↓		↓		↓	↑
Pancreatic or intestinal fluid loss	Loss	↓	↓		↓		↓	↓
Diarrhea		↓	↓		↓		↓	↓
Starvation	Loss	↑	↑↓	↓	↓		↓	
Acute hemorrhagic pancreatitis	Loss	↓↑	↑	↓↓	↓	↑↓	↑	↓
Malabsorption syndrome	Loss	↓↑	↑↓	↓	↓	↑↓	↑	↓
Acute renal failure (oliguric)	Excess	↑	↑↑	↑		↑	↑	↓
Renal tubular dysfunction	Loss	↓↑	↑				↓	
Chronic renal disease	Loss	↑↓↑	↑↓	↓	↑	↑	↓	↑
Diabetes insipidus	Loss	↑↓		↑			↑	↑
Burns	Loss	↑↓						
Primary aldosteronism	Excess	↑	↓	↓	↑	↑	↑	↑
Stress, surgery, including ADH	Excess	↑						
Hypoadrenocorticalism (Addison's disease)	Loss	↓	↑	↑	↓			
Hypopituitarism	Excess	↑↓						
Hyperadrenocorticalism (Cushing's disease)	Excess		↓	↑↓↑	↓↓			
Excess citrated blood				↓		↑		
Hyperparathyroidism								
Excess lactation (milk fever)			↑↓				↑	
Acidosis (metabolic)								↓
Alkalosis (metabolic)								↑

↑, Increased serum concentration; ↓, decreased serum concentration; —, normal serum concentration.

      c. Depress minute ventilation; respiratory acidosis may occur

      d. Decrease urine formation and renal concentrating ability

   2. General anesthesia usually depresses the sympathoadrenal response to hypercapnea and decreases effective circulating blood volume

  C. Imbalances caused by surgery

   1. Blood loss

   2. Evaporative loss from exposed tissues

   3. Removal of effusions

II. Fluid losses leading to a decrease in effective circulating blood volume usually cause metabolic acidosis

III. Blood loss is replaced with crystalloid fluids when the hematocrit is 20% and total protein is above 3.5 g/dl

  A. Colloids, 6% dextran 70, or hetastarch can be administered as alternatives to crystalloids, especially when the total protein is less than 4 g/dl

  B. Blood substitutes or blood are indicated if the packed cell volume (PCV) is acutely decreased below 20% during surgery or in patients with a PCV less than 15% as a result of chronic anemia

IV. Fluid administration to young or small patients should be supplemented with a source of calories (dextrose) and monitored closely to prevent overhydration

V. The administration of large quantities of room-temperature fluids can produce hypothermia and hemodilution; PCV and total protein should be monitored

VI. Fluid administration (Tables 25-3, 25-4)

  A. Most fluid administration sets deliver 10 drops/ml (regular drip) or 60 drops/ml (mini-drip)

  B. Larger-diameter needles or intravenous catheters offer less resistance to fluid flow and increase the rate of fluid administration

  C. Occasionally, fluids are administered at extremely rapid rates with fluid pumps

  D. Infusion pumps and syringe infusion pumps facilitate delivery of accurate volumes of fluid (Figs. 25-1, 25-2)

TABLE 25-3
GUIDELINES FOR CRYSTALLOID FLUIDS FOR SURGICAL PATIENTS

Step 1

Start intravenous fluids, replace insensible loss with maintenance-type solutions, 2-5 ml/kg/hr, during interval since last oral intake

Step 2

Change to replacement-type solution for intraoperative insensible losses. Administer LRS, Normosol-R, or in some cases 0.9% NaCl, 2 ml/kg/hr

Step 3

Estimate surgical trauma and add appropriate volume of replacement-type solution to that given in **Step 2:**
  Minimal trauma, add 5 ml/kg/hr
  Moderate trauma, add 10 ml/kg/hr
  Extreme trauma, add 15 ml/kg/hr
  Replace 1 ml of blood loss with 3 ml of crystalloid
  Administer appropriate fluid; when in doubt give balanced electrolyte solution

Step 4

Give appropriate colloid solution for each volume of blood lost over 20% of the patient's estimated blood volume

Step 5

Monitor vital signs and urine output. Adjust fluids to keep urine output at 1 ml/kg/hr

Modified from Glesecke AH, Egbert LD: Perioperative fluid therapy—crystalloids. In Miller RD, editor: *Anesthesia,* ed 2, New York, 1986, Churchill Livingstone, p. 1315.

NORMAL BODY WATER DISTRIBUTION

   I. Total body water represents 55% to 75% of body weight (BW) (use 60%), primarily depending on age and body fat
  II. Extracellular water constitutes 23% to 33% of body weight (use 30%); the percentage is greater in very young animals
 III. Intracellular water constitutes 35% to 45% of body weight
  IV. Plasma water constitutes approximately 5% of body weight
   V. Blood volume constitutes 8% to 10% of body weight (approximately 40 ml/lb or 90 ml/kg), depending on the hemat-

TABLE 25-4

GUIDE TO MONITORING FLUID THERAPY IN SURGICAL PATIENTS

1. Auscultation: normal bronchovesicular lung sounds
2. Packed cell volume > 20%
3. Total protein > 3.5 g/dl
4. Electrolytes
   a. Sodium 145-155 mEq/L
   b. Chloride 95-110 mEq/L
   c. Potassium 4.0-5.0 mEq/L
   d. Calcium 8.0-10.0 mg/dl
5. Blood pH 7.3-7.45; $PaCO_2$ 35-45 mm Hg
6. Urine output > 1 ml/kg/hr
7. Hemodynamics
   a. Central venous pressure 0-5 cm H_2O
   b. Pulmonary capillary wedge pressure 5-10 mm Hg
   c. Mean arterial blood pressure 70-90 mm Hg

---

   ocrit level; blood volume equals plasma water plus red blood
   cell (RBC) volume

  VI. Interstitial water constitutes 15% to 25% of body weight

 VII. Extracellular water equals plasma plus interstitial water

ELECTROLYTE DISTRIBUTION

   I. Extracellular water contains large quantities of sodium and chloride ions

  II. Intracellular water contains large quantities of potassium ions

 III. Table 25-1 shows the normal electrolyte composition of serum

PRINCIPLES OF FLUID ADMINISTRATION

   I. Correct dehydration and electrolyte and acid-base imbalances before anesthesia

  II. Do not attempt to replace chronic fluid losses acutely; severe dilution of plasma proteins, blood cells, and electrolytes may be produced (see Table 25-2)

 III. Monitor pulmonary, renal, and cardiac function when administering fluids rapidly (e.g., for shock)

     A. Pulmonary function; overhydration can lead to pulmonary edema

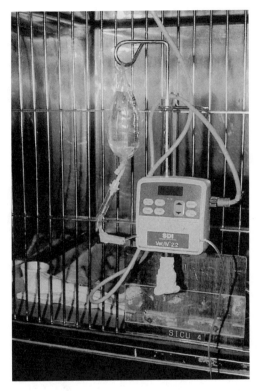

Fig. 25-1
Volumetric infusion pump.

  B. Renal function
    1. Improve or reestablish glomerular perfusion rate (renal perfusion) before anesthesia
    2. Administer mannitol at 0.5 to 1 g/lb over 30 minutes after hydration has been restored
    3. Monitor urine output: 1 to 2 ml/kg/hr
  C. Cardiac function
    1. Monitor central venous pressure (CVP) to prevent acute fluid overload

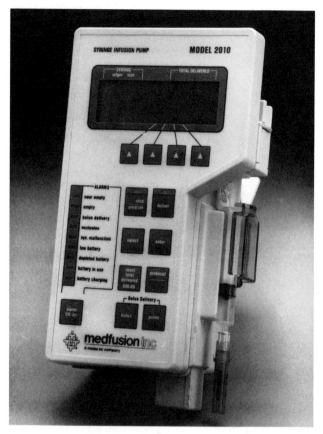

Fig. 25-2
Syringe infusion pump.

2. Auscultate the chest; if the total protein (TP) drops below 3.5 g/dl from fluid administration, pulmonary edema may occur
3. In cases of left-sided heart failure, monitor pulmonary capillary wedge pressures, if possible

FLUID ADMINISTRATION DURING ANESTHESIA
(SEE TABLES 25-3, 25-4)

   I. Fluids administered during anesthesia are usually polyionic isotonic crystalloid solutions (Table 25-5)

  II. Rate of initial crystalloid fluid administration depends on fluid loss during surgery

    A. Initial minimum rates of fluid administration:

Small animals	5 to 10 ml/lb/hr
Large animals	3 to 5 ml/lb/hr

    B. Increase this rate if significant hypotension develops

    C. Monitor PCV and TP for hemodilution

 III. Estimate blood loss and administer 3 ml of crystalloid solution for each milliliter of blood loss (unless blood transfusion is indicated) over and above the basic fluid rate provided during anesthesia

    A. Crystalloids are rapidly redistributed from the blood (8% to 10% BW) into the extracellular fluid (23% to 33% BW), which is approximately three times larger than the blood volume

 IV. Maximum rate of safe administration of fluids during shock therapy varies considerably; the rule of thumb is 40 ml/lb/hr

  V. Colloids (Table 25-6, 25-7)

    A. Intravascular volume-replacing fluids

    B. Duration of effect ($t\frac{1}{2}$) determined by molecular size; larger size, longer duration

    C. Colloids produce acute and lasting increases in the following:

      1. Intravascular volume

      2. Arterial blood pressure

      3. Cardiac output

      4. Tissue perfusion and oxygen delivery

    D. Small volumes (5 to 10 ml/lb IV) produce immediate increases in arterial blood pressure and cardiac output

      1. Helps to maintain plasma oncotic value and delay fluid extravasation

    E. May prolong bleeding time

TABLE 25-5
CHARACTERISTICS AND CONTENTS OF COMMONLY USED CRYSTALLOIDS AND NATURAL COLLOIDS

NAME	FLUID COMPART-MENT	OSMOLARITY (mOsm/L)	pH	Na$^+$ (mEq/L)
Crystalloids				
Maintenance				
2.5% Dextrose in half-strength Lactated Ringer's Solution	Extra-cellular	264 (isotonic)	4.5-7.5	65.5
ProcalAmine*	Extra-cellular	735 (hypertonic)	6-7	35
3% Freamine III*	Extra-cellular	405 (hypertonic)	6-7	35
Replacement				
0.9% Saline	Extra-cellular	308 (isotonic)	5.0	154
Lactated Ringer's Solution	Extra-cellular	275 (isotonic)	6.5	130
Plasmalyte-A pH 7.4†	Extra-cellular	294 (isotonic)	7.4	140
Normosol-R‡	Extra-cellular	295 (isotonic)	5.5-7	140
7.0% saline	Extra-cellular	2396 (hypertonic)	—	1197
5% Dextrose in H$_2$O	Intra-cellular	252 (hypotonic)	4.0	0
Colloids				
Natural				
Whole blood	Extra-cellular	300 (isotonic)	Variable	140
Frozen plasma	Extra-cellular	300 (isotonic)	Variable	140

*McGaw Inc.
†Baxter Healthcare, Corp.
‡Abbott Laboratories

Cl$^-$ (mEq/L)	K$^+$ (mEq/L)	Mg^{++} (mEq/L)	Ca^{++} (mEq/L)	DEX-TROSE (g/L)	BUFFER	COP (mm Hg)
55	2	0	1.5	25	Lactate	0
41	24	5	0	30	Acetate, Phosphate	0
41	24	5	0	0	Acetate, Phosphate	0
154	0	0	0	0	None	0
109	4	0	3	0	Lactate	0
98	5	3	0	0	Acetate, Gluconate	0
98	5	3	0	0	Acetate, Gluconate	0
1197	0	0	0	0	None	0
0	0	0	0	50	None	0
100	4	0	0	0-4	None	20
110	4	0	0	0-4	None	20

Continued

TABLE 25-6

CHARACTERISTICS AND CONTENTS OF COMMONLY USED SYNTHETIC COLLOIDS AND BLOOD SUBSTITUTE

Name	FLUID COMPART-MENT	OSMOLARITY (mOsm/L)	pH	Na⁺ (mEq/L)
Synthetic colloids				
6% Hetastarch	Extra-cellular	310 (isotonic)	5.5	154
10% Pentastarch	Extra-cellular	326 (isotonic)	5.0	154
Dextran 40	Extra-cellular	311 (isotonic)	3.5-7.0	154
Dextran 70	Extra-cellular	310 (isotonic)	3-7	154
Oxypolygelatin	Extra-cellular	200 (hypotonic)	7.4	155
Blood substitute (O_2 carriers)				
Oxyglobin	Extra-cellular	300 (isotonic)	7.7	150

VI. Hypertonic saline (see Table 25-5)

    A. Normal saline contains 0.9% NaCl

        1. Commonly used hypertonic saline solutions contain 3%, 5%, and 7% (70 mg/ml) NaCl

    B. Hypertonic fluids increase vascular volume by pulling water from the extracellular fluid space into the vascular space

    C. Hypertonic fluids produce acute increases in the following:

        1. Arterial blood pressure

        2. Cardiac output

        3. Renal perfusion and diuresis

    D. 7% NaCl is used as acute fluid therapy for hypotension or shock; 3 ml/lb IV

    E. Overdose produces hypernatremia, hyperchloremia, and nonrespiratory acidosis; cardiac arrhythmias are also a possibility

VII. Blood substitutes (see Table 25-6)

    A. Oxygen-carrying solutions that are ultra-purified and hemoglobin-based can be used to replace volume and im-

Cl⁻ (mEq/L)	K⁺ (mEq/L)	Mg⁺⁺ (mEq/L)	Ca⁺⁺ (mEq/L)	DEXTROSE (g/L)	BUFFER	COP (mm Hg)
154	0	0	0	0	None	70
154	0	0	0	0	None	25
154	0	0	0	0	None	40
154	0	0	0	0	None	60
100	0	0	1	0	None	45-47
110	4.0	—	1.0	—	None	17

TABLE 25-7
CHARACTERISTICS OF COMMON COLLOID SOLUTIONS

COLLOID	MOLECULAR WEIGHT (RANGE)	MOLECULAR WEIGHT (AVERAGE)	COP (mm Hg)	OSMOLARITY (mOsm/L)
Saline	0	0	0	310
Plasma	66-400	119	22	285
Dextran 40	10-80	40	82	310
Dextran 70	15-160	70	62	310
Hetastarch	10-1000	450	32	310
Pentastarch	150-350	264	—	310
Gelatins	5-100	35	—	—

COP, Colloid oncotic pressure.

prove tissue oxygen delivery following trauma and hemorrhage; they can also be used in anemic patients

B. Uses
    1. Improve oxygen delivery by increasing oxygen content of the blood and expanding vascular volume

2. Immediate improvement in clinical signs of anemia
3. Immediate availability and ready to use
4. Not 2,3-DPG-dependent; chloride-ion dependent
5. 2-year shelf life
6. Stored at room temperature
7. No typing and crossmatching
8. No transfusion reaction
9. No disease transmission
10. No need for donor dog
11. Saves time, labor, and materials

C. Polymerized bovine hemoglobin (Oxyglobin Hb = 13 g/dl) in modified lactated Ringer's solution is a colloid solution that carries oxygen
   1. Dose: 30 ml/kg at 10 ml/kg/hr

D. Clinical issues
   1. Temporary interference with some serum chemistries
   2. Transient discoloration of urine, sclera, and mucous membranes
   3. Potential for overexpansion of vascular volume in normovolemic patients

E. Contraindications
   1. Plasma volume expanders, such as Oxyglobin, are contraindicated in dogs with advanced cardiac disease (i.e., congestive heart failure) or otherwise severely impaired cardiac function or renal impairment with oliguria or anuria
   2. Use during sepsis and endotoxemia has been questioned
   3. Warnings
      a. Overdosage or an excessively rapid administration rate (more than 10 ml/kg/hr) may result in circulatory overload; see the product's package insert for complete information

PERIOPERATIVE FLUID THERAPY

I. When continued intravenous fluid therapy is necessary before or after surgery, the normal daily fluid maintenance rates are as follows:

A. 20 to 30 ml/lb/24 hr (mature animal)

B. 30 to 45 ml/lb/24 hr (young animal)

II. Calculation of replacement fluid volume in dehydrated animals
  A. Body weight (kg) $\times$ % dehydration (figured as a decimal): fluid deficit (L) (e.g., 20 kg $\times$ 10% dehydration = 2 L fluid deficit); reassess periodically to determine the response to volumes administered
  B. Replacement fluids to correct dehydration can be administered over a 4- to 6-hour period or added to the maintenance fluid volume and administered over a 24-hour period

CLINICAL ASSESSMENT OF HYDRATION

	MINIMAL (4%)	MODERATE (6% TO 8%)	SEVERE (10% TO 12%)
Skin resiliency	Pliable	Leathery	Absolutely no pliability
Skin tenting	Twist disappears immediately and tent persists up to 2 seconds	Twist disappears immediately and tent persists up to 3 seconds or more	Twist and tent persists indefinitely
Eye	Bright Slightly sunken	Duller than normal Obviously sunken	Cornea dry Deeply sunken, 2- to 4-mm space between eyeball and bony orbit
Mouth	Moist, warm	Sticky to dry, warm	Dry, cyanotic, warm to cold

BLOOD TRANSFUSION—MAJOR BLOOD GROUPS

  I. Dogs
  A. At least eight specific antigens have been identified on the dog erythrocyte
    1. Dog erythrocyte antigen $(DEA)_1$, DEA_2, and DEA_7 have the greatest potential to induce hemolytic antibody production in recipients; dogs negative for these RBC antigens are desirable as donors
    2. Transfusion reactions related to the remaining blood-group antigens are usually clinically insignificant
    3. Donor dogs should test negative for heartworms

II. Cats
- A. Three major antigens have been identified on the cat erythrocyte
  1. Transfusion reactions are rare in cats; blood typing is rarely performed
  2. RBC survival time may decrease after multiple transfusions

III. Horses
- A. At least nine specific blood group antigens have been identified in the horse
  1. Compatibility testing should be done in the horse erythrocyte before transfusion
     a. Blood typing
     b. Major and minor antigen agglutination
     c. Lysis cross-matching test
  2. When compatibility cannot be tested, a healthy male horse that has never had a transfusion is the most suitable donor

IV. Cows: at least 11 antigenic blood groups are recognized

V. Swine: at least 15 antigenic blood groups are recognized

VI. Sheep: at least 8 antigenic blood groups are recognized

INDICATIONS FOR BLOOD OR BLOOD SUBSTITUTES

I. Restoration of oxygen-carrying capacity
- A. Anemia
  1. PCV is less than 20%; Hb is less than 5 g/dl in a normally hydrated patient being prepared for surgery
  2. Nonsurgical, chronically anemic patients may not require transfusion unless PCV is less than 15 in dogs or less than 10 in cats
- B. Hemorrhage
  1. Crystalloid infusion may adequately treat 15% to 30% total blood volume loss
  2. Colloids should be considered when blood loss exceeds 25%
  3. Whole blood or blood substitutes are necessary for replacement of more than 50% total blood volume loss
     a. Stored blood is a poor source of oxygen because the Hb cannot off-load oxygen

      b. Fresh whole blood or blood substitutes should be administered to replace acute blood loss and improve oxygen delivery to tissues
II. Restoration of blood volume
III. Coagulation factor replacement
    A. Poor viability of platelets and coagulation factors in stored blood
    B. Choose fresh blood (stored for less than 12 hours) when treating coagulopathies

COLLECTING AND STORING BLOOD FOR TRANSFUSION

  I. Obtain blood from the jugular vein or with a cardiac puncture
  II. Anticoagulant solutions used
    A. Acid citrate dextrose (ACD)
    B. Citrate phosphate dextrose (CPD) maintains higher pH, adenosine triphosphate (ATP), and 2,3-diphosphoglycerate (DPG) content during storage
    C. Heparin
      1. Heparin activates platelet aggregation and inhibits thrombin formation by inhibiting factor IX activation
      2. Do not use blood collected with heparin as the anticoagulant if it has been stored longer than 48 hours
III. Plastic containers are recommended for blood collection; they are less likely to activate platelet and coagulation factors
IV. Suggested guidelines for blood storage
    A. Maintain temperature between 1° and 6° C for the following storage times:
      1. ACD anticoagulant: 21 days
      2. CPD anticoagulant: 28 days
      3. Feline blood: 30 days
    B. 70% to 75% RBCs are viable at the end of the storage times listed above

MODIFICATIONS OF STORED BLOOD

  I. RBCs become less deformable because of the following conditions:
    A. Hypertonicity of anticoagulant solution
    B. Decreasing erythrocyte ATP content

II. Erythrocyte 2,3-DPG content is decreased

    A. The oxygen dissociation curve shifts to the left; decreased oxygen is released at the tissue level

        1. Stored blood is a poor choice when increased oxygen delivery to tissues is required; blood substitutes (Oxyglobin) are recommended in these circumstances

    B. 2,3-DPG content in RBCs is restored within hours of transfusion

III. pH decreases (less than 6.5 after 3 weeks of storage); citrate anticoagulants are converted to bicarbonate within minutes by the liver; bicarbonate therapy with blood transfusion is not necessary unless inadequate liver blood flow or altered liver metabolism is suspected

IV. Platelet numbers decrease; functional platelets are nonexistent after 2 to 3 days of storage

V. Ammonia content increases; this may be detrimental for patients with impaired hepatic function

VI. Plasma potassium concentration increases because of progressive hemolysis during storage

VII. Metabolic transformations in stored blood are largely reversed during the first 24 hours following transfusion

VIII. Blood administration

    A. Blood administration sets

        1. Use a set with a filter to remove aggregated debris

            a. Micropore filter with pore size 20 to 40 μm

            b. Cloth filter of administration set with pore size 170 μm

        2. Flush tubing before introducing blood

            a. This reduces resistance to blood flow

            b. Isotonic saline is the recommended fluid

            c. Lactated Ringer's or other calcium-containing solutions may re-calcify blood and trigger coagulation

            d. Dextrose solutions may cause agglutination and/or hemolysis

ADVERSE, IMMUNE-MEDIATED EFFECTS OF BLOOD TRANSFUSION

I. Nonhemolytic hypersensitivity reactions
   A. Activation of kallikrein-kinin system or immunoglobulin E
   B. Release of biogenic amines
   C. Clinical signs are muscle tremor, pyrexia, hypotension, tachycardia, and urticaria
II. Hemolytic reactions
   A. Hemolysis results from the following:
      1. Recipient antibodies interacting with incompatible antigen of donor
      2. Antibodies of a previously sensitized donor interacting with recipient antigen
   B. Immediate transfusion reactions are unlikely during a first transfusion
   C. Clinical signs usually develop within an hour after a transfusion and include hypotension, pyrexia, muscle tremor, emesis, convulsions, hemoglobinemia or hemoglobinuria, and bilirubinemia or bilirubinuria
   D. Shock, renal failure, and disseminated intravascular coagulation may ensue
   E. Delayed transfusion reactions can occur up to 2 weeks after a transfusion
      1. The recipient mounts an immune response to incompatible erythrocytes
      2. Clinical signs include pyrexia, anorexia, jaundice, and bilirubinuria
   F. Hemolysis in neonates resulting from previous sensitization of the mother (neonatal isoerythrolysis) can be avoided by preventing colostrum absorption; withhold mother's milk from the neonate in the first 48 hours of life

NONIMMUNOLOGIC ADVERSE TRANSFUSION REACTIONS

I. Sepsis: improper collection, storage, or handling may result in bacterial contamination and overgrowth
II. Transmission of infectious or parasitic diseases

III. Circulatory overload
IV. Citrate toxicity
    A. Citrate toxicity is rarely seen because of the rapid metabolism of citrate by the liver; it is more likely in animals with liver dysfunction or excessively rapid blood administration
    B. Excessive circulating citrate causes chelation of serum ionized calcium

PLASMA TRANSFUSION

I. Indications
    A. Hypoproteinemia: total protein ≤ 4 g/dl; albumin ≤ 1.5 g/dl
    B. Failure of passive transfer; inadequate colostral antibody absorption
    C. Thrombocytopenia: use fresh plasma
    D. Coagulopathies: use fresh plasma
II. Plasma can be stored in a conventional freezer for up to 1 year

ROUTES AND VOLUME OF FLUID ADMINISTRATION

I. A peripheral or jugular vein
II. Intraperitoneal administration
    A. Administer slowly
    B. RBCs are poorly recovered into the system; approximately 40% of blood is absorbed in 24 hours
III. Medullary cavity of femur, tibia, or humerus
    A. Adequate for neonatal small animals
    B. Use a 20-gauge needle or a bone-marrow aspiration needle
    C. 95% of the blood is absorbed within 5 minutes
IV. Rewarm stored blood to decrease viscosity and prevent hypothermia in recipients; immerse transfusion tubing in water that is maintained at a temperature below 40° C; autoagglutination occurs at higher temperatures
V. Volume of colloid or blood to be administered
    A. General rule: 1 milliliter of colloid or blood per milliliter of blood lost
    B. General rule: 1 milliliter of whole blood per pound raises the PCV by 1% (assuming there is a donor PCV of 40%)

C. Blood volume needed to obtain target PCV

Amount of donor blood needed =
$$\frac{\text{Desired PCV} - \text{Actual patient PCV}}{\text{PCV of anticoagulated donor blood}} \times \text{Recipient blood volume}$$

Estimate total blood volume at 40 ml/lb (30 ml/lb in cats)
D. The amount of blood lost in aspirated fluids

Volume of blood in suction fluid =
$$\frac{\text{PCV of fluid} \times \text{Volume of fluid}}{\text{PCV of animal}}$$

E. Plasma volume needed to attain a target total protein (TP)

Amount of donor plasma needed (ml) =
$$\frac{\text{Desired TP} - \text{Actual TP}}{\text{Donor plasma TP}} \times \text{Recipient plasma volume}$$

VI. Fluid administration rate depends on clinical circumstances
   A. Administer rapidly following massive hemorrhage
   B. In other cases
      1. Transfuse blood slowly at 0.1 ml/lb during the first 30 minutes; observe for adverse reactions
      2. Afterward, the rule of thumb is 5 ml/lb/hr, until the desired PCV is achieved
      3. Monitor for signs of fluid overload (e.g., CVP, thoracic auscultation)

CHAPTER TWENTY-SIX

Shock

"I'm late, I'm late for a very important date" (early recognition and treatment is essential to prevent death).

LEWIS CARROLL

OVERVIEW

Traditional approaches to the classification of shock stress the importance of various etiologies (hemorrhage, trauma, sepsis, allergies, and drug reactions) or emphasize the functional relationship between the effective circulating volume, the heart, and peripheral vasculature. The latter rationalization ascribes shock to hypovolemia, cardiac failure, obstruction (high resistance) to blood flow, or the abnormal distribution (low resistance) of blood flow. Although instructive, these attempts at categorization do not provide the necessary knowledge required for a rational approach to therapy. Rather, an appropriate clinical approach to shock emphasizes the temporal pathophysiologic processes responsible for the circulatory changes that may potentially lead to patient decompensation and death. Shock can be perpetuated or caused by bacterial infection leading to systemic inflammatory response syndrome (SIRS), while local infections shift to uncontrolled systemic reactions. The development of SIRS can result from opportunistic infections in depressed, debilitated, or severely stressed animals. This chapter defines shock and discusses current thoughts regarding the pathophysiology of shock, circulatory compensation and decompensation, signs and symptoms, the relevance of monitored physiologic variables, and the treatment of shock syndromes.

DEFINITION OF SHOCK

I. Definition: shock is a disease syndrome best characterized by impaired tissue perfusion and oxygenation

II. Etiology (Table 26-1)

TABLE 26-1
CAUSES OF SHOCK

CATEGORY	CAUSE
Hypovolemic shock	
Exogenous	Blood loss caused by hemorrhage
	Plasma loss caused by thermal or chemical burns and inflammation
	Fluid and electrolyte loss caused by dehydration, vomiting, diarrhea, renal disease, severe exercise, heat stress, or excessive diuresis
Endogenous	Extravasation of fluids, plasma, or blood into a body cavity or tissues (third-space losses) caused by trauma, endotoxins, hypoproteinemia, anaphylaxis, or burns
Cardiac shock	
	Myocardial mechanical problems caused by regurgitant or obstructive defects
	Myopathic defects caused by inheritable traits, chemicals, or toxins
	Cardiac arrhythmias
Distributive shock	
High resistance	Distribution of blood volume and flow to vital organs caused by endotoxins, anesthetic drug overdose, CNS trauma, anaphylaxis
Low resistance	Distribution of blood away from vital organs caused by severe infections, abscesses, or arterio-venous fistulas
Obstructive shock	
	Obstruction to blood flow through the heart (pericardial tamponade, neoplasia, embolism), aorta (embolism, aneurysm), vena cava (gastric bloat, heartworm, neoplasia), lungs (embolism, heartworm, positive-pressure ventilation)

CNS, Central nervous system.

    A. Hypovolemic
    B. Cardiogenic
    C. Distributive
    D. Obstructive
III. Pathophysiology (Fig. 26-1)
    A. Poor tissue perfusion can result from the following (Table 26-2):
        1. Endotoxin
           a. Endotoxin-induced extravasation of fluids (third space loss)
           b. Release of vasoactive substances (histamine, catecholamines, serotonin, bradykinins, prostaglandins, tumor necrosis factor, interleukins)

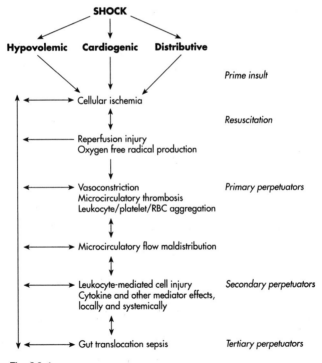

Fig. 26-1
Progressive pathophysiologic processes in shock.

TABLE 26-2
COMPENSATORY AND CORRECTIVE RESPONSES TO A DECREASE IN THE EFFECTIVE CIRCULATING BLOOD VOLUME

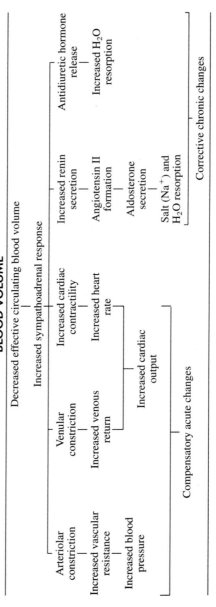

  c. Generalized vasoconstriction (occurs early in septic shock)

  d. Capillary damage with loss of volume

  e. Selective capillary dilatation

  f. Relative hypovolemia

  g. The opening of arteriovenous shunts may result in blood flow bypassing capillary beds, regardless of cardiac output

2. Traumatic, hemorrhagic (see Table 26-2)

  a. Blood loss

   (1) 20% loss: mild signs of shock

   (2) 30% loss: obvious signs of shock

  b. Release of catecholamines

  c. Vasoconstriction

  d. Hypovolemia

3. If untreated, septic, traumatic, hemorrhagic, or cardiogenic shock eventually leads to the following:

  a. Ischemic anoxia can be caused by decreased circulatory volume, decreased venous return, reduced cardiac output, increased total peripheral resistance, decreased tissue perfusion, and increased catecholamines

  b. Hypoxia, ischemia, and acidosis activate monocytes, macrophages, and leukocytes, which then trigger the release of cellular reactant substances

   (1) Various interleukins (1, 6, 8, and others); products of activated monocytes and macrophages:

    (a) Stimulate fever by initiating prostaglandin synthesis

    (b) Stimulate activation and release of neutrophils

    (c) Initiate proteolysis in skeletal muscles

    (d) Stimulate insulin and glucagon production

    (e) Activate the immune system

   (2) Activated leukocytes release lytic enzymes (proteases, lipases) and oxygen free radicals, resulting in:

    (a) Initiation of the complement cascade

    (b) Damage to cell membranes by lysosomal enzymes

      (c) Production of autocoids (histamine, brady-kinin, and serotonin)

      (d) Increased capillary membrane permeability

  (3) Arachidonic acid metabolism is activated, producing a number of biologically active cyclo-oxygenase and lipoxygenase products (prostaglandins)

      (a) Prostacyclin relaxes vascular smooth muscle and inhibits platelet aggression

      (b) Thromboxane A_2 constricts vascular smooth muscle, releases lysosomes, and causes platelet and leukocyte activation and aggregation

      (c) Leukotrienes (e.g., the slow-reacting substance of anaphylaxis) produce many detrimental effects such as vasoconstriction, bronchoconstriction, and increased capillary membrane permeability

  (4) Cellular damage causes the production of cardiac depressant substances and vasoactive peptides; factor XII is produced, which converts kallikreinogen to kallikrein, bradykinin, and other active peptides, resulting in vasodilation and increased capillary membrane permeability

      (a) Factor XII initiates the intrinsic system in the coagulation cascade

        • Fibrin thrombi are formed, perpetuating hypoxia, acidosis, and tissue damage; fibrin split products are formed, thrombocytopenia develops, and hemorrhage occurs

c. Stagnant anoxia can be caused by anoxia, stagnation, acidosis, microthrombosis, and arteriovenous shunting (admixture): bacteria-tissue interaction and/or atelectasis in the lungs may contribute to shunting

  (1) Same as above, but without significant production of oxygen-dependent by-products

d. Time: ischemic anoxia to stagnant anoxia may take hours to occur in hemorrhagic shock; it occurs in seconds to minutes in anaphylactic or septic shock

e. The ultimate outcome is cell damage and death

B. Cellular events
   1. Reduced oxygen and nutrient supply
   2. Anaerobic metabolism
   3. Decreased adenosine triphosphate (ATP) and energy
   4. Increased membrane permeability
   5. Influx of sodium and water
   6. Efflux of intracellular potassium
   7. Cellular edema
   8. Mitochondrial damage (swelling)
   9. Intracellular acidosis
   10. Lysosomal membrane rupture
   11. Extracellular lytic enzymes
   12. Extracellular acidemia
   13. Cell damage and death
IV. Compensation and decompensation
   A. Most compensatory changes are initiated in an attempt to sustain tissue oxygen supply and preserve cellular metabolic functions (see Table 26-2; Fig. 26-2)
      1. Hemorrhage decreases blood volume, cardiac output, arterial blood pressure, and oxygen delivery; the sympathetic nervous system is activated
         a. Compensatory mechanisms include tachycardia, systemic and pulmonary vasoconstriction, and increased myocardial contractility
         b. Blood flow is preferentially redistributed to the heart, brain, lungs, and liver at the expense of the kidneys, gut, and skin
         c. Continued or severe untreated hemorrhage (more than 50% blood volume) causes cardiac output and arterial blood pressure to decrease until death
         d. Prolonged intense vasoconstriction predisposes the patient to tissue ischemia, hypoxia, and cellular acidosis
      2. Trauma (surgical stress), with or without major blood loss, increases sympathetic neural activity; this stimulates the cardiorespiratory centers
         a. Compensatory mechanisms include tachycardia, increased cardiac output, and increased arterial pressure and peripheral vascular resistance
         b. If hypovolemia occurs, cardiac output decreases

DECREASED TISSUE PERFUSION

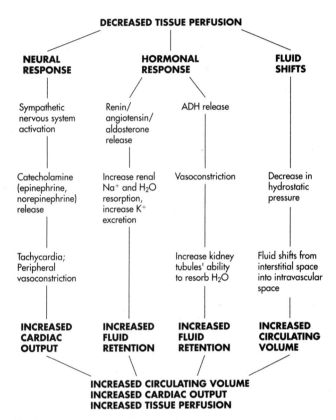

Fig. 26-2

Compensatory mechanisms activated in shock.

c. Respiratory alkalosis occurs secondary to increased ventilation

d. The duration and magnitude of the traumatic event determine the onset of various decompensatory events

(1) Persistent tachycardia

(2) Decreased cardiac output (less than 90 ml/kg/min)

(3) Decreased arterial pressure (less than 60 mm Hg)

      (4) Activation of neuroendocrine, immune comple-
ment, and arachidonic acid systems by cellular
breakdown products

3. Heart failure and severe cardiac arrhythmias (ventricular tachycardia) decrease cardiac output, which activates
various neuroendocrine and renal mechanisms designed
to restore blood flow

   a. Compensatory mechanisms include tachycardia,
vasoconstriction, and increased total blood volume

   b. Peripheral vascular resistance increases

   c. Cardiac decompensation produced by progressive
heart failure results in reduced cardiac output, tachycardia, arterial hypotension, elevated venous pressures, pulmonary edema, and ascites

4. Sepsis activates neuroendocrine, immune, arachidonic
acid (prostaglandin), and complement systems

   a. Compensatory responses include fever, chills, leuko-
cytosis with or without hypotension, and tachycardia; cardiac output and alveolar ventilation are initially increased

   b. Cardiac output is increased and systemic vascular resistance is decreased early during sepsis to meet the
increased metabolic demands for oxygen

   c. The hyperthermic response increases metabolic
(oxygen) and circulatory demands

   d. Decompensation, which can take hours or minutes,
is an extension of the hyperdynamic state; progressive increases in tissue oxygen demand and mal-
distribution of blood flow eventually lead to tissue
ischemia, hypoxia, and acidosis

   e. Endotoxins damage endothelial cells and cause the
release of vasoactive peptides, which result in the following:

      (1) Activation of the complement cascade

      (2) Activation of the coagulation system

      (3) Activation of factor XII, which produces
bradykinin and the release of other autocoids

      (4) Activation of the fibrinolytic system

         (a) Formation of fibrin split products

         (b) Consumption of coagulation factors

         (c) Thrombocytopenia

5. Extreme dehydration, hemorrhage, or trauma can cause redistribution of body water from plasma, interstitial, and intracellular compartments

   a. Body fluid shifts occur following hemorrhage in an attempt to refill the plasma compartment and result in a delayed reduction in hemoglobin concentration (packed cell volume [PCV])

   b. Inappropriate fluid shifts following trauma, surgery, and depletional states lead to hypovolemia, excessive interstitial water, reduced intracellular water, and increased total body water

     (1) Peripheral edema may occur

     (2) Pulmonary edema may occur

V. Signs

  A. The signs of shock are indicative of exaggerated adrenergic responses and the products of tissue ischemia, hypoxia, and acidosis

    1. Hemorrhage causes activation of the autonomic nervous system; redistribution of blood to the heart, brain, and lungs; and a shift of body fluids to the plasma volume

     a. Depression, unconsciousness

     b. Pale or white mucous membranes

     c. Decreased skin temperature

     d. Prolonged capillary refill time

     e. Tachycardia

     f. Oliguria

     g. Delayed reduction in PCV

    2. Severe physical or surgical injury increases autonomic neural activity, which stimulates central cardiac and respiratory centers and activates humoral mechanisms

     a. History of trauma or surgery

     b. Physical evidence of injury (fractures, lacerations)

     c. Depression, collapse

     d. Signs of hemorrhage (see above)

     e. Tachypnea, respiratory distress

    3. Heart failure reduces cardiac output, which activates the autonomic and neuroendocrine systems; this results in retention of electrolytes (Na^+, Cl^-) and water

     a. Reduced exercise tolerance, depression, or fainting

     b. Pale and cold mucous membranes

     c. Prolonged capillary refill time

     d. Tachycardia and arrhythmias

     e. Weak peripheral pulses

     f. Cardiac murmurs

     g. Oliguria

     h. Pulmonary edema and ascites

4. Localized or systemic infection (SIRS), with or without bacteremia and endotoxemia, is associated with sympathetic activation of the cardiorespiratory centers and the immune, coagulation, complement, and kinin systems as well as the release of various hormones, prostaglandins, and vasoactive peptides

     a. Depression

     b. Fever, chills

     c. Warm skin and mucous membranes

     d. Normal or red mucous membranes

     e. Tachycardia

     f. Strong or weak pulse

     g. Tachypnea

     h. Oliguria

     i. Leukocytosis or leukopenia

     j. Thrombocytopenia

CLINICAL AND LABORATORY FEATURES

I. Shock is divided into early (reversible) and late (irreversible) stages (Table 26-3)

II. Laboratory findings: laboratory data vary greatly and in many instances depend on the cause of the shock syndrome and the stage of shock (Fig. 26-3)

  A. Packed cell volume (PCV)

    1. In hemorrhagic shock

      a. Below normal in hypovolemic and progressive phases of oligemic shock; plasma volume increases as interstitial fluid moves into the vascular system during the first 30 minutes after hemorrhage (0.25 ml/kg/min); in many species (particularly horses), the spleen serves as a blood reservoir and buffers the effects of acute blood loss on PCV; because of the ability of splenic contraction to restore blood volume, hemorrhage must be severe to produce PCV decreases

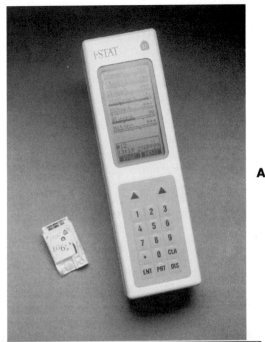

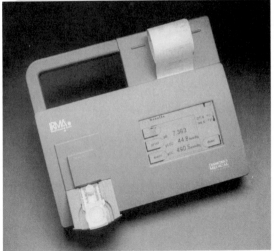

Fig. 26-3
A, B, Portable point-of-care analyzers can provide valuable acid-base and electrolyte data in approximately 120 seconds.

TABLE 26-3
STAGES OF SHOCK

CHARACTERISTIC	EARLY STAGE	LATE STAGE
Cardiovascular		
Heart rate	Moderately increased	Markedly increased
Heart rhythm	Regular, rapid, normal	Regular or irregular
Pulse pressure	Normal	Reduced (weak, thready pulse)
Capillary refill time	Minimally prolonged	Markedly prolonged (>3 sec)
Mucous membrane color	Pale pink (injected in septic shock)	White (red or blue in septic shock)
CVP	Minimally reduced	Markedly reduced (<1 cm H_2O) <60 mm Hg)
Arterial blood pressure	Normal or decreased (elevated in septic shock)	Decreased (mean pressure)
ECG	Normal, tachycardia	Tachycardia, arrhythmic, S-T segment deviation
Respiratory		
Respiratory rate	Increased	Rapid, shallow breathing
Pattern of respiration	Regular	Normal, intermittent dyspnea

Auscultation	Normal, increased tracheal sounds	Increased bronchovesicular sounds, crackles
Tidal volume	Increased	Decreased
Arterial oxygen tension	Normal	Normal or decreased
Arterial carbon dioxide	Decreased	Normal, decreased or increased
Central nervous system		
Level of consciousness	Alert, anxious, minimally depressed	Depressed, semiconscious, coma
Laboratory evaluation		
Packed cell volume	Normal or increased	Normal or decreased
Total protein	Normal or increased	Decreased
Blood lactate	Normal	Increased
Serum K^+	Normal or decreased	Increased
BUN and creatinine	Normal	Normal or increased
Urine volume and Na^+	Decreased	Markedly decreased
White blood cell count	Increased (left shift)	Decreased (left shift)

CVP, Central venous pressure; *ECG*, electrocardiogram; *BUN*, blood urea nitrogen.

      b. With traumatic burns, endotoxic shock, and colic, PCV increases and hemoconcentration occurs

2. Blood glucose is elevated; epinephrine is released
3. Blood serum protein concentration may be normal or increased at first, but it is generally reduced during later stages of shock
4. Platelet count is usually decreased
5. Blood urea nitrogen and creatinine are elevated, and creatinine clearance is reduced
6. Urinalysis generally shows no specific abnormalities
7. Electrolyte patterns vary considerably, but there is a tendency toward a low serum sodium level and a low serum chloride level
8. Serum potassium may be high, low, or normal
9. Plasma bicarbonate is usually low, and blood lactate is elevated
10. Respiratory alkalosis occurs early in shock and is manifested by a low $PaCO_2$
11. Hypoxia and metabolic acidosis develop as shock progresses; $PaCO_2$ values are below 70 mm Hg (normal values are 75 to 100 mm Hg)

B. The lungs in shock: respiratory failure is the most frequent cause of death in patients with shock, particularly after the hemodynamic alterations have been corrected; this syndrome is characterized by pulmonary congestion, hemorrhage, atelectasis, edema, and the formation of capillary thrombi; pulmonary surfactant decreases, and pulmonary compliance becomes progressively compromised

MONITORING

Monitoring provides vital information for evaluating patient trends and guiding the course of therapy. A global monitoring approach is necessary, including a detailed medical history and a meticulous physical examination supplemented by physiologic, laboratory, and radiographic or other imaging information (e.g., ultrasound). Serial measurements are mandatory (Table 26-4).

I. Circulatory system monitoring should stress tissue perfusion but must emphasize variables reflecting oxygen transport
    A. Heart rate
    B. Heart and lung sounds

TABLE 26-4
CLINICALLY USEFUL VARIABLES FOR ASSESSING SHOCK

	UNIT	NORMAL VALUE OR CONDITION
Mucous membrane color	—	Pink
Capillary refill time	Sec	<2
Respiratory rate	Breaths/min	
Dog		<20
Cat		<30
Arterial oxygen tension, PaO_2	mm Hg	100-120
Arterial oxygen saturation	%	>85
Central venous oxygen saturation, SvO_2	%	>70
Heart rate	Beats/min	
Dog		70-180
Cat		15-210
Urine output	ml/kg/hr	2-5
Blood glucose concentration	mg/dl	70-150
Potassium	mEq/L	4-5
Packed cell volume	%	30-45
Hemoglobin	g/dl	12-16
Temperature	° F	100-102
Lactic acid concentration	mM/L	<1.0
Central venous pressure	mm Hg	<1.0
Arterial blood pressure (AP)	mm Hg	
Systolic		100-150
Diastolic		60-110
Mean		80-120

    C. Pulse pressure measurement

    D. Mucous membrane capillary refill time (less than 2 seconds)

    E. Mucous membrane color (pink)

    F. Temperature (more than 100° F; less than 101.5° F)

    G. Packed cell volume and hemoglobin (more than 20%; 7 g/dl)

    H. Blood pressure measurement (more than 60 mm Hg)

       1. Direct arterial or venous (central venous pressure [CVP]) catheters

       2. Indirect blood pressure cuffs (oscillometric or Doppler blood pressure monitors)

    I. Electrocardiogram

    J. Pulse oximetry for noninvasive assessment of tissue oxygenation and heart rate

    K. Blood gas and pH measurements

        1. Arterial blood gases are indicative of adequate oxygenation and ventilation

        2. Venous blood gases and pH reflect tissue metabolic status and adequacy of blood flow (cardiac output)

II. Respiratory system monitoring should evaluate alveolar ventilation and must stress arterial oxygenation

    A. Mucous membrane color: cyanotic (blue) mucous membrane color suggests low hemoglobin saturation with oxygen

    B. Respiratory rate

    C. Thoracic radiographs

    D. Effort of breathing (dyspnea)

    E. Tidal volume

        1. Subjectively assessed by rebreathing from a bag (anesthetic machine)

        2. Ventilometer

    F. End tidal CO_2 determination noninvasively assesses the adequacy of ventilation

    G. Blood gases and pH

        1. Arterial blood gases are used to assess oxygenation (P_{O_2}) and ventilation (P_{CO_2})

III. Extracellular fluid volume should be assessed continuously to ensure adequate tissue perfusion and to prevent overhydration

    A. Skin turgor

    B. Mucous membrane color and capillary refill time

    C. Urinary output

    D. Urine sodium concentration

    E. Urine and plasma osmolality

    F. Responses of CVP to a fluid challenge

        1. Sudden increases in CVP (more than 5 mm Hg) with small fluid infusions indicate poor cardiac function, an infusion rate that is too rapid, or a transfusion that is too large

IV. Laboratory evaluation may provide insights regarding tissue damage, infection, and prognosis

    A. Hemogram (hematocrit, total protein, platelets)

    B. White cell counts

   C. Electrolytes (Na^+, K^+, Cl^-, Ca^{2+}), anion gap, strong ion difference

   D. Blood urea nitrogen and creatinine to evaluate renal function

   E. Tests of visceral organ damage

      1. For possible liver damage: alanine transaminase (ALT) and alkaline phosphatase (ALP) measurements

      2. For possible general tissue damage: aspartate transaminase and lactic dehydrogenase measurements

      3. For possible pancreatic damage: lipase or amylase measurements

   F. Lactate

      1. Excellent indicator of the severity of tissue acidosis and prognosis (normal value less than 15 mmol/L)

   G. Blood gases and pH

   H. Coagulation screening tests

      1. Clotting time

      2. Fibrin split products

THERAPY (TABLES 26-5, 26-6, 26-7)

   I. Support of respiration: in many patients with shock, arterial PO_2 is significantly depressed; oxygen may be administered nasally or by mask; endotracheal intubation and the use of a positive-pressure respirator may be helpful in achieving proper ventilation

  II. Volume replacement: with the CVP or pulmonary wedge pressure as a guide, blood volume should be replaced with appropriate fluids; oliguria in the presence of hypotension is not a contraindication for continued vigorous fluid therapy

 III. In addition to fluids, inotropes, antiarrhythmics, antibiotics, and glucocorticosteroids may be indicated; small volumes (3 to 4 ml/kg) of hypertonic saline (7%) in 6% solution help restore and maintain cardiovascular function

   A. Hypertonic (3%, 5%, 7%) saline solutions mixed with 6% dextran 70 solution can be used to treat hemorrhagic, traumatic, and endotoxic shock with remarkably good response; 3 to 4 ml/kg of 7% saline solution produces a beneficial hemodynamic response

 IV. Antibiotics: blood cultures and cultures of relevant body fluids or exudates should be taken before the administration of

TABLE 26-5

THERAPEUTIC MANAGEMENT OF PROBLEMS ASSOCIATED WITH SHOCK

PROBLEM	TREATMENT	TRADE NAME	DOSAGE	SIDE EFFECTS OR CONTRAINDICATIONS
Hypovolemia				
Fluid loss	Crystalloid	Lactated Ringer's	50-100 ml/kg/hr IV	Hypervolemia, pulmonary edema, hypoproteinemia
Plasma loss	Colloid expander	6% Dextran 70 Hetastarch	10-20 ml/kg IV	Hypervolemia, pulmonary edema, allergic reactions
Blood loss	Whole blood	—	10-40 ml/kg IV	Hypervolemia, allergic reactions
	Blood substitute	Oxyglobin	150-30 mg/kg	Hypervolemia
	Hypertonic saline	7% crystalloid	3-4 mg/kg IV until effective	Adjunct to fluid therapy once hemorrhage has been controlled
Hypotension	Correct hypovolemia first			
	Dopamine	Intropin (Arnar-Stone)	3-10 μg/kg/min IV	Hypertension, tachycardia
	Dobutamine	Dobutrex (Lilly)	3-10 μg/kg/min IV	Hypertension, tachycardia

			5 mg IV	Hypertension, tachycardia
Ephedrine		Ephedrine sulfate		
Epinephrine		Adrenaline (Parke-Davis)	3-5 µg/kg IV	Hypertension, tachycardia, arrhythmias

Cardiac arrhythmias

Bradycardia	Atropine	—	0.01-0.02 mg/kg IV	Tachycardia
	Glycopyrrolate	Robinul (Robins)	0.005-0.01 mg/kg IV	Tachycardia
Tachycardia	Digoxin	Lanoxin (Burroughs-Wellcome)	0.01-0.02 mg/kg IV slowly	Bradycardia, cardiac arrhythmias
	Propranolol	Inderal (Ayerst)	0.05-0.01 mg/kg IV	Bradycardia, cardiac failure
	Esmolol	Brevibloc	10-50 µg/kg/min IV	Bradycardia, hypotension
Atrial arrhythmias	Quinidine	Quinidine gluconate (Lilly)	4-8 mg/kg/10 min IV	Hypotension
Ventricular arrhythmias	Lidocaine	Xylocaine (Astra)	2-4 mg/kg IV	CNS excitement
	Procainamide	Pronestyl (Squibb)	4-8 mg/kg/5 min IV	Hypotension

Continued

TABLE 26-5

THERAPEUTIC MANAGEMENT OF PROBLEMS ASSOCIATED WITH SHOCK—cont'd

PROBLEM	TREATMENT	TRADE NAME	DOSAGE	SIDE EFFECTS OR CONTRAINDICATIONS
Acute heart failure				
	Dopamine	Intropin (Amar-Stone)	3-10 µg/kg/min IV	Hypertension, tachycardia, cardiac arrhythmias
	Dobutamine	Dobutrex (Lilly)	3-10 µg/kg/min IV	
	Epinephrine	Adrenaline (Parke-Davis)	3-5 µg/kg IV	
Respiratory failure				
Hypoxia	O$_2$, nasal catheter; oxygen cage		2-4 L/min	Decreased venous return, respiratory alkalosis
Hypercarbia	Doxapram	Dopram V (Robins)	1-2 mg/kg	CNS excitement
	Ventilation		V$_T$ = 14 ml/kg	Decreased venous return, respiratory alkalosis
Dyspnea	Tracheostomy			
	Chest tubes	Heimlich valve		
	Ventilation		V$_T$ = 14 ml/kg	Decreased venous return, respiratory alkalosis
Sepsis	Surgery			
	Gentamicin	Gentocin (Schering)	4 mg/kg qid IM	Muscle weakness, renal toxicity

Metabolic acidosis			
	Sodium lactate*	Bicarbonate dose = Base deficit × 0.3 × wt (kg) or 0.5 mEq/kg/10min IV, give to effect	Metabolic alkalosis, hyperosmolarity, CSF acidosis, hyperkalemia, hypocalcemia
	Sodium acetate*		
	Sodium bicarbonate		
Hyperkalemia	Sodium bicarbonate	0.5-1 mg/kg IV	As above
	0.9% NaCl solution	10-40 ml/kg/hr IV	Hypervolemia, hypoproteinemia
	Calcium gluconate	0.5 ml/kg of 10% solution IV	Tachycardia
	Hyperventilation	$V_T = 14$ ml/kg	Decreased venous return, respiratory alkalosis
Hypoglycemia	50% dextrose	1-2 ml/kg IV	Hyperosmolarity
		0.5-1 g/kg/hr 10% glucose	
Renal ischemia	Fluids		
	Lactated Ringer's	10-40 ml/kg/hr IV	Hypervolemia, hypoproteinemia, pulmonary edema
	Mannitol (20%) (Osmitrol (Travenol))	0.5-2 mg/kg IV	Hyperosmolality
	Furosemide (Lasix (National))	1-2 mg/kg IM, IV	Decreased cardiac output

Continued

*Questionable efficacy during severe low-flow states.

TABLE 26-5

THERAPEUTIC MANAGEMENT OF PROBLEMS ASSOCIATED WITH SHOCK—cont'd

PROBLEM	TREATMENT	TRADE NAME	DOSAGE	SIDE EFFECTS OR CONTRAINDICATIONS
Hypothermia	Fluids	Lactated Ringer's	10-40 ml/kg/hr warmed to 37° C	Hypervolemia, hypoproteinemia, pulmonary edema
	H₂O-filled heating pad		Warmed slowly to 38° C	
Disseminated intravascular coagulation	Correct hypotension Correct hypoxemia	Lactated Ringer's Nasal catheter Ventilation	10-40 mg/kg/hr IV 2-4 L/min V_T = 14 ml/kg	Hypervolemia, hypoproteinemia, pulmonary edema Decreased venous return, respiratory alkalosis
	Correct acidosis	Sodium bicarbonate	0.5-1 mg/kg IV	
	Heparin		Dog: 500 U/kg tid SQ Cat: 250-400 U/kg tid SQ	Bleeding
Cellular ischemia	Fluids	Lactated Ringer's	10-40 ml/kg/hr IV	Hypervolemia, hypoproteinemia, pulmonary edema
	Oxygen Dexamethasone sodium phosphate	Nasal catheter Azium SP (Schering)	2-4 L/min 4-6 mg/kg IV	
	Prednisolone sodium succinate	Solu-Delta-Cortef (Upjohn)	>10 mg/kg	

IV, Intravenously; *CNS,* central nervous system; *IM,* intramuscularly; *CSF,* cerebrospinal fluid; *SQ,* subcutaneously.

TABLE 26-6
ANTIBIOTICS USED TO TREAT SEVERE BACTERIAL INFECTIONS

DRUG	IV DOSAGE
Gentamicin	6 mg/kg/24 hr
Amikacin	10 mg/kg/8 hr
Tobramycin	2-4 mg/kg/8 hr
Ampicillin	20-40 mg/kg/8 hr
Clindamycin	11 mg/kg/8 hr
Metronidazole	10 mg/kg/8 hr
Cefazolin	20 mg/kg/8 hr

antimicrobial therapy, but they do not usually provide substantial information (Table 26-6)

V. Surgical intervention: many patients with shock may have an abscess or other local situation that requires surgical drainage and excision; immediate surgical intervention is of paramount importance; the patient will continue to deteriorate unless surgical intervention is undertaken

VI. Nutritional support should be considered for chronically debilitated patients and those that do not respond well to initial therapies (Table 26-7)

SUGGESTED READINGS

Muir WW, Bonagura J: Cardiovascular emergencies. In Sherding RG, editor: *Medical emergencies,* New York, 1985, Churchill Livingstone, 1985, pp. 37-94.

Muir WW, DiBartola SP: Fluid therapy. In Kirk RW, editor: *Current veterinary therapy,* Philadelphia, 1983, WB Saunders, pp. 28-40.

Geller ER: *Shock and resuscitation,* St Louis, 1993, McGraw-Hill, pp. 1-580.

Muir WW: Shock, *The Compendium* 20(5):549-567, 1998.

TABLE 26-7

ENTERAL FEEDING ALTERNATIVES FOR PATIENTS WITH SEPSIS

SPECIES	CONDITION	PROTEIN REQUIREMENT (g/100 kcal)	EXAMPLE DIETS	CALORIES (kcal/ml)	PROTEIN (g/100 kcal)
Dog	Normal protein	4.0-8.0	312 g Prescription Diet a/d* + 50 ml water	1.0	9
			CliniCare Canine†	0.9	5.5
	Protein loss	>8.0	312 g Prescription Diet a/d* + 50 ml water	1.0	9
			237 ml Sustacal‡ + 24 g ProBalance Max Stress Feline§	1.2	8.8
Cat	Normal protein	6.0-9.0	Blenderized 224 g Prescription Diet Feline p/d* + 170 ml water	0.9	9.3
			50 ml Sustacal‡ + 50 ml Pulmocare§ + 4.8 g ProBalance Max Stress Feline§	1.3	6.4
	Protein loss	>9.0	312 g Prescription Diet a/d* + 50 ml water	1.0	9
			237 ml Sustacal ‡ + 24 g ProBalance Max Stress Feline§	1.2	8.8

Choose a diet that meets the protein requirement of the animal.
Calculate the volume of diet required: (kcal/day)/(kcal/ml) = ml of formula/day.
Calculate the volume of each feeding: (ml of formula/day)/(number of feedings/day).
*Hills Pet Nutrition, Inc., Topeka, Kansas.
†PetAg, Hampshire, Ill.
‡Bristol-Meyers Squibb, Princeton, N.J.
§Pfizer Animal Health, Exton, Penn.

CHAPTER TWENTY-SEVEN

Respiratory Emergencies

"Each person is born to one possession which out values all
his others—his last breath."

MARK TWAIN

OVERVIEW

Respiratory depression occurs during almost all chemical restraint
and anesthesia. Respiratory depression leads to hypoventilation
($\uparrow$PaO$_2$), hypoxemia ($\downarrow$PaO$_2$), and respiratory emergencies. Hypoventilation cannot always be determined by visual inspection but
can be assessed by arterial blood gas analysis or capnography. Although potentially devastating, respiratory depression, if recognized
early, is easily treated by establishing a patent airway and providing
adequate inflation of the lungs to ensure appropriate gas exchange.

GENERAL CONSIDERATIONS

I. Definition: a respiratory emergency is the inability to maintain
adequate ventilation (PaCO$_2$) and normal blood gas (PaO$_2$,
PaCO$_2$) values

II. Clinical causes

   A. Major causes

   1. Hypoventilation caused by drug-induced respiratory depression
   2. Improper placement (e.g., esophageal) of the endotracheal tube
   3. Parenchymal pulmonary disease (diffusion impairment)
   4. Pleural cavity disease
   5. Airway obstruction
      a. Laryngeal spasm with intubation
      b. Small or plugged endotracheal tubes

      c. Improper physical restraint or positioning for surgery

      d. Nasal obstruction or edema

         (1) Oxygen flow turned off on anesthetic machine

         (2) Low inspired O_2 (FIO_2)

    6. Low inspired O_2 (FIO_2)

      a. Oxygen flow turned off on anesthetic machine

III. Patient age and size determine respiratory frequency, rate of lung inflation, inflation pressure, and tidal volume delivered; large adult patients generally require slower inflation rates, lower frequencies of breathing, and larger volumes

    A. Pneumothoraces should be corrected immediately to ensure adequate lung expansion and prevent tension pneumothorax

    B. Intrathoracic air or fluid should be removed

IV. Signs of respiratory difficulty or emergency

    A. Lack of respiration (apnea)

    B. Increased respiratory frequency using the accessory muscles of respiration (particularly the abdominal muscles)

      1. Open mouth breathing

    C. Cyanosis

    D. Change in mentation

      1. Agitation

      2. Loss of consciousness

 V. Support of ventilation (assisted or controlled ventilation) should be continued until the patient can maintain consciousness, normal mucous membrane color, and normal blood gases

CLINICAL SIGNS OF RESPIRATORY DISTRESS

    I. Apnea or dyspnea

   II. Respiratory rate, depth, and effort are generally increased in animals with respiratory disease

  III. Stridor or sonorous breathing sounds are associated with airway obstruction

  IV. Cyanosis: bluish discoloration of the mucous membranes

    A. Cyanosis may be absent in severely anemic animals (Hb less than 5 g/dl)

   V. Abnormal upper airway and lung sounds (wheezes, crackles)

  VI. Deformities of the head, neck, and thorax

VII. Abnormal positions
   A. Open mouth breathing
   B. Extension of the head and neck
   C. Abduction of the forelimbs

TREATMENT OF RESPIRATORY DISTRESS

   I. Treat the primary cause
  II. Control or assist breathing when necessary
   A. Use a volume-cycled ventilator with a standing bellows (see Chapter 15)
 III. Use respiratory stimulants when necessary
   A. Doxapram: 0.05 to 0.2 mg/lb intravenously (IV); repeat if necessary; or 5 to 10 μg/kg/min IV infusion

AIRWAY OBSTRUCTION

   I. Partial airway obstruction may be associated with respiratory disease or endotracheal intubation
  II. Anatomic conformations that predispose animals to airway collapse
   A. Stenotic nares in brachycephalic breeds
   B. Edema of the nasal turbinates in horses
   C. Elongated or displaced soft palate
      1. Brachycephalic breeds
      2. Beagles and cocker spaniels
      3. Horses
   D. Collapsing arytenoid cartilages
      1. Congenital in Bouvier des Flandres, bull terriers, and Siberian huskies
      2. Acquired in giant-breed dogs (e.g., St. Bernards)
   E. Everting laryngeal ventricles
      1. Brachycephalic breeds
      2. English bulldogs
      3. May be associated with hypothyroidism
   F. Collapsing trachea
      1. Middle-aged to older, obese toy-breed dogs, especially miniature Poodles, Yorkshire terriers, and Chihuahuas
      2. Calves

    G. Laryngeal paralysis
        1. Congenital, especially in Bouvier des Flandres, bull terriers, and Siberian huskies
        2. Acquired in giant-breed dogs, especially St. Bernards
        3. Hemiplegia or postsurgical paralysis in horses
    H. Hypoplasia of the trachea
        1. Congenital in brachycephalic breeds
        2. English bulldog
III. Other causes of airway obstruction
    A. Foreign bodies
    B. Nasal disease (e.g., tumor, fungal)
    C. Mucus or blood
    D. Other causes
        1. Cat: asthma
        2. Horse: nasal edema, displaced soft palate, guttural pouch infections or tympany, ethmoidal hematoma, tumors
        3. Sheep: nasal parasites
        4. Pig: atrophic rhinitis
        5. Llamas, alpacas: congenital choanal atresia
    E. Clinical signs
        1. Noisy, stridorous, or labored breathing (snoring)
           a. Loudest at larynx and pharynx during upper airway obstruction
           b. Low-pitched honking sound during tracheal collapse
        2. History of exercise intolerance, cyanosis, and/or collapse
        3. Choking, retching, and vomiting
        4. Severely distressed animals may paw or claw at the face and throat
        5. Abnormal body positions
        6. Diagnosis (consider establishing a patent airway before attempting a diagnosis)
        7. History of facial injuries, epistaxis, or wounds to the neck
        8. The presence of stenotic nares, foreign bodies or tumors, and soft tissue swelling
        9. Radiography
           a. Survey
           b. Contrast

      c. Fluoroscopy

      d. Bronchoscopy or endoscopy to confirm airway obstruction

  F. Electromyography to confirm denervation of laryngeal muscles

IV. Treatment

  A. Establish patent airway

    1. Intubate

    2. Remove oral, nasal, or tracheal foreign material or blood using forceps, suction, and postural drainage

    3. Perform nasotracheal intubation or tracheotomy, if necessary, to relieve or bypass obstruction (Fig. 27-1)

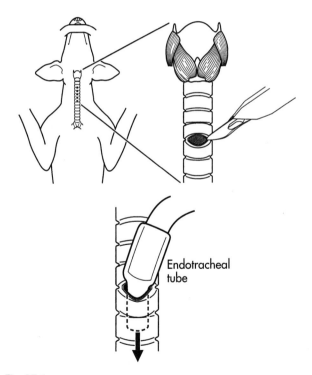

Endotracheal tube

Fig. 27-1
A tracheotomy can be easily performed in most species.

      4. Apply local anesthetic creams (lidocaine) to prevent laryngospasm
- B. Provide oxygen
- C. Avoid stress
- D. If the animal is apneic, institute artificial ventilation with air or oxygen; oxygen is preferable
  1. Mouth-to-mouth
  2. Mouth-to-nose
  3. Nasal intubation with oxygen administration
  4. Face mask and oxygen
  5. Deliver oxygen to endotracheal or tracheotomy tube
- E. Control breathing rate if apneic; assist ventilation if breathing
  1. Rate: 6 to 15 breaths per minute
  2. Inspiratory time: 1 to 3 seconds, depending on size of the patient
  3. Maintain proper inspiratory/expiratory ratio of 1:2, 1:3, or 1:4
  4. Inflate lungs to 15 to 20 cm water if chest is closed (up to 30 to 40 cm water in large animals)
  5. Inflate lungs to 20 to 30 cm water if chest is open or atelectasis of lungs has occurred (up to 40 cm water in large animals)
  6. Tidal volume
     a. Approximately 5 to 7 ml/lb
     b. 7 to 10 ml/lb if mechanical ventilator is used
- F. Supportive care
  1. Oxygen
  2. Intravenous fluid therapy
  3. Bronchodilators
  4. Respiratory stimulants, if necessary
  5. Sedation
  6. Antibiotics
  7. Corticosteroids
  8. Maintain normal body temperature
- G. Treat coexisting problems; prepare for surgery
  1. Remove foreign bodies or tumors
  2. Repair fractures and wounds of the respiratory system
  3. Drain chest
  4. Correct anatomic defects when necessary

H. Care of tracheotomy tube
   1. Apply suction every 2 hours using aseptic technique
   2. Nebulize with saline or acetylcysteine diluted with saline
   3. Maintain normal hydration
   4. Monitor body temperature
   5. Take periodic chest radiographs

PARENCHYMAL EXCHANGE DISEASES

I. Classification
   A. Life-threatening pneumonia
      1. Acute, fulminating bronchopneumonia
      2. Smoke inhalation
      3. Aspiration pneumonia
   B. Pulmonary contusion
   C. Pulmonary edema
II. Diagnosis
   A. Physical signs, including lethargy
   B. Radiographs of the chest
   C. Laboratory tests
      1. Complete blood count
      2. Transtracheal aspirate
      3. Bronchoscopy
      4. Blood gas determination
III. Treatment
   A. Remove aspirated material, if present
   B. Maintain the patency and function of the airways
   C. Apply positive end-expiratory pressure
   D. Treat infection
   E. Enhance removal of secretions (suction, acetylcysteine, guaifenesin)
   F. Supportive care
      1. Administer oxygen (40% or more) using the following methods:
         a. Face mask
         b. Nasal catheter
         c. Pediatric incubator
         d. Oxygen cage

      e. Tracheotomy and positive-pressure ventilation (if laryngeal spasm or airway obstruction with secretions persist)

2. Humidify the air by nebulization with normal saline to improve removal of secretions
3. Maintain normal body hydration with fluids intravenously or subcutaneously (SQ) to prevent drying and thickening of secretions
4. Perform periodic coupage (percussion of the chest)
5. Provide physiotherapy with deep breathing; this aids in removal of secretions, increases lymphatic drainage of the lungs, and activates surfactant
6. The use of diuretics, corticosteroids, and antiprostaglandins in pneumonia is controversial
7. Bronchodilators are helpful in reversing bronchial spasm and constriction (e.g., aminophylline)
8. Pneumonia with viscous secretions may require expectorants (e.g., guaifenesin)
9. Antibiotic use should be based on culture and sensitivity results
10. Analgesics may be used for pain and apprehension in selected patients
     a. Monitor blood gases to detect respiratory depression
11. Medical therapy of pulmonary edema
     a. Confine the animal to a cage to decrease the workload of its heart; administer oxygen and sedation (low-dose opioids)
     b. Improve ventilation by endotracheal suctioning
     c. Nebulize with 40% alcohol
     d. Eliminate excessive fluids with diuretics and vasodilators

PLEURAL CAVITY DISEASE

I. Definition: pleural cavity disease includes problems that decrease the functional capacity of the lungs because of fluid, masses or inflammation in the thoracic cavity, or damage to the integrity of the thoracic wall

II. Classification
  A. Pneumothorax
    1. Open
    2. Closed
    3. Spontaneous
    4. Tension
  B. Pleural effusion
    1. Chylothorax
    2. Pyothorax
    3. Hydrothorax
    4. Hemothorax
    5. Neoplastic effusion
    6. Infectious, inflammatory effusion
  C. Diaphragmatic hernia
  D. Flail chest
III. Causes
  A. Pneumothorax: accumulation of free air in the pleural cavity
    1. Pneumothorax—occurs spontaneously in Afghan hounds (Fig. 27-2, *A*)
    2. Tension pneumothorax: air accumulates in pleural space during inspiration and is not expelled during expiration; intrapleural pressure increases, collapsing the lungs and great vessels (Fig. 27-2, *B*)
    3. Trauma, resulting in pleural or parenchymal lacerations or tracheobronchial ruptures, is the most common cause of pneumothorax
    4. Other causes
      a. Penetrating injuries from bite wounds and projectiles
      b. Rupture of congenital bullous emphysematous or granulomatous lung lesions (blebs or bullae)
      c. Rupture of parasitic cysts *(Paragonimus);* neoplasia
      d. Hardware disease in cattle
      e. Pleuritis
      f. Iatrogenic causes
        (1) Overzealous intermittent positive-pressure ventilation (particularly in cats)
        (2) Following pneumomediastinum from trauma, air migrates from the trachea or esophagus to the chest

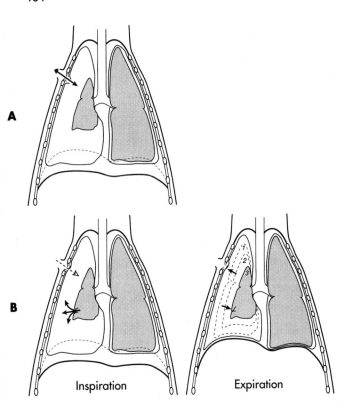

Fig. 27-2
A, Open pneumothorax. Air moves into the chest. The lung collapses due to loss of negative pressure. **B,** Tension pneumothorax. During inspiration, air moves one way into the chest, gradually increasing intrathoracic pressure and collapsing the lung. Note: since the mediastinum is incomplete in most species, the effects discussed are usually bilateral.

Inspiration   Expiration

         (3) Intrathoracic surgical procedures
         (4) Cardiopulmonary resuscitation
   B. Pleural effusion: abnormal fluid accumulation within the pleural cavity
     1. Hemothorax
       a. Rupture of cardiac and intrathoracic blood vessels from trauma

      b. Clotting disorders

      c. Bleeding neoplasms (e.g., hemangiosarcoma)

      d. Lung-lobe torsion

      e. Pleuritis

  2. Chylothorax

      a. Accumulation of lymphatic fluid in the pleural space

        (1) Rupture of the thoracic duct

        (2) Idiopathic lymphatic obstruction

  3. Hydrothorax

      a. Hypoproteinemia

      b. Heart failure and cardiomyopathy

  4. Pyothorax (pleuritis)

      a. Penetrating wounds of the thorax or esophagus

      b. Migrating foreign bodies

      c. Spread of pulmonary infection and pleuritis

      d. Organisms: *Escherichia coli, Staphylococcus,* β-*streptococcus, Pasteurella, Nocardia*

C. Chest wall abnormalities

      a. Diaphragmatic hernias displace the lungs with abdominal viscera

      b. Flail chest is caused by proximal and distal fractures of several consecutive ribs

        (1) Chest wall is drawn inward with inspiration and blown outward with inspiration (paradoxic movement [see Fig. 27-2, *B*])

        (2) Lung contusion and hemopneumothorax may be present, precipitating acute respiratory distress

IV. Diagnosis

  A. Auscultation and percussion

  B. Thoracic radiography

  C. Ultrasound examination

  D. Thoracocentesis

V. Treatment

  A. Establish a patent airway

  B. Oxygen therapy

  C. Shock therapy (fluids)

  D. Bandage penetrating wounds, flail chest

  E. Assess animal's status

F. Remove the cause
1. Needle aspiration (air or liquid)
2. Tube thoracostomy (Fig. 27-3)
   a. Indications
      (1) Acute severe pneumothorax
      (2) Tension pneumothorax
      (3) Pneumothorax associated with rib fractures, emphysema, or hemothorax
      (4) Fluid accumulation
      (5) In situations where repeated needle evacuations are necessary
   b. Methods of drainage
      (1) Intermittent aspiration using a syringe and three-way stopcock

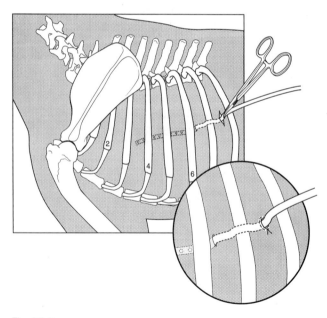

Fig. 27-3
A chest tube is placed to restore negative intrathoracic pressure by connecting it to a Heimlich valve (see Fig. 27-4) or a three-bottle negative pressure system (see Fig. 27-5).

      (2) Unidirectional flutter (Heimlich) valves (Fig. 27-4)

      (3) Intermittent connection of the chest tube to a suction pump (10 to 15 cm water negative pressure)

      (4) Connection of the chest tube to underwater seal units (Fig. 27-5)

         (a) Commercially available thoracic drainage units

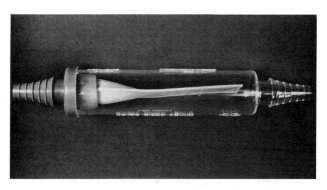

Fig. 27-4
Heimlich (one-way) valve.

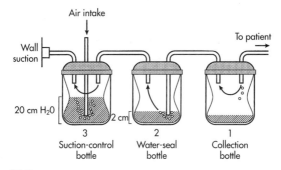

Fig. 27-5
Underwater seal system (three-bottle) for connection to a chest tube and creating negative intrathoracic pressure.

       (b) One-bottle system

       (c) Two-bottle system

       (d) Three-bottle system (Fig. 27-5)

  3. Complications

    a. Chest tube attaches to an underwater seal and requires constant monitoring (disconnection causes pneumothorax)

    b. Accumulation of fibrin and blood

    c. Displacement of tube

    d. Kinking of tube

    e. Subcutaneous emphysema

    f. Lung tissue entrapment and infarction after vigorous suction

    g. Infection

IATROGENIC CAUSES OF RESPIRATORY EMERGENCIES

  I. Inadequate patient evaluation

  II. Faulty anesthetic techniques

    A. Anesthetic overdose (e.g., barbiturates)

    B. Excessive dead space in anesthetic equipment

    C. Lack of oxygen delivery

      1. Nitrous oxide on; oxygen off

      2. Excessive use of N_2O (more than 70%)

      3. Oxygen supply depleted

      4. Anesthetic system not connected properly

      5. Endotracheal tube too small

      6. Overdistended endotracheal tube cuff

        a. Collapse of tracheal tube within cuff

        b. Postsurgical stenosis of trachea

      7. Inappropriately placed endotracheal tube

        a. In esophagus

        b. In pharynx

        c. At or caudal to bifurcation of trachea

    D. Kinked or obstructed anesthetic delivery hoses and tubes

    E. Overdistention of lungs during mechanical ventilation

    F. Neuromuscular paralysis of diaphragm and intercostal muscles without ventilatory support

III. Restrictive bandages

IV. Inadequate monitoring of the patient

    A. Patterns of respiration

        1. Eupnea: normal rate and rhythm

        2. Tachypnea: increased respiratory rate; caused by fever, hypoxia, hypercapnea, pneumonia, or lesions of the central nervous system (CNS) respiratory centers

        3. Bradypnea: slow but regular respirations; caused by sleep, anesthesia, opiates, hypothermia, neoplasia, or respiratory decompensation

        4. Apnea: absence of respiration; may be periodic; caused by drug depression, muscle paralysis, overventilation, obstruction, shock, increased cerebral blood pressure (BP), or surgical manipulation of vagus and splanchnic nerves

        5. Hyperpnea: large respirations (increased tidal volume); rate normal; caused by excitement, pain, surgical stimulation, hypoxia, hypercarbia, heat, or cold

        6. Cheyne-Stokes respiration: respirations become faster and larger, then slower, followed by an apneic pause; caused by increased intracranial pressure from head trauma or neoplasia, meningitis, renal failure, severe hypoxia, anesthetic drug overdose, or high altitude

        7. Biot's respiration: respirations that are faster and deeper than normal, with abrupt pauses between them; each breath has approximately the same tidal volume; caused by anesthesia in normal, athletic horses and greyhounds; spinal meningitis; or drugs that cause generalized CNS depression

        8. Kussmaul's respiration: regular and deep respirations without pauses; patient's breathing usually sounds labored, with breaths that resemble sighs; caused by renal failure, metabolic acidosis, or diabetic ketoacidosis

        9. Apneustic: prolonged gasping inspiration, followed by extremely short, inefficient expirations; caused by high doses of drugs (e.g., ketamine in cats and horses or excessive doses of guaifenesin in horses) or lesions in the pons and thalamus

OTHER CAUSES OF PULMONARY INSUFFICIENCY

I. Ventilation-perfusion inequalities
  A. Hypoventilation
  B. Decreased cardiac output
  C. Atelectasis
    1. Absorption: absorption of oxygen from behind blocked small airways
    2. Compression: compression of lungs by distended abdominal viscera pressing against the diaphragm (colic in horses; rumen in cattle, sheep, and goats; bloat in dogs)
    3. Gravitational effects
II. Increased venous admixture (shunts)
  A. Pulmonary arteriovenous shunts
  B. Bronchial vessel shunts
  C. Atelectasis (physiologic shunt)
  D. Pulmonary neoplasia

RESPIRATORY ARREST

  I. Cessation of breathing from any of the previously discussed causes
  II. Correct immediately (within 1 to 3 minutes)
  III. Treatment
    A. Establish a patent airway
      1. Remove the obstruction or foreign material
      2. Intubate
      3. Consider a tracheostomy if unable to orotracheally intubate (see Fig. 27-1)
    B. Provide artificial ventilation
      1. Room air delivered through Ambu-bag (Fig. 27-6)
      2. 100% oxygen delivered through anesthetic system
      3. Transtracheal insufflation of O_2; 3 to 6 L/min in dogs
    C. Proceed with cardiopulmonary resuscitation, if necessary (see Chapter 28)
    D. Acupuncture resuscitative techniques have been used successfully in emergency situations
      1. Use 25- to 28-gauge hypodermic needle, 25 to 50 mm long

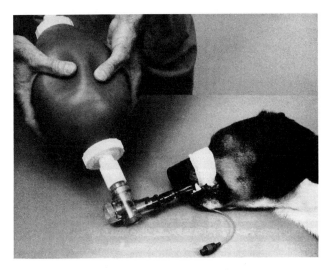

Fig. 27-6
Ventilation with an Ambu-Bag.

2. Insert the needle 10 to 20 mm into the nasal septum at point GV 26, along the midline of the nasolabial cleft at the left of the lower canthi of the nostril
3. Twirl the needle strongly and move it up and down
4. Use this technique as an adjunct to, but not a replacement for, conventional techniques

PREVENTION OF RESPIRATORY EMERGENCIES

I. Proper preanesthetic evaluation
  A. Clinical signs
  B. Auscultation
  C. Radiography
  D. Blood gas analysis (i-Stat; IRMA)
II. Use of proper anesthetic and monitoring equipment (see Chapter 16)
III. Adequate inspection of anesthetic equipment

  IV. Proper administration of preanesthetic and anesthetic agents
   V. Careful and continuous monitoring during anesthesia
 VI. Awareness of possible problems

USE OF ANALEPTICS, BICARBONATE, AND BRONCHODILATOR DRUGS

   I. Doxapram hydrochloride (0.5 to 0.2 mg/lb in small animals; 0.1 to 0.3 mg/lb IV in large animals) is a general CNS and respiratory center stimulant and can be administered by infusion (5 to 10 μg/kg/min) until effective; a centrally acting respiratory stimulant; increases tidal volume and, in larger doses, respiratory rate; causes small elevations in arterial BP and heart rate and may cause arousal from anesthetic depression

  II. Sodium bicarbonate (0.5 to 2 mEq/lb); used to correct metabolic (nonrespiratory) acidosis, which may occur during hypoxia, or complete respiratory and cardiac arrest; excessive administration may produce hypokalemic metabolic alkalosis or paradoxic cerebrospinal fluid acidosis

 III. Aminophylline: up to 2 mg/lb IV slowly over 30 minutes, 1 to 2 mg/lb IM; dilates bronchial smooth muscle and may be useful in asthmatics and bronchospasm; has inotropic action on the heart

 IV. Specific antagonists (see Chapter 3)
    A. Narcotic antagonists (naloxone, nalorphine, levallorphan); Nalline (nalorphine): 1 mg/5 lb; acts by competitively displacing narcotic analgesics from opiate and nonopiate receptors
    B. Neostigmine, edrophonium: reversal of nondepolarizing neuromuscular blocking drugs (see Chapter 12)
    C. α_2-antagonists (yohimbine, tolazoline, atipamazole); reversal of xylazine, medetomidine, or detomidine (see Chapter 3)

TREATMENT OF PULMONARY EDEMA

   I. Measures to improve ventilation-gas exchange
    A. Reduction of activity (cage rest): to decrease oxygen demand

    B. Sedation, relief of anxiety
       1. Morphine (dogs): 0.2 to 0.5 mg/kg SC, IM, IV
       2. Acepromazine: 0.1 to 0.2 mg/kg SC, IM (maximum of 4 mg)
       3. Xylazine (horses): 0.1 mg/lb IV, IM
    C. Oxygen therapy (40% to 50%)
    D. Endotracheal suctioning in severe cases to clear foam from airways
    E. Ethyl alcohol nebulization (40%) into O_2 (prevents foaming in airways)
    F. Positive-pressure ventilation through an endotracheal tube
       1. Manual or mechanical
          a. Criteria for ventilation: PaO_2 less than 60 mm Hg, $PaCO_2$ more than 50 mm Hg, persistent cyanosis, dyspnea, or tachypnea (all while breathing 60% O_2)
       2. Use only as a last resort when life-threatening respiratory failure persists despite other measures
       3. Positive end-expiratory pressure (PEEP), 5 to 10 cm water, is used to ventilate stiff lungs (e.g., pulmonary edema, pneumonia)
II. Measures to reduce capillary hydrostatic pressure and pulmonary fluid accumulation
    A. Decrease circulating blood volume
       1. Diuretics: furosemide 2 to 4 mg/kg IV, IM, SC, PO q6 to 8h
       2. Phlebotomy: remove 6 to 10 ml/kg; rarely used
    B. Redistribute pulmonary blood flow to other circulatory beds
       1. Morphine; in addition to sedative effects, increases systemic venous capacitance
       2. Furosemide (Lasix); in addition to diuresis, redistributes pulmonary blood flow by increasing systemic venous capacitance
       3. Vasodilators
          a. Sodium nitroprusside, nitroglycerine
          b. Peripheral vasodilation redistributes circulation away from pulmonary beds (noncardiogenic) and decreases resistance to left ventricular outflow (afterload; cardiogenic)

    C. Improve cardiac function (cardiac output); mostly used in cardiogenic edema
       1. Positive inotropes (dopamine, dobutamine)
       2. Antiarrhythmics to control arrhythmias, if present
III. Other therapy
    A. Corticosteroids (e.g., prednisolone sodium succinate: 10 to 15 mg/lb IV)
IV. Monitoring the response to therapy
    A. Physical examination (including rate and depth of breathing, auscultation, mucous membrane color)
    B. Sequential arterial blood gas analyses (see Chapter 16)
    C. Thoracic radiography
    D. Pulmonary capillary wedge pressure

CHAPTER TWENTY-EIGHT

Cardiac Emergencies

"It is by presence of mind in untried emergencies that the native metal of a man is tested."

JAMES RUSSELL LOWELL

OVERVIEW

Bradycardia, hypotension, and decreased peripheral perfusion leading to shock can occur following the administration of chemical restraining drugs and anesthetics. The potential for these emergencies is increased in severely debilitated or traumatized patients. A variety of physical and pharmacologic approaches have been developed to prevent further deterioration of the circulation or to reestablish normal hemodynamics. Because it is difficult to perform external or internal cardiac massage in animals weighing more than 400 pounds, one should have a working knowledge of the various pharmacologic approaches to cardiopulmonary resuscitation. Generally, most therapeutic responses to acute cardiovascular crises must be followed by continued care and close patient monitoring.

GENERAL CONSIDERATIONS

I. Definition: a cardiac emergency is any condition involving the heart that results in the inability to maintain an adequate cardiac output

II. Common causes
   A. Respiratory failure (hypoxia)
      1. Hypoventilation
      2. Low inspired PO_2
      3. Ventilation-perfusion abnormalities
      4. Shunt
      5. Diffusion abnormalities

  B. Acid-base imbalance
      1. Respiratory acidosis
      2. Metabolic acidosis leading to myocardial depression
      3. Respiratory alkalosis
      4. Metabolic alkalosis leading to myocardial irritability
      5. Mixed metabolic and respiratory alkalosis or acidosis
  C. Electrolyte imbalance
      1. Hyperkalemia (bradycardia; poor contractility, vasodilation)
      2. Hypokalemia (tachycardia)
      3. Hypocalcemia (hypocontractility, hypotension)
  D. Autonomic imbalance
      1. Increased sympathetic tone; increased myocardial automaticity and irritability
      2. Increased parasympathetic tone; predisposition to bradycardia and various forms of heart block; predisposition to atrial arrhythmias, including atrial fibrillation
  E. Hypothermia
  F. Air embolism
  G. Toxicity
      1. Myocardial depressant factors produced by ischemic organs (e.g., pancreas)
      2. Any hypersensitivity or drug overdose such as a hypotensive crisis secondary to drug administration
          a. Most commonly observed after intravenous drug administration
          b. Treatment includes fluids, steroids, and occasionally vasopressors
  H. Excessive or inappropriate drug administration
      1. Administration of catecholamines during inhalation anesthesia with halothane (ventricular arrhythmias, tachycardia)
      2. Accidental intraarterial drug administration (e.g., accidental intracarotid administration of preanesthetic drugs [phenothiazines, xylazine] in horses and cattle); treatment should include adequate padding, anticonvulsants (diazepam), fluids, and steroids
  I. Cardiac disease and/or arrhythmias (Table 28-1)
      1. Cardiovascular collapse
          a. Cardiac failure that is unresponsive to therapy

TABLE 28-1

DISTINGUISHING CHARACTERISTICS OF SEVERAL TYPES OF CARDIAC FAILURE OR ARREST

CAUSE	PERIPHERAL PULSE	AUSCULTATION OF HEART SOUNDS	ELECTROCARDIOGRAM	VISUAL OBSERVATIONS
Bradycardia	Slow; may be irregular	Slow	Infrequent or irregular QRS complexes	Infrequent coordinated ventricular contractions
Ventricular tachycardia	Rapid, irregular Pulse deficits	Muffled; may be variable intensity	Wide QRS complexes; absence of P-QRS relationship	Disorganized, rapidly beating heart
Ventricular fibrillation	None	None	Absence of QRST complexes; fibrillation waves	Fine-to-coarse rippling of the ventricular myocardium
Ventricular asystole	None	None	Absence of QRST complexes; straight-line ECG	No cardiac movement
Electromechanical dissociation*	None	None	Normal PQRST complexes	Feeble or absent cardiac contractions

ECG, Electrocardiogram.
*Results clinically in pulseless electrical activity.

      b. Occurs primarily in patients who have chronic heart disease or are extremely toxic

2. Bradycardia
   a. Increased parasympathetic tone
   b. Hypothermia
   c. Hyperkalemia
   d. Specific medications (opioids, α_2-agonists)
   e. Conduction disease (sick sinus syndrome, atrioventricular block)
   f. Drug overdose

3. Tachycardia
   a. Increased sympathetic tone
      (1) Pain
      (2) Excitement, stress
      (3) Hypotension
      (4) Hypoxia
      (5) Hypokalemia
   b. Specific drug administration (catecholamines, atropine, ketamine)

4. Atrial or ventricular arrhythmias (atrial tachycardia, ventricular tachycardia); associated with conditions that include ischemia, hypoxia, hypotension, hypercarbia, metabolic acidosis or alkalosis, hypothermia, hypotension, surgical manipulation, anesthetic drugs, and cardiac catheterization

5. Atrial fibrillation
   a. Variable-intensity heart sounds
   b. Variable-strength pulses
   c. Irregular heart rates

6. Ventricular fibrillation
   a. Most likely to occur during hypoxia because of the instability of autonomic reflexes and the endogenous release of catecholamines
   b. May be associated with too rapid an infusion of thiobarbiturate or high initial concentrations of inhalation anesthetics
   c. May follow severe hypercarbia, hypoxia, hypovolemia, or acidosis

    7. Ventricular asystole (lack of ventricular contraction)
       a. Usually associated with anesthetic overdose
       b. Seen during shock or in toxic animals that must be anesthetized
    8. Electromechanical dissociation (EMD) and pulseless electrical activity (PEA); electrocardiogram (ECG) is present, but poor contraction produces low arterial blood pressure
       a. Hypoxia and ischemia
       b. Drug overdose

INDICATORS OF POOR CARDIAC FUNCTION

  I. Weak or absent peripheral pulses
    A. Weak cardiac apex beat
  II. Irregular pulses or heart sounds
  III. Poor perfusion; prolonged refill time (more than 2 seconds)
  IV. Cardiac arrhythmias
  V. Cyanosis (not seen in anemic patients)
  VI. Abnormal breathing pattern or apnea
  VII. Dilated pupils
  VIII. Depression or loss of consciousness
    IX. No bleeding from cut surfaces
    X. Signs of shock (see pp. 439-440) {later section on shock}

EQUIPMENT NEEDED FOR CARDIAC EMERGENCIES

I. Equipment should be readily accessible in the event of cardiovascular collapse
   A. Cuffed endotracheal tubes and stylet (for small dogs and cats)
     1. Small
     2. Medium
     3. Large
   B. Lighted laryngoscope with blades
   C. Ambu-bag, demand valve, or anesthetic machine (Fig. 28-1)
   D. Tongue depressors
   E. Syringes
     1. Five 3-ml
     2. Five 5-ml

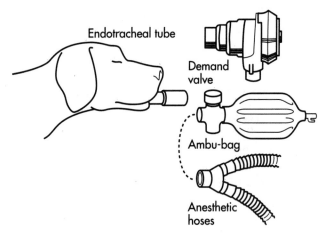

Fig. 28-1
Methods to provide breathing to an apneic animal.

      3. Five 12-ml
      4. Five 30-ml
  F. Three-way stopcock
  G. One roll of 1-inch adhesive tape
  H. One roll of 2-inch gauze
   I. One pack of sterile 4- × 4-inch gauze pads
  J. One roll of elastic bandage
  K. Blood administration set
  L. Needles
      1. Five 20-gauge
      2. Five 18-gauge
      3. Two 16-gauge
  M. Butterfly administration needles
      1. Two 21-gauge
      2. Two 19-gauge
  N. Intravenous fluid administration set
  O. Sterile emergency surgery pack
      1. Scalpel handle
      2. Blades: two No.10, two No. 15
      3. Two small hemostats
      4. Thumb forceps

  5. One pair of Metzenbaum scissors
  6. One pair of curved forceps
  7. Several packages suture of preference swaged to needles
  8. Needle holders
  9. One set of medium-sized rib retractors
 P. Intravenous catheters: 16-gauge to 22-gauge
 Q. Chest tube: Heimlich valve
 R. Defibrillator/ECG

TREATMENT (Tables 28-2, 28-3, 28-4; Fig. 28-2)

  I. Airway (see Chapter 27)
 II. Breathing (Table 28-3)
III. Circulation (Tables 28-4 and 28-5)
 IV. Drugs (Table 28-6)
  V. ECG
 VI. Defibrillation (Table 28-5)

TABLE 28-2
TREATMENT OF CARDIOPULMONARY ARREST

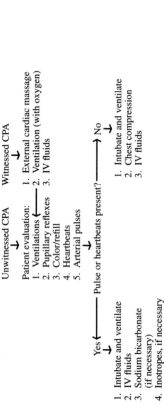

Unwitnessed CPA   Witnessed CPA

↓   ↓

Patient evaluation: 1. External cardiac massage
1. Ventilations   2. Ventilation (with oxygen)
2. Pupillary reflexes   3. IV fluids
3. Color/refill
4. Heartbeats
5. Arterial pulses

↓

Pulse or heartbeats present? ⟶ No

Yes ⟵   ↓

↓   1. Intubate and ventilate
1. Intubate and ventilate   2. Chest compression
2. IV fluids   3. IV fluids
3. Sodium bicarbonate
   (if necessary)
4. Inotropes, if necessary
5. Reevaluate

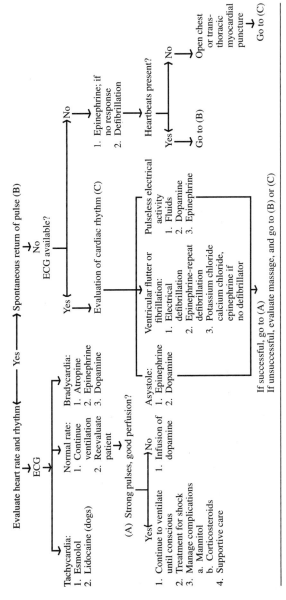

Evaluate heart rate and rhythm ← Yes → Spontaneous return of pulse (B)

↑No

ECG available?
→No

ECG

Yes →
Evaluation of cardiac rhythm (C)

Tachycardia:
1. Esmolol
2. Lidocaine (dogs)

Normal rate:
1. Continue ventilation
2. Reevaluate patient

Bradycardia:
1. Atropine
2. Epinephrine
3. Dopamine

(A) Strong pulses, good perfusion?

Yes↙   ↘No

Yes:
1. Continue to ventilate until conscious
2. Treatment for shock
3. Manage complications
   a. Mannitol
   b. Corticosteroids
4. Supportive care

No:
1. Infusion of dopamine

Ventricular flutter or fibrillation:
1. Electrical defibrillation
2. Epinephrine-repeat defibrillation
3. Potassium chloride calcium chloride, epinephrine if no defibrillator

Asystole:
1. Epinephrine
2. Dopamine

Pulseless electrical activity
1. Fluids
2. Dopamine
3. Epinephrine

If successful, go to (A)
If unsuccessful, evaluate massage, and go to (B) or (C)

→No

1. Epinephrine; if no response
2. Defibrillation

Heartbeats present?

Yes↙   ↘No

Go to (B)

Open chest or transthoracic myocardial puncture → Go to (C)

CPA, Cardiopulmonary arrest; *IV,* intravenous.

TABLE 28-3
GUIDELINES FOR VENTILATING PATIENTS

PARAMETER	GUIDELINES
Respiratory rate	6-18/min
Tidal volume	15-20 ml/kg
Inspiratory time	<1.5 sec
Inspiratory/expiratory ratio	1:2–1:3
Peak inspiratory pressure	20-25 cm H_2O
Positive-end expiratory pressure	3-5 cm H_2O
Sigh (every 5-10 min)	30 cm H_2O
Assessment of ventilatory adequacy	1. Observe chest wall excursions
	2. Monitor blood gases; preferred method (maintain $Paco_2$ at 40 mm Hg)

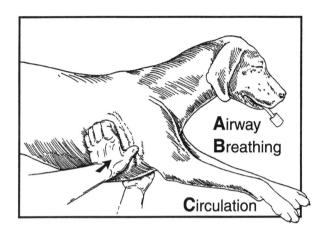

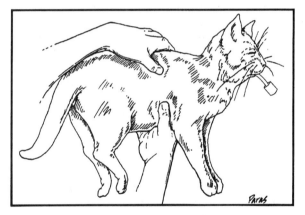

Fig. 28-2
Chest compression (approximately 100 compressions/minute) in dogs and cats.

TABLE 28-4
RECEPTOR ACTIVITY OF INOTROPIC AND VASOACTIVE AGENTS

	ALPHA$_1$	ALPHA$_2$	BETA$_1$	BETA$_2$	DOPAMINERGIC
Isoproterenol	0	0	++++	++++	0
Dobutamine	++/+++	?	++++	++	0
Dopamine	+	+	++++	++	+++
Ephedrine	+	?	++	+	
Epinephrine	++++	++++	++++	+++	0
Norepinephrine	+++	+++	+/++	+/++	0
Phenylephrine	++/+++	+	?	0	0

TABLE 28-5
TREATMENTS FOR VENTRICULAR FIBRILLATION

Direct-current defibrillators

- 0.5 to 2 Ws/kg internal
- 5 to 10 Ws/kg external
- Small patient (<7 kg)
  5 to 15 Ws internal
  50 to 100 Ws external
- Large patient (>10 kg)
  20 to 80 Ws internal
  100 to 400 Ws external

Alternating-current defibrillators

Small patient
- 30 to 50 V internal
- 50 to 100 V external

Chemical defibrillation

1 mg potassium chloride and 6 mg acetylcholine/kg followed by 1 ml/10 kg of 10% calcium chloride

Unresponsive ventricular fibrillation

- Evaluate ventilation
- Evaluate chest or cardiac compression
- Repeat epinephrine and consider calcium chloride administration
- Administer sodium bicarbonate
- Administer lidocaine
- Repeat electrical defibrillation

TABLE 28-6
ESSENTIAL DRUGS USED IN THE MANAGEMENT OF CARDIOPULMONARY ARREST

GENERIC NAME	TRADE NAME	BENEFICIAL EFFECTS (RECOMMENDED USE)	ADVERSE OR SIDE EFFECTS	DOSE AND ROUTE OF ADMINISTRATION
Vasoactive and cardiostimulatory agents				
Epinephrine HCl	Adrenaline	Positive inotrope; initiates heartbeats; increases heart rate and cardiac output; initially increases, then decreases mean arterial blood pressure and coronary blood flow	Intense vasoconstriction of renal and splanchnic vasculature; causes decreased perfusion of these tissues; increases myocardial oxygen consumption and cardiac work; arrhythmogenic; may cause ventricular fibrillation	6-10 µg/kg IC 10-30 µg/kg IV 0.1-0.2 ml/20 kg, small animals 1-3 ml/450 kg, large animals
Dopamine HCl	Inotropin	Positive inotrope; increases heart rate, cardiac output, and mean arterial blood pressure; improves blood flow to coronary, renal, and mesenteric circulation	May produce severe tachycardia if given rapidly; arrhythmogenic; vasoconstriction at higher doses	Give to effect, add 6 mg to 250 ml 5% dextrose; drip slowly at rate of 2-10 µg/kg/min

Dobutamine HCl	Dobutrex	Positive inotrope; has lower chronotropic and vasopressor effect than dopamine	Tachyarrhythmias, vasoconstriction, and arrhythmias at higher dosages	Give to effect, 1-10 μg/kg/min
Ephedrine sulphate	Ephedrine	Vasopressor; positive inotrope, chronotrope, vasoconstrictor	Tachycardia, hypertension	5-10 μg/kg
Drugs used specifically to increase contractility				
Calcium chloride		Positive inotrope; used to treat hyperkalemia and electromechanical dissociation	May cause asystole; myocardial calcium overload; "stone" heart	0.05-1 ml/kg of the 10% solution IV, IC
Digoxin	Lanoxin	Positive inotrope; increased vagal tone; used in cases of CPA caused by congestive heart failure; treat supraventricular tachycardia	Arrhythmogenic; increases oxygen consumption; causes vasoconstriction when given IV	0.01-0.02 mg/kg IV; given in four divided doses; dosed every hour give to effect; monitor ECG

Continued

IC, Intracardiac; *IV*, intravenously; *CPA*, cardiopulmonary arrest; *IM*, intramuscularly.

TABLE 28-6
ESSENTIAL DRUGS USED IN THE MANAGEMENT OF CARDIOPULMONARY ARREST—cont'd

GENERIC NAME	TRADE NAME	BENEFICIAL EFFECTS (RECOMMENDED USE)	ADVERSE OR SIDE EFFECTS	DOSE AND ROUTE OF ADMINISTRATION
Drugs used to combat acidosis				
Sodium bicarbonate		Buffer acidosis; allows more effective defibrillation	Excessive administration may produce alkalosis, hyperosmolarity, paradoxical cerebrospinal fluid acidosis	1-2 mEq/kg IV, give to effect
Drugs used to treat acute cardiac arrhythmias				
Atropine sulfate		Parasympatholytic effects; may correct supraventricular bradycardia or a slow ventricular rhythm by stimulating supraventricular pacemakers	May cause excessive tachycardia; increases myocardial oxygen consumption; lowers ventricular fibrillatory threshold; may predispose to sympathetic-induced arrhythmias	0.1-0.2 mg/kg IV

Glycopyrrolate	Robinul-V	Parasympatholytic (anticholinergic); may correct supraventricular bradycardia	May cause excessive tachycardia	0.005-0.01 mg/kg IV
Esmolol	Brevebloc	β_1-adrenergic blocker; treat supraventricular and ventricular tachycardia	Hypertension, bradycardia, heart failure	10-50 µg/kg/min IV bolus dose
Propanolol HCl	Inderal	β-adrenergic blocker; antiarrhythmic; may correct supraventricular and ventricular tachycardia	Decreases contractility, an important adverse effect; may increase airway resistance	1 mg diluted in 1 ml saline; this dilution is given as 0.05-0.1 ml boluses IV give to effect
Lidocaine	Xylocaine	Ventricular antiarrhythmic	Dosage must be considerably decreased when used in cats	2-6 mg/kg dogs IV 0.5-1 mg/kg; cats IV
Diltiazem	Cardiazem	Calcium channel blocker; treat supraventricular arrhythmias	Bradycardia hypotension	1-2 mg/kg PO
Sotalol	Betapase	Ventricular arrhythmias	Hypotension, proarrhythmia	5 mg/kg IV
Acetylcholine KCl cocktail		Chemical defibrillator?	Parasympathomimetic side effects	6 mg/kg ACh + 1 mEq/kg KCl, IC

Continued

TABLE 28-6

ESSENTIAL DRUGS USED IN THE MANAGEMENT OF CARDIOPULMONARY ARREST—cont'd

GENERIC NAME	TRADE NAME	BENEFICIAL EFFECTS (RECOMMENDED USE)	ADVERSE OR SIDE EFFECTS	DOSE AND ROUTE OF ADMINISTRATION
Drugs used to stimulate ventilation				
Doxapram HCl	Dopram	Direct action on centers in the medulla	Respiratory alkalosis, hyperkalemia	1-4 mg/kg IV 10 μg/kg/min give to effect
Drugs used to combat cerebral edema				
Oxygen		Prevents vasodilation	May cause pulmonary edema with prolonged administration; may suppress ventilatory drive	2-4 L/min (small animal) 15 L/min (large animal)
Mannitol	20% Osmitrol	Osmotic diuretic; reduces cerebral edema	May overload the volume of the circulatory system, causing edema	1-2 g/kg IV
Dexamethasone	Azium	(See section on shock)		

Drugs used to combat acute pulmonary edema

Furosemide	Lasix	Potent loop diuretic promoting loss of Na^+, Cl^-, and H_2O	May cause dehydration or lead to hypokalemic metabolic alkalosis if used excessively	1-2 mg/kg IV, 2-4 mg/kg IM
Steroids				
Prednisolone sodium	Solu-Delta-Cortef	Stabilizes lysosomal membranes; induces vasodilation; regulated fluid and electrolyte homeostasis		30 mg/kg IV
Dexamethasone	Azium SP	Increases cardiac output		8 mg/kg IV
Isotonic IV fluids Lactated Ringer's 0.9% saline		Expand the blood volume; hypotension; increase tissue perfusion	May increase edema in cats with congestive heart failure; fluid administration rate generally should not exceed 90 ml/kg/min; administer at high rates initially to improve venous return	20-40 mg/kg hr until effective

Continued

TABLE 28-6
ESSENTIAL DRUGS USED IN THE MANAGEMENT OF CARDIOPULMONARY ARREST—cont'd

GENERIC NAME	TRADE NAME	BENEFICIAL EFFECTS (RECOMMENDED USE)	ADVERSE OR SIDE EFFECTS	DOSE AND ROUTE OF ADMINISTRATION
Specific drug antagonists				
Naloxone	Narcan	Narcotic antagonist	None	50 µg/kg
Neostigmine	Protigimine Stiglyn	Cholinesterase inhibitor; used to reverse nondepolarizing neuromuscular blocking agents	Cholinergic effects; a parasympatholytic must be given before drug administration (e.g., atropine, glycopyrrolate)	0.02 mg/kg
Pyridostigmine	Regonol	Cholinesterase inhibitor; used to reverse nondepolarizing neuromuscular blocking agents	Cholinergic effects; a parasympatholytic must be given before drug administration (e.g., atropine, glycopyrrolate)	0.1 mg/kg

Edrophonium	Tensilon	Cholinesterase inhibitor; used to reverse nondepolarizing neuromuscular blocking drugs	Same as neostigmine	0.2-1 m/kg IV
Yohimbine	Yobine	α_2-antagonist; used to reverse α_2-agonists	Excitement, disorientation	0.2-0.4 mg/kg IV
Tolazoline Antipamazole	Tolezine	Same as yohimbine but more selective for α_2-receptors	Excitement	2-4 mg/kg IV 0.1-0.2 mg/kg IV
Flumazenil	Mazicon	Benzodiazepine antagonist	—	0.1 mg/kg IV

CHAPTER TWENTY-NINE

Euthanasia

"Sweet is true love though given in vain, and sweet is death
that puts an end to pain."

ALFRED LORD TENNYSON

OVERVIEW

Euthanasia is a personal and emotional decision often made in the
face of incurable disease or uncontrollable pain. Almost all drugs
used for chemical restraint and anesthesia have the capability of producing death, as long as a sufficient amount of the drug is administered. Anesthetic drugs offer the advantage of producing total unconsciousness before cardiopulmonary arrest and the elimination of
brain electrical activity. This chapter does not presume to identify
what technique of anesthesia is the best but describes the various
techniques applied to produce euthanasia.

GENERAL CONSIDERATIONS

I. Euthanasia is the act of inducing painless death in animals; death
   may be defined as permanent abolition of central nervous system
   (CNS) function
   A. Euthanasia often requires the animal to be physically re-
      strained
   B. In many species, capturing and immobilizing the animal for
      euthanasia may cause a variety of aesthetically unpleasant re-
      sponses
      1. Vocalization
      2. Avoidance or aggressive behavior
      3. Immobility (the animal may be "frozen with fear")
      4. Urination and defecation

  5. Sweating, salivation
  6. Skeletal muscle tremors, spasms, or shivering
C. Selection of a method of euthanasia depends on the following factors:
  1. Species of animal
  2. Size and weight
  3. The animal's behavior
  4. Type of physical restraint necessary
  5. Owner preference
  6. Skill of personnel and risk involved
  7. Number of animals to be euthanatized
  8. Economics
  9. Facilities available
D. Tranquilizers or other depressant drugs (e.g., α_2-agonists, opioids) are recommended before the administration of euthanatizing drugs in excitable or vicious animals
E. Pain perception requires a functional cerebral cortex; an unconscious animal does not experience pain; pain-provoking stimuli in an unconscious animal may evoke a reflex motor or sympathetic response

AVAILABLE METHODS

  I. Euthanatizing agents include mechanical, chemical, electrical, and gaseous methods of producing death (Table 29-1)
 II. Euthanatizing agents produce death by three mechanisms
   A. Hypoxia; direct or indirect
   B. Depression of the CNS
   C. Physical damage or concussion of the brain
III. The most common drug used for euthanasia of dogs, cats, horses, and cattle is pentobarbital sodium, 50 mg/lb IV (100 mg/kg)

EVALUATION CRITERIA

I. Criteria for evaluation of acceptable methods of euthanasia
   A. Production of death without pain
   B. Immediate loss of consciousness, breathing, heart beat (peripheral pulse)

TABLE 29-1
METHODS FOR PRODUCING EUTHANASIA

AGENT	SITE OF ACTION	ADVANTAGES	DISADVANTAGES	GENERAL COMMENTS
Hypoxic agents				
Carbon dioxide (CO_2)	Produces CNS anesthetic effect	Unconsciousness occurs rapidly; analgesia; inexpensive	Chamber required	Acceptable
Carbon monoxide (CO)	Carbon monoxide combines with hemoglobin, preventing combination with O_2	Unconsciousness occurs rapidly; inexpensive	Motor activity persists after unconsciousness until death; hazardous to personnel	Acceptable
Nitrogen argon inhalation	Reduced partial pressure of oxygen (PaO_2)	Available, safe for personnel	Motor activity remains until death, may be distressing	Not preferred Accepted if animal is anesthetized

Direct central nervous system depression

Anesthetic gases* Methoxyflurane Enflurane Halothane Isoflurane Sevoflurane Desflurane	Direct depression of cerebral cortex; death from respiratory and cardiovascular failure	Unconsciousness; analgesia; No venipuncture Rapid	Potential pollution of environment; expensive; requires closed chamber, motor activity	Acceptable
Barbituric acid derivatives	Direct depression of cerebral cortex; respiratory and cardiovascular failure	Unconsciousness; inexpensive	Transient excitement; requires IV injection of controlled substances	Acceptable
Chloral hydrate and chloral hydrate combinations	Direct depression of cerebral cortex; respiratory and cardiovascular failure	Unconsciousness; inexpensive	Transient anxiety; requires IV injection	Acceptable for large animals Use prior sedation

Continued

Modified from AVMA Panel on Euthanasia, *J Am Vet Med Assoc* 202:229-249, 1993.

*Although effective, inhalation or gaseous agents is not only expensive but also hazardous to personnel if adequate precautions are not taken against atmospheric pollution. To avoid pollution, scavenging devices are recommended. Because of the high percentage of concentrations and high gas-flow rates of inhalation anesthetic agents necessary to produce death, their use is not recommended in large animals.

IV, Intravenous.

TABLE 29-1
METHODS FOR PRODUCING EUTHANASIA—cont'd

AGENT	SITE OF ACTION	ADVANTAGES	DISADVANTAGES	GENERAL COMMENTS
Physical or mechanical agents				
Gunshot or penetrating captive bolt	Direct concussion of brain	Inexpensive; immediate unconsciousness	Motor activity may continue after death	Acceptable under appropriate circumstances
Decapitation; cervical dislocation	Elimination of brain blood supply and central nervous system input	Inexpensive; immediate	Aesthetically unpleasant	Acceptable for rodents and some fowl
Electrocution (current through brain)	Direct depression of brain; death from hypoxia	Inexpensive; immediate unconsciousness	Violent muscle contractions	Acceptable; should be used after anesthesia
Pithing	Hypoxia due to brain damage	Inexpensive; immediate	Aesthetically unpleasant	Acceptable under appropriate circumstances

C. Restraining capabilities of the method used; ability to minimize physical and psychologic stress

D. Time required to produce loss of consciousness and death

E. Reliability

F. Safety to personnel

G. Emotional effect on observers

H. Economic considerations

I. Compatibility with histopathologic evaluation

J. Equipment or drug availability and abuse potential

UNACCEPTABLE DRUGS AND TECHNIQUES

I. Unacceptable drugs: strychnine, magnesium sulfate, and nicotine are intravenous drugs that were commonly used for euthanasia in the past; their individual use as the sole euthanatizing agent is absolutely unwarranted

   A. Strychnine produces violent muscular contractions associated with extreme pain

   B. Magnesium sulfate causes death from asphyxia

   C. Nicotine produces convulsions before death and is extremely hazardous to personnel

   D. Neuromuscular blocking drugs (e.g., succinylcholine, atracurium) cause paralysis without anesthesia

   E. Do not use drugs that exhibit the following characteristics:

      1. Do not produce unconsciousness

      2. Do not produce analgesia

      3. Have no anesthetic effect

      4. Lead to specific problems

      5. Produce death by hypoxia

II. Unacceptable techniques

   A. Exsanguination

   B. Rapid freezing

   C. Air embolism

   D. Decompression (slow to unreliable)

   E. Drowning

   F. Electrocution (stunning)

NOTE: techniques A, B, and C have been used in anesthetized animals under special circumstances

Partial Listing of Commonly Used Drugs, Anesthetic and Monitoring Equipment, and Their Manufacturers

ANTICHOLINERGICS

Atropine *(atropine)*
Elkins-Sinn, Inc.
Cherry Hill, N.J.

Robinul-V *(glycopyrrolate)*
Fort Dodge Laboratories, Inc.
Fort Dodge, Iowa

TRANQUILIZERS/SEDATIVES

Dormosedan *(detomidine)*
Pfizer Animal Health, Inc.
West Chester, Pa.

Domitor *(medetomidine)*
Pfizer Animal Health, Inc.
Exton, Pa.

Prom Ace *(acepromazine maleate)*
Fort Dodge Laboratories, Inc.
Fort Dodge, Iowa

Rompun *(xylazine)*
Bayer Corporation
Shawnee, Kan.

Tranquived Injection *(xylazine)*
Vedco, Inc.
St. Joseph, Mo.

OPIOID ANALGESICS

Astramorph/PS *(preservative-free morphine sulfate)*
Astra Pharmaceuticals, Inc.
Westborough, Mass.

Buprenex *(buprenorphine)*
Reckitt & Coleman Pharmaceuticals, Inc.
Richmond, Va.

Demerol *(meperidine)*
Winthrop Pharmaceuticals
New York, N.Y.

Dolophine *(methadone)*
Roxane Laboratories, Inc.
Columbus, Ohio

Morphine
Elkins-Sinn, Inc.
Cherry Hill, N.J.

Nubain *(nalbuphine)*
DuPont Pharmaceuticals, Inc.
Wilmington, Del.

Oxymorphone
Schering Plough Animal Health
Liberty Corner, N.J.

Sublimaze *(fentanyl)*
Abbott Laboratories
North Chicago, Ill.

Sufenta *(sufentanil)*
Janssen Pharmaceutica, Inc.
Titusville, N.J.

Talwin *(pentazocine)*
Sanofi-Winthrop Pharmaceuticals
New York, N.Y.

Torbugesic *(butorphanol)*
Fort Dodge Laboratories, Inc.
Fort Dodge, Iowa

LOCAL ANESTHETICS

Carbocaine-V *(mepivacaine)*
Sterling Drug, Inc.
McPherson, Kan.

Lidocaine HCl 2%
Butler
Dublin, Ohio

Naropin *(ropivacaine)*
Astra Pharmaceuticals
Westborough, Mass.Z

Xylocaine MPF *(lidocaine)*
Astra Pharmaceuticals
Westborough, Mass.

INTRAVENOUS ANESTHETICS

Amidate *(etomidate)*
Abbott Laboratories
North Chicago, Ill.

Brevital *(methohexital)*
Jones Medical
St. Louis, Mo.

Etomidate
Bedford Laboratories
Bedford, Ohio

Ketaset/Vetalar *(ketamine)*
Fort Dodge Laboratories, Inc.
Fort Dodge, Iowa

Pentobarbital *(pentobarbital)*
Butler
Dublin, Ohio

Pentothal *(thiopental)*
Abbott Laboratories
North Chicago, Ill.

Propoflo *(propofol)*
Abbott Laboratories
North Chicago, Ill.

Rapinovet *(propofol)*
Schering Plough Animal Health
Liberty Corner, N.J.

Telazol *(tiletamine-zolazepam)*
Fort Dodge Laboratories
Fort Dodge, Iowa

INHALANT ANESTHETICS

Aerrane *(isoflurane)*
Anaquest, Inc.
Liberty Corner, N.J.

Halothane *(halothane)*
Halocarbon Laboratories
River Edge, N.J.

Isoflo *(isoflurane)*
Abbott Laboratories
North Chicago, Ill.

Metofane *(methoxyflurane)*
Abbott Laboratories
Abbott Park, Ill.

Suprane *(desflurane)*
Ohmeda Pharmaceuticals
Liberty Corner, N.J.

Ultane *(sevoflurane)*
Abbott Laboratories
North Chicago, Ill.

MUSCLE RELAXANTS
Central

Diazepam
Elkins-Sinn, Inc.
Cherry Hill, N.J.

Guaifenesin
Vedco Injection
Phoenix Scientific, Inc.
St. Joseph, Mo.

Butler guaifenesin (manufactured by
Phoenix Scientific for Butler)
Columbus, Ohio

Guailaxin (powder)
Fort Dodge Laboratories
Fort Dodge, Iowa

Valium *(diazepam)*
Roche Laboratories, Inc.
Nutley, N.J.

Versed *(midazolam)*
Roche Laboratories, Inc.
Nutley, N.J.

Peripheral

Norcuron *(vecuronium)*
Organon, Inc.
West Orange, N.J.

Pavulon *(pancuronium)*
Organon, Inc.
West Orange, N.J.

Sucostrin *(succinylcholine chloride)*
Burroughs-Welcom Co.
Research Triangle Park, N.C.

Tracrium *(atracurium)*
Abbott Laboratories
North Chicago, Ill.

ANTAGONISTS
Alpha-2

Antisedan *(atipamazole)*
Pfizer Animal Health
Exton, Pa.

Priscoline HCl *(tolazoline HCl)*
Ciba-Geigy Corp.
Ardsley, N.Y.

Yobine *(yohimbine)*
Lloyd Laboratories
Shenandoah, Iowa

Benzodiazepine

Romazicon *(flumazenil)*
Hoffman-La Roche, Inc.
Nutley, N.J.

Opioid

Revex *(nalmefene)*
Ohmeda Pharmaceuticals
Liberty Corner, N.J.

Narcan *(naloxone)*
Schering Plough Animal Health
Liberty Corner, N.J.

Peripheral Acting Muscle Relaxants

Reversol *(edrophonium)*
Organon, Inc.
West Orange, N.J.

Prostigmin *(neostigmine)*
Astra Pharmaceuticals
Westborough, Mass.

Regonol *(pyridostigmine)*
Organon, Inc.
West Orange, N.J.

RESPIRATORY STIMULANTS

Dopram-V *(doxapram)*
Fort Dodge Laboratories
Fort Dodge, Iowa

CARDIAC STIMULANTS

Calcium Chloride
Astra Pharmaceuticals
Westborough, Mass.

Calcium Gluconate
Luitpold Pharmaceuticals
Shirley, N.Y.

Dobutrex *(dobutamine)*
Gensia Laboratories, Ltd.
Irvine, Calif.

Ephedrine
UDL Laboratories, Inc.
Rockford, Ill.

Epinephrine (1:1000)
Vedco, Inc.
St. Joseph, Mo.

Inotropin *(dopamine)*
Abbott Laboratories
North Chicago, Ill.

Magnesium Chloride
American Regent
Shirley, N.Y.

Magnesium Sulfate
American Regent
Shirley, N.Y.

Procainamide
Elkins-Sinn, Inc.
Cherry Hill, N.J.

EUTHANASIA SOLUTION

Beuthanasia *(pentobarbital)*
Schering-Plough Animal Health
Kenilworth, N.J.

OTHER PRODUCTS

Azium-SP *(dexamethasone sodium phosphate)*
Steris Laboratories, Inc.
Phoenix, Ariz.

Benadryl *(diphenhydramine)*
Steris Labs, Inc.
Florham Park, N.J.

Dextrose Inj USP
Abbott Laboratories
North Chicago, Ill.

Potassium Chloride
American Reagent
Shirley, N.Y.

Lasix 5% *(furosemide)*
Hoechst Roussel
Warren, N.J.

Nitropress *(sodium nitroprusside)*
Abbott Laboratories
North Chicago, Ill.

HypoTears
CIBA Vision Ophthalmics
Atlanta, Ga.
IOLAB Corp., Johnson & Johnson Co.
Claremont, Calif.

Mannitol Inj
Abbott Laboratories
North Chicago, Ill.

Sodium Bicarbonate Inj
Vedco, Inc.
St. Joseph, Mo.
Abbott Laboratories
North Chicago, Ill.

Solu-Delta Cortef
Pharmacia & Upjohn
Kalamazoo, Mich.

EMLA Cream
Astra Pharmaceuticals, Inc.
Westborough, Mass.

ANESTHETIC AND RELATED EQUIPMENT

Allied Health Care Products, Inc.
St. Louis, Mo.

Bivona, Inc.
Gary, Ind.

Engler Engineering Corp.
Hialeah, Fla.

Hallowell EMC Engineering and Manufacturing Corp.
Pittsfield, Mass.

Henry Schein, Inc.
Florham Park, N.J.

Hudson Oxygen Therapy Sales Co.
Temecula, Calif.

Isotec: Clover Medical
Buffalo, N.Y.

Life Medical Technologies, Inc.
Houston, Tex.

Mallard Medical
Redding, Calif.

Matrix Medical, Inc.
Orchard Park, N.J.

North American Drager
Telford, Pa.

Ohio Medical Products
Division of Airco, Inc.
Madison, Wis.

Parts Medical Electronics, Inc.
Aloha, Ore.

Spectrum Anesthesia Services
Louisville, Ky.

SurgiVet, Inc.
Waukesha, Wis.

Timeter Instrument Corp.
St. Louis, Mo.

ANESTHETIC MONITORING AND RELATED EQUIPMENT
Anesthetic Agent Monitoring

Biochem
Model 8100
Waukesha, Wis.

Handheld Electrocardiogram Monitors

Heska
Vet/ECG 2000
Ft. Collins, Colo.

Micromedical Industries, Inc.
Biolog
Northbrook, Ill.

Technology Transfer, Inc.
PAM Cardiac Monitor
Lafayette, Ind.

Blood Pressure/Electrocardiogram Monitors

Cormetrics
Wallingford, Conn.

Datascope Corp.
Paramus, N.J.

Gould, Inc.
Dayton, Ohio

Hewlett Packard
McMinnville, Ore.

Space Labs Medical
Redmond, Va.

Indirect Blood Pressure Monitors

Critikon, Inc.
Tampa, Fla.

Heska
Ft. Collins, Colo.

Nellcor, Inc.
Pleasanton, Calif.

Parks Medical Equipment, Inc.
Aloha, Ore.

Pulse Oximetry

Heska
Ft. Collins, Colo.

Nellcor, Inc.
Pleasanton, Calif.

Nonin Medical, Inc.
Minneapolis, Minn.

Palco Labs, Inc.
Santa Cruz, Calif.

SurgiVet, Inc.
Waukesha, Wis.

Respiratory Monitors

Spencer Instruments
Irvine, Calif.

Syringe/Fluid Infusion Pumps

Autosyringe, Inc.
Hooksett, N.H.

Heska
Ft. Collins, Colo.

Medex, Inc.
Duluth, Ga.

Pro Products, Inc.
Sparks, Nev.

Travenol Labs, Inc.
Deerfield, Ill.

Stat Electrolytes

Gem-Stat
Mallinckrodt
Ann Arbor, Mich.

IRMA
Diametrics Medical
St. Paul, Minn.

i-STAT
Heska
Ft. Collins, Colo.

Stat Blood Gases and pH

IRMA
Diametrics Medical
St. Paul, Minn.

i-STAT
Heska
Ft. Collins, Colo.

PPG Industries, Inc.
Biomedical Systems Division, Sensors
La Jolla, Calif.

ABL 500
Radiometer America
Cleveland, Ohio

Defibrillators

Datascope Corp.
Montvale, N.J.

Hewlett Packard
McMinnville, Ore.

Temperature Monitors

Yellow Springs Instruments
Yellow Springs, Ohio

Oxygen Cages

Isollette: Air Shields, Inc.
Hatboro, Pa.

Spectrum Anesthesia Services, Inc.
Louisville, Ky.

Heating Devices

Baxter K-Module
Baxter Health Care Co.
Deerfield, Ill.

Thermadrape
Vital Signs, Inc.
Totowa, N.J.

Bair Hugger
Augustine Medical, Inc.
Eden Prairie, Minn.

Hotline (fluid warmer)
Level 1–Smiths Industries Medical Systems
Rockland, Mass.

Physical Principles of Anesthesia

I. Laws

A. Boyle's law

$$\text{Volume} = \frac{k}{\text{Pressure}}; \quad V \times P = k$$

$$P_1 V_1 = P_2 V_2$$

B. Charles' law

$$V = k + T \qquad T = {}^\circ\text{Kelvin (K)}$$

$$\frac{V_1}{V_2} = \frac{T_1}{T_2}$$

C. Gay-Lussac's law

$$P = k \times T \qquad T = {}^\circ\text{K}$$

$$\frac{P_1}{P_2} = \frac{T_1}{T_2}$$

From above:

$$\frac{P_1 V_1}{T_1} = \frac{P_2 V_2}{T_2}$$

D. Ideal Gas law

$$\frac{PV}{T} = n \frac{(1 \text{ atm})(22.412)}{273\text{K}}$$

$$PV = nRT \qquad R = 0.08206 \qquad 1 \text{ atm/}^\circ\text{K} \qquad n = \text{g moles}$$

E. Henry's law

$$V = \alpha P \qquad \begin{aligned} &V = \text{volume of gas dissolved} \\ &\alpha = \text{solubility coefficient} \\ &P = \text{partial pressure} \end{aligned}$$

The solubility of a gas or vapor in a liquid (α) decreases as the temperature increases

517

F. Law of partial pressure (Dalton's law): each gas in a mixture exerts the same pressure as it would exert if it alone occupied the same volume at the same temperature; since pressure measurements cannot distinguish different molecules in a mixed sample, the contribution to total pressure made by a given constituent is in proportion to the number of molecules of that constituent

G. Graham's law: the velocity or rate of diffusion is inversely proportional to the square root of the density

II. Terms

A. Vapor pressure
1. Tendency for a liquid to evaporate
2. When a liquid and its vapor are in equilibrium, the partial pressure that the vapor exerts

B. Heat of vaporization: the amount of heat required for a liquid to evaporate

C. Volumes of a vapor

$$\frac{\text{Vapor pressure}}{\text{Total pressure}} \times 100 = \text{Vol \%}$$

D. Boiling point of a liquid: that temperature at which its vapor pressure is equal to the prevailing atmospheric pressure; generally stated for 760 mm Hg

E. Critical temperature: when a liquid is confined in a strong container, the temperature at which the contents of the container consists of vapor only

F. Critical pressure: when a liquid is confined in a strong container, the pressure that exists when the container has reached its critical temperature; liquid volumes may be converted to weight by the formula: volume (ml) $\times$ density (g/ml) = grams of liquid

G. Latent heat of vaporization: the amount of heat necessary to evaporate a quantity of liquid to its vapor state without any changes in temperature; expressed in calories/g liquid; this heat is stored in the vapor

III. **Specific partition coefficients; the solubility coefficient may be expressed as follows:**

    A. Bunsen's absorption coefficient: amount of gas (volume) at standard temperature and pressure that dissolves in one volume of liquid when the partial pressure of the gas above the liquid is 1 atm

    B. Ostwald's solubility coefficient: the volume of gas absorbed by a unit volume of liquid when the partial pressure of the gas is 1 atm, the volume of gas being expressed at the temperature of the experiment

    C. The partition coefficient

        1. May be expressed as the ratio of concentration of a substance in the gas phase and in the liquid phase (e.g., milligrams per milliliter)

        2. Partition coefficients are also used to relate the ratios of concentrations in any two phases that are in equilibrium

           a. Liquid-liquid (oil-water)

           b. Liquid-solid

           c. Gas-solid

IV. **Useful tables (Tables 1, 2, 3, and 4)**

TABLE 1
STANDARD VALUES AND EQUIVALENTS*

METRIC WEIGHTS		
1 gram (1 g)	=	weight of 1 cc water at 4°C
1000 g	=	1 kilogram (kg)
0.1 g	=	1 decigram (dg)
0.01 g	=	1 centigram (cg)
0.001 g	=	1 milligram (mg)
0.001 mg	=	1 microgram (μg)
METRIC VOLUMES		
1 liter (L)	=	1 cubic decimeter or 1000 cubic centimeters (cc)
0.001 liter	=	1 milliliter (ml)

*International System (SI) units.

TABLE 2
CONVERSION FACTORS

		CONVERSION FACTORS	
SI UNIT	OLD UNIT	TO SI (EXACT)	SI TO OLD (APPROX)
kPa	mm Hg	0.133	7.5
kPa	1 standard atmosphere (approx. 1 Bar)	101.3	0.01
kPa	cmH$_2$O	0.0981	10
kPa	lb/sq inch	6.89	0.145

			CONVERSION FACTORS	
MEASUREMENT	SI UNIT	OLD UNIT	TO SI (EXACT)	SI TO OLD (APPROX)
Blood				
Acid-base				
Pco$_2$	kPa	mm Hg	0.133	7.5
Po$_2$	kPa	mm Hg	0.133	7.5
Base excess	mmol/liter	mEq/liter	Numerically equivalent	
Plasma				
Sodium	mmol/liter	mEq/liter	Numerically equivalent	
Potassium	mmol/liter	mEq/liter	Numerically equivalent	
Magnesium	mmol/liter	mEq/liter	0.5	2.0
Chloride	mmol/liter	mEq/liter	Numerically equivalent	
Phosphate (inorganic)	mmol/liter	mEq/liter	0.323	3.0
Creatinine	μmol/liter	mg/100 ml	88.4	0.01
Urea	mmol/liter	mg/100ml	0.166	6.0
Serum				
Calcium	mmol/liter	mg/100 ml	0.25	4.0
Bilirubin	μmol/liter	mg/100 ml	17.1	0.06
Total protein	g/liter	g/100 ml	10.0	0.1
Albumin	g/liter	g/100 ml	10.0	0.1
Globulin	g/liter	g/100 ml	10.0	0.1

TABLE 3
EQUIVALENTS OF CENTIGRADE AND FAHRENHEIT THERMOMETRIC SCALES

CENTIGRADE DEGREE	FAHRENHEIT DEGREE	CENTIGRADE DEGREE	FAHRENHEIT DEGREE
−17	+1.4	14	57.2
−16	3.2	15	59.0
−15	5.0	16	60.8
−14	6.8	17	62.6
−13	8.6	18	64.4
−12	10.4	19	66.2
−11	12.2	20	68.0
−10	14.0	21	69.8
−9	15.8	22	71.6
−8	17.6	23	73.4
−7	19.4	24	75.2
−6	21.2	25	77.0
−5	23.0	26	78.8
−4	24.8	27	80.6
−3	26.6	28	82.4
−2	28.4	29	84.2
−1	30.2	30	86.0
0	32.0	31	87.8
+1	33.8	32	89.6
2	35.6	33	91.4
3	37.4	34	93.2
4	39.2	35	95.0
5	41.0	36	96.8
6	42.8	37	98.6
7	44.6	38	100.4
8	46.4	39	102.2
9	48.2	40	104.0
10	50.0	41	105.8
11	51.8	42	107.6
12	53.6	43	109.4
13	55.4	44	111.2
		45	113.0

TABLE 4

ALVEOLAR AND ARTERIAL GAS PRESSURES IN HEALTHY SUBJECTS AT ALTITUDE

ALTITUDE (FEET)	ATMOSPHERIC PRESSURE (mm Hg)	PIO_2 (mm Hg)	SEA LEVEL FIO_2	ALVEOLAR GAS TENSIONS (mm Hg)				ARTERIAL GAS TENSIONS (mm Hg)			INSPIRED FIO_2 NEEDED TO YIELD SEA LEVEL PIO_2
				H_2O	CO_2	N_2	O_2	CO_2	O_2	SpO_2	
Sealevel	760	149	20.9	47	37	574	102	40	95	97	20.9
6000	609	118	16.6	47	36	452	74	—	—	—	26.5
8000	565	108	15.1	47	37	416	65	38	56	89	28.8
10,000	523	100	14.0	47	36	379	61	—	—	—	31.3

PIO_2, Inspired oxygen tension; FIO_2, fraction of inspired oxygen concentration.

Drug Schedules

Controlled substances are obtained by prescription and must be used for legitimate medical purposes. Practitioners may not dispense prescriptions from their own offices. The prescriber must have authorization from appropriate legal authorities (usually the attorney general) to prescribe a controlled substance. State and other local regulations must be followed.

CLASSES I AND II

Class I and II drugs must be dispensed by filling out an official order form, which is usually obtained by contacting the Drug Enforcement Agency (DEA). Power of attorney may also be given to one or more people to obtain and use the forms; any theft or loss of these forms must be reported.

If prescriber registration expires, all unused forms must be returned.

All or part of an order may be canceled if both buyer and supplier are informed.

For all controlled substances, the prescription must be dated and signed (as any legal document) on the date of issue. The full name and address of the patient's and prescriber name, address, and DEA number must be on the written prescription.

CLASS II

These drugs may be dispensed or administered without a prescription (subject to the above rules).

Oral orders for Class II drugs are permitted in emergencies, but only for the amount needed for the emergency period; oral orders must be followed up within 72 hours with a written, signed prescription, issued to the providing pharmacy for the emergency quantity dispensed. The date of the oral order and "authorization for emergency dispensing" must be written on the follow-up prescription. Failure to do this will cause action to void all "dispensing without a written prescription" rights.

Oral orders are not permitted in nonemergency situations. Indelible pencil, ink, or typewriter may be used; the prescription should be signed by hand. Prescriptions may be prepared by a secretary or agent, but the prescriber is responsible for all statements.

Class II drugs may not be refilled. A new prescription is required for each filling.

CLASSES III, IV, AND V

Class III, IV, and V drugs may be dispensed by written or oral prescription or may be dispensed or administered from the office without a prescription.

An institutional practitioner may directly administer or dispense (but not prescribe) Class III, IV, or V drugs only if the prescribing physician has done the following:
1. Written and signed the prescription
2. Given an oral order or had the pharmacist make it into a written order
3. Ordered the prescription for immediate administration to the ultimate user

REFILLS

Class III and Class IV drugs may not be filled or refilled more than 6 months after the original date of issue of the prescription. They may not be refilled more than five times. Refills must be entered on the back of the original prescription or other appropriate document (medication record).

When retrieving the prescription number, the following information should be available: patient's name, dosage form, date filled or refilled, quantity dispensed, initials of the registered pharmacist for each refill, total number of refills for that prescription to date.

ORAL REFILLS (CLASSES III AND IV)

The total number of refills (quantity) allowed, including the amount of the original, may not exceed five refills or 6 months from the original date.

SCHEDULED DRUGS	CONTROLLED SUBSTANCES (OR CLASSES)	DESCRIPTIONS	EXAMPLES
Schedule I	C-I	No accepted medical use High potential for abuse	Heroin, dihydromorphine
Schedule II	C-II	Accepted medical uses in United States (may include severe restrictions) High potential for abuse, which may lead to severe psychologic or physical dependence	Morphine, meperidine, butorphanol, oxymorphone, etorphine, pentobarbital
Schedule III	C-III	Accepted medical uses in United States Lesser degree of abuse potential than C-II Abuse may lead to moderate or low physical dependence or high psychologic dependence.	Thiopental, tiletamine-zolazepam, ketamine
Schedule IV	C-IV	Accepted medical uses in United States Low potential for abuse of C-III Abuse of C-III may lead to limited physical or psychologic dependence	Chloral hydrate, diazepam, pentazocine
Schedule V	C-V	Accepted medical uses in United States Low potential for abuse of C-IV Abuse of C-IV may lead to limited physical or psychologic dependence Some over-the-counter items included in this class (as determined by the Federal Food, Drug and Cosmetic Act) may be dispensed without prescription subject to overriding state regulation and provisions of the buyer	Buprenorphine

All references and laws from Code of Federal Regulations and selected provision and Controlled Substance Act, in *Ohio Drug Laws* Handbook, 1987.

The quantity of each refill must be less than or equal to the original quantity authorized.

A new and separate prescription must be issued for any more than five refills or after 6 months.

All of the above information may be kept on computer. The physician's name, telephone number, DEA number, and the patient's name and address must also be kept on computer.

Class IV drugs may only be refilled if the prescription is authorized by the prescribing physician.

PARTIALS (CLASSES III, IV, AND V)

Partial prescriptions must be recorded in the same manner as refills.

The total quantity of partials may not exceed the total quantity prescribed.

Class III, IV, and V drugs may not be dispensed more than 6 months past the original date of the prescription.

LABELING

All controlled substances must be labeled with the pharmacy's name and address, serial number and date of initial filling, the patient's and physician's names, directions for use, and any cautionary statements.

DISPOSAL

If you are required by the DEA to make reports for all controlled substances, these can be submitted in triplicate on part b of the report form DEA 222 and directed to the Special Agent in Charge of Administration. If no report is required, list the controlled substances on DEA form 41 and submit three copies to the Special Agent in Charge of Administration.